T0231580

Paediatric Rehabilitation Engineering

From Disability to Possibility

REHABILITATION SCIENCE IN PRACTICE SERIES

Series Editors

Marcia Scherer, Ph.D.

President
Institute for Matching Person and Technology

Professor
Orthopaedics and Rehabilitation
University of Rochester Medical Center

Dave Muller, Ph.D.

Executive
Suffolk New College

Editor-in-Chief
Disability and Rehabilitation

Founding Editor
Aphasiology

Published Titles

Paediatric Rehabilitation Engineering: From Disability to Possibility, *edited by*
Tom Chau and Jillian Fairley

Forthcoming Titles

Multiple Sclerosis Rehabilitation: From Impairment to Participation, *edited by*
Marcia Finlayson

Assistive Technology Assessment Handbook, *edited by*
Marcia Scherer and Stefano Federici

Rehabilitation Goal Setting: Theory, Practice and Evidence, *edited by*
Richard Siegert and William Levack

Ambient Assisted Living, *edited by*
Nuno M. Garcia, Joel Jose P. C. Rodrigues, Dirk Christian Elias, Miguel Sales Dias

Paediatric Rehabilitation Engineering

From Disability to Possibility

Edited by

Tom Chau

Jillian Fairley

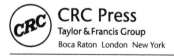

CRC Press
Taylor & Francis Group
Boca Raton London New York

CRC Press is an imprint of the
Taylor & Francis Group, an **informa** business

CRC Press
Taylor & Francis Group
6000 Broken Sound Parkway NW, Suite 300
Boca Raton, FL 33487-2742

First issued in paperback 2019

© 2011 by Taylor and Francis Group, LLC
CRC Press is an imprint of Taylor & Francis Group, an Informa business

No claim to original U.S. Government works

ISBN-13: 978-1-4398-0842-9 (hbk)
ISBN-13: 978-1-138-37415-7 (pbk)

This book contains information obtained from authentic and highly regarded sources. Reasonable efforts have been made to publish reliable data and information, but the author and publisher cannot assume responsibility for the validity of all materials or the consequences of their use. The authors and publishers have attempted to trace the copyright holders of all material reproduced in this publication and apologize to copyright holders if permission to publish in this form has not been obtained. If any copyright material has not been acknowledged please write and let us know so we may rectify in any future reprint.

Except as permitted under U.S. Copyright Law, no part of this book may be reprinted, reproduced, transmitted, or utilized in any form by any electronic, mechanical, or other means, now known or hereafter invented, including photocopying, micro-filming, and recording, or in any information storage or retrieval system, without written permission from the publishers.

For permission to photocopy or use material electronically from this work, please access www.copyright.com (http://www.copyright.com/) or contact the Copyright Clearance Center, Inc. (CCC), 222 Rosewood Drive, Danvers, MA 01923, 978-750-8400. CCC is a not-for-profit organization that provides licenses and registration for a variety of users. For organizations that have been granted a photocopy license by the CCC, a separate system of payment has been arranged.

Trademark Notice: Product or corporate names may be trademarks or registered trademarks, and are used only for identification and explanation without intent to infringe.

Library of Congress Cataloging-in-Publication Data

Paediatric rehabilitation engineering : from disability to possibility / edited by Tom Chau, Jillian Fairley.
    p. ; cm. -- (Rehabilitation science in practice series)
    Includes bibliographical references and index.
    Summary: "Written by international experts, this book provides an up-to-date synopsis of advances in pediatric rehabilitation engineering research. Offering a single comprehensive resource on the latest research findings, each chapter presents a different area of technology or the developments of particular clinical relevance to pediatric rehabilitation. The material within each chapter also includes a conceptual description of the technology or underlying scientific principles, followed by a synthesis of relevant literature, recent research advances, selected clinical case studies (where applicable), and perspectives for future directions"--Provided by publisher.
    ISBN 978-1-4398-0842-9 (hardcover : alkaline paper)
    1. Children with disabilities--Rehabilitation. 2. Biomedical engineering. I. Chau, Tom, editor. II. Fairley, Jillian, editor. III. Title. IV. Series: Rehabilitation science in practice series.
    [DNLM: 1. Biomedical Engineering--methods. 2. Rehabilitation. 3. Adolescent. 4. Disabled Children. 5. Self-Help Devices. WS 368]
    RJ138.P26 2011
    618.9200028'4--dc22
                                                       2010044862

**Visit the Taylor & Francis Web site at
http://www.taylorandfrancis.com**

**and the CRC Press Web site at
http://www.crcpress.com**

This book is dedicated to Eric Wan, who as a bright and musically gifted 18-year-old was rendered a quadriplegic without the ability to ventilate independently as a consequence of transverse myelitis secondary to vaccination. Although his life was turned upside down, Eric never lost his love for learning nor his enormous sense of service to his neighbour. A year after his injury, Eric returned to finish high school and in 2010 completed his bachelor's degree in computer engineering. He will be commencing graduate school in the fall of 2010. Over the last 5 years, Eric has devoted his energies to augmenting possibilities for children and youth with disabilities, by applying his superior software engineering skills and know-how to develop virtual reality therapy applications, assistive technologies, and embedded systems for paediatric rehabilitation. He is an inspirational example of the defiant power of the human spirit and a testimony to the engineering of possibilities from disability.

Contents

Acknowledgements

The editors are deeply indebted to CRC Press/Taylor & Francis for the opportunity to assemble this contributed volume. It has been both an educational and an immensely rewarding journey. This work would not have been possible without the tremendous editorial assistance of Tasnim Kamani, who spent countless hours formatting references, retrieving information for incomplete references, tracking different versions of manuscript files for the various chapters, and coordinating timely communications with the contributing authors. We are also grateful for the efforts of Xiao Jin Chen, who helped to distribute initial materials and instructions to the authors and collect signed agreements. We would also like to acknowledge the graphic and visualization creativity of Steven Bernstein, who collaborated with the various authors to develop the chapter roadmaps.

Contributors

An international cast of authors devoted time and energy to the writing of this book. The editors cannot adequately thank the authors for their time, specialized expertise and precious contributions.

Natasha Alves
Holland Bloorview Kids Rehabilitation
    Hospital
Bloorview Research Institute
and
Institute of Biomaterials and
    Biomedical Engineering
University of Toronto
Toronto, Ontario, Canada

Jan Andrysek
Holland Bloorview Kids Rehabilitation
    Hospital
Bloorview Research Institute
and
Institute of Biomaterials and
    Biomedical Engineering
University of Toronto
Toronto, Ontario, Canada

Gabriella Basili
Department of Pediatrics
Senigallia General Hospital
Senigallia, Italy

Elaine Biddiss
Holland Bloorview Kids Rehabilitation
    Hospital
Bloorview Research Institute
and
Institute of Biomaterials and
    Biomedical Engineering
University of Toronto
Toronto, Ontario, Canada

Stefanie Blain
Holland Bloorview Kids Rehabilitation
    Hospital
Bloorview Research Institute
and
Graduate Department of Rehabilitation
    Science
University of Toronto
Toronto, Ontario, Canada

Tom Chau
Holland Bloorview Kids Rehabilitation
    Hospital
Bloorview Research Institute
and
Institute of Biomaterials and
    Biomedical Engineering
University of Toronto
Toronto, Ontario, Canada

T. Claire Davies
Department of Surgery
University of Auckland
Auckland, New Zealand

Jillian Fairley
Holland Bloorview Kids Rehabilitation
    Hospital
Bloorview Research Institute
Toronto, Ontario, Canada

Tiago Falk
Holland Bloorview Kids Rehabilitation
    Hospital
Bloorview Research Institute
and
Institute of Biomaterials and
    Biomedical Engineering
University of Toronto
Toronto, Ontario, Canada

Giulio E. Lancioni
Department of Psychology
University of Bari
Bari, Italy

Yocheved Laufer
Department of Physical Therapy
University of Haifa
Haifa, Israel

Brian Leung
Holland Bloorview Kids Rehabilitation
    Hospital
Bloorview Research Institute
and
Institute of Biomaterials and
    Biomedical Engineering
University of Toronto
Toronto, Ontario, Canada

Negar Memarian
Holland Bloorview Kids Rehabilitation
    Hospital
Bloorview Research Institute
and
Institute of Biomaterials and
    Biomedical Engineering
University of Toronto
Toronto, Ontario, Canada

Francois Michaud
Department of Electrical Engineering
    and Computer Engineering
Université de Sherbrooke
Sherbrooke, Quebec, Canada

Doretta Oliva
Lega F. D'Oro Research Center
Osimo, Italy

Mark F. O'Reilly
Meadows Center for Preventing
    Educational Risk
Department of Special Education
University of Texas at Austin
Austin, Texas

Tamie Salter
Department of Electrical Engineering
    and Computer Engineering
Université de Sherbrooke
Sherbrooke, Quebec, Canada

Jeff Sigafoos
School of Educational Psychology and
    Pedagogy
Victoria University of Wellington
Wellington, New Zealand

Nirbhay N. Singh
ONE Research Institute
Midlothian, Virginia

N. Susan Stott
Department of Surgery
University of Auckland
Auckland, New Zealand

Cynthia Tam
Department of Occupational Science
    and Occupational Therapy
University of Toronto
Toronto, Ontario, Canada

Eric Tam
Department of Health Technology and
    Informetics
Jockey Club Rehabilitation Engineering
    Centre
The Hong Kong Polytechnic University
Hong Kong, China

Gail Teachman
Graduate Department of Rehabilitation
    Science
and
Department of Occupational Science
    and Occupational Therapy
and
Holland Bloorview Kids Rehabilitation
    Hospital
University of Toronto
Toronto, Ontario, Canada

Naomi Weintraub
School of Occupational Therapy
Hadassah and the Hebrew University
Jerusalem, Israel

Patrice L. (Tamar) Weiss
Department of Occupational Therapy
University of Haifa
Haifa, Israel

1 Introduction

Tom Chau and Jillian Fairley

CONTENTS

"You are the bows from which your children as living arrows are sent forth."

Khalil Gibran, 1883–1931
Lebanese-American artist, poet and writer

It is probably reasonable to assume that paediatric rehabilitation engineering was not the inspiration for Khalil Gibran's eloquent philosophical prose about children, written nearly a century ago in his most well-known and treasured work, *The Prophet* (Gilbran 1923). Nonetheless, the above quotation is a strikingly appropriate metaphor for paediatric rehabilitation engineering. Our intuitive notions of paediatric rehabilitation engineering would converge on the idea of technology, that is, the "practical application of knowledge," in this case, to the specialised needs of children and youth with disabilities. The bow and arrow *is a technology*, many thousands of years old, that has played many critical roles (e.g., hunting for food) in the development of civilization. The technology itself draws on the physics of springs and kinetic projectiles, and the mechanics of materials (e.g., tensile and compressive strength). As an elegant, enduring and functional technology, the bow and arrow is a fitting icon for paediatric rehabilitation engineering. The bow's elastic limbs and string provide the potential energy for the swift and distant propulsion of the arrow. In a similar vein, paediatric rehabilitation engineering as a flexibly minded discipline can launch children and youth with disabilities on a flight path to a promising future; engineering innovations can serve as a springboard to education, and psychosocial, social, physical and cognitive development. While the angling of the bow can determine the direction of the arrow, appropriate engineering supports can also align children and youth with disabilities to targets of success and achievement. This book is an international sampling of the diverse bows with which paediatric rehabilitation engineering research is propelling children and youth forward towards new possibilities.

Instead of providing an overview of rehabilitation engineering, which exists in stellar expositions elsewhere (e.g., Cooper, Ohnabe and Hobson 2007), in this introduction we shall focus on establishing the uniqueness of the paediatric subspecialty, thereby offering a 'raison d'être' for this volume. The introduction closes with a preview of the contributed chapters contained herein.

PAEDIATRIC REHABILITATION ENGINEERING: A UNIQUE SUB-SPECIALTY

The Institute of Electrical and Electronic Engineers has defined rehabilitation engineering as a branch of biomedical engineering that deals with 'the application of science and technology to improve the quality of life of individuals with disabilities' (IEEE EMBS 2003). This definition generally encompasses the current research in paediatric rehab engineering, although one might replace the words "quality of life" with "health and well-being" to imply an even broader potential impact of the field. Paediatric rehab engineering can be considered a sub-specialty of the larger rehab engineering field, given the unique or exacerbated challenges of working with children and youths with disabilities, as discussed in the following sections.

MOVING TARGETS

Fundamentally, children are extremely dynamic individuals. Here, we use the term 'dynamic' in the systems engineering sense to connote something that is evolving over time. Indeed, children are developing physically, cognitively, emotionally and socially, often at an alarming pace. Herein lies a fundamental challenge for paediatric rehabilitation engineering: the target is not stationary. Rehabilitation technologies designed to meet a child's functional or therapy needs at one instance in time may no longer be relevant 6 months down the road due to, for example, physical growth, disease progression (e.g., Duchenne muscular dystrophy), environmental change associated with progression through the educational system, evolving recreational interests, or regaining of function (e.g., post-brain injury). The economic challenge for paediatric rehabilitation engineers is to design technologies, whether they be therapeutic, assistive or compensatory, that are metamorphic, capable of changing as the child changes (Chau 2007). In the lingo of the *International Classification of Functioning, Disability and Health: Children and Youth Version* (World Health Organization 2007), a mismatch between the dynamic needs of a child and the static affordances of the technological support leads to a gap between individual performance (what the child does in his or her current environment) and capacity (the highest probable level of functioning a child may reach in an appropriately adjusted environment). Indeed, highly configurable technologies with cross-age appeal such as autonomous robots (Chapter 8) and virtual reality (Chapter 9) may be practical solutions to the elusive problem of meeting the needs of dynamic paediatric clients.

DEVELOPMENTAL URGENCY

There is an inherent urgency when working with children; there are critical periods for the acquisition and development of various abilities, such as language and gesture (Bates and Dick 2002), motor proficiencies (Vereijken 2005) and visual acuity (Lewis and Maurer 2005). Thus, while the condition that a child may have is often life-long, the window of opportunity for the most impactful intervention is comparatively very small. Missed opportunities to promote healthy development may bear life-long deficits for which remediation later in life may have limited effectiveness (Newberger 1997). For example, a severely disabled child who is not provided a means of communication and social interaction may develop learned helplessness (Basil 1992), an acquired pattern of passivity and decreased motivation to respond. This perceived lack of control and non-responsiveness often persists even when appropriate instruments are available and the environment has become more supportive. Once presented with a case for need, paediatric rehabilitation engineers are thus challenged to arrive at time-sensitive solutions, which can be a tall order within a resource-constrained environment. Modular technologies that facilitate turn-key solutions (Chapter 7) and response-oriented microswitch programs (Chapter 2) appear to be viable approaches to address the predicament of developmental urgency.

CAPRICIOUS TEMPERAMENT

The most well-planned experimental data collection or assessment can unexpectedly go afoul when the paediatric participant has a 'bad day' or simply does not 'feel like' participating. The manifestation of these sentiments may range from challenging behaviour to lackadaisical effort, or from constant crying and yelling to a state of partial or total unconsciousness (i.e., simulating or actually falling asleep). Further, the paediatric participant may be highly distractible, inattentive and difficult to engage, and may have fears about certain equipment, or unfamiliar environments or people, resulting in general non-compliance with experimental protocol. Some children may have hypersensitivities to ambient noise, lighting, temperature (e.g., too hot due to multiple layers of clothing), or superficial attachment of sensors to certain parts of the body (e.g., near the mouth of a child who does not feed orally) and exaggerated reactions to thirst and hunger, or discomfort from remaining in a seated posture for an extended period of time. Thus, paediatric rehabilitation engineering researchers are frequently confronted with the seemingly unpredictable child temperament (Zentner and Bates 2007). Optimised seating (Chapter 6), multisensory, engaging robots (Chapter 8) and virtual environments (Chapter 9) may present innovative options to the weary rehabilitation engineering researcher.

INCONSISTENT INTERACTION

Children and youth with disabilities necessarily spend time in multiple environments, including but not limited to their homes, schools and rehabilitation facilities. In each environment, there is typically a different set of caregivers, each having a unique comfort level with assistive technologies. While expert knowledge and on-site technical assistance is usually available through paediatric rehabilitation centres, parents, grandparents and extended family who support the child in the home environment may have varying levels of technical expertise. Several studies have reported that teachers and educational assistants in the school environment generally feel that they do not have adequate assistive technology training or awareness of specialised applications to offer suitable support to students with disabilities (Copley and Ziviani 2004). Further, in the school setting, teachers may have limited time for individual technology setup for each student. As a consequence, technological supports may be inconsistently deployed across environments or applied in some environments and not others. This lack of consistent interaction can encumber the child's learning, say, of a new switch interface or an electronic communication aid. Further exacerbating the issue is the fact that traditional assistive technology assessments have often been geared towards specific school activities rather than independent functioning of a child in multiple environments (Judge 2000). The dissonant nature of interaction across environments may be particularly detrimental to the paediatric client given that response efficiency plays a likely pivotal role in assistive technology abandonment (Johnston and Evans 2005). There are four tenets of response efficiency: (1) response effort — the physical effort required to produce a behaviour, (2) rate of reinforcement — the frequency at which the user receives reinforcement, (3) quality of reinforcement — the level at which the user is engaged by the reinforcement, and (4) immediacy of reinforcement — the latency between the use of the technology and the delivery of reinforcement. These components of response interact to determine a user's choice behaviour, which may be to interact or to withdraw and become increasingly passive. Hence, when the response effort and the rate, quality and immediacy of reinforcement are inconsistent across natural milieus, there may be a heightened risk of developing learned helplessness. The call to paediatric rehabilitation engineers is thus to conceive of technologies that are easy for a wide variety of caregivers to support and that are usable in multiple ecologically salient child settings. These are clearly the goals of technologies facilitating communication (Chapter 4) and Web access (Chapter 5) described in this volume.

UNCOVERING THE CHILD'S OPINION

According to postmodern perspectives of childhood, children are considered as social actors, worthy of investigation in their own right, apart from their parents and caregivers (Einarsdóttir 2007). Children are recognised as knowledgeable experts in their own lives (Clark and Moss 2001) and competent witnesses to speak for themselves about their experiences, preferences and opinions (Barker and Weller 2003). Various techniques have been proposed and implemented for discovering the views and experiences of children, including, for example, photo elicitation (Epstein et al. 2006),

drawings, collages and mappings (Hart 1997). The challenge for paediatric rehabilitation engineering is to capture children's perspectives in the assessment for and
design of appropriate assistive technology. However, this is often not a straightforward
undertaking. Paediatric clients may be pre-literate or delayed in the development of
language and expressive communication. There may also be sensory deficits and significant motor impairments that may preclude the application of the aforementioned
techniques. Despite this quagmire of complicated data collection issues, it is necessary
to explore innovative, perhaps unconventional methods of physical access (Chapters 2
and 3) and communication (Chapter 4); evidence from the literature strongly indicates
that omitting the child's input verily leads to device abandonment (e.g., Judge 2000;
Copley and Ziviani 2004; Colorado Consortium on Assistive Technology 2001).

Hopefully, this discussion has (1) given the reader an appreciation of the unique
challenges faced by paediatric rehabilitation engineers, and (2) piqued the reader's
curiosity about how the work described within the ensuing chapters is addressing
some of these issues.

FROM DISABILITY TO POSSIBILITY

Contents-at-a-Glance

This book is a sampling of the landscape of paediatric rehabilitation engineering. Each
chapter introduces a different aspect of clinically motivated paediatric rehabilitation
engineering research. As depicted in Figure 1.1, we have organised the chapters into three
major conceptual blocks, namely, Interfacial Technologies, Physical Compensatory
Technologies, and Multisensory Interactive Machines and Environments.

Interfacial Technologies

The first block of chapters is broadly concerned with connecting individuals with
disabilities to their environment and the people around them, whether physically
face-to-face or virtually via the Internet. Chapter 2 is an international effort describing microswitch-based occupational, recreational and rehabilitation programs for
children with severe and multiple disabilities. The clinical goal is to establish and
shape constructive physical responses that can be used for communication and environmental interaction, while suppressing problematic postures and behaviours. In
a comprehensive critical appraisal of evidence by clinical goal and response type,
Dr. Giulio Lancioni and colleagues exemplify the application of a broad spectrum
of microswitch technology, including, for example, pressure, position, vibration,
tilt, and optical sensors, custom sound switches, and creative combinations thereof.
Through their appraisal, the authors highlight the importance of selecting suitable
responses for each child and ensuring that each response produces preferred effects,
so as to offset the physical and mental costs of generating that response. Compelling
evidence is presented for the clinical potential of microswitch therapy programs that
target multiple responses; children with severe disabilities can be taught to augment
multiple responses and exhibit preference among available stimuli. Two highly innovative paradigms in microswitch-driven habilitation are presented. One is the stra-
tegic integration of intervention for both positive and negative behaviours within a

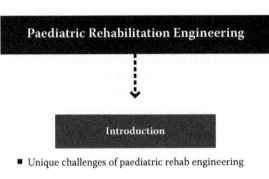

FIGURE 1.1   Conceptual roadmap of book content.

unified treatment program and the other is the application of microswitches to mobility devices to encourage step responses as precursory skills to basic locomotion. The latest research on these emerging fronts is presented. The reader walks away with a greater appreciation of the concrete potential of carefully crafted microswitch rehabilitation programs for children with severe and multiple disabilities.

Focusing on the technical facilitation of physical access to a computer or other external machine, Chapter 3 introduces a handful of nascent access technologies, each targeting a very specific extant physical ability or physiological response. The technologies and the corresponding targeted ability or response (indicated in parentheses) are infrared thermal imaging (mouth opening and closing), multicamera fusion (tongue protrusion), vocal cord vibration detection (silent vocalizations), mechanomyography (residual voluntary muscle twitches) and electrodermal monitoring (sympathetic nervous response). In a series of descriptive case studies, this chapter introduces the different technologies, profiles at least one exemplary client for the technology and describes experimental evaluation of the access pathway. The key take-home message is that advances in body-machine interfacing have greatly expanded the potential of harnessing the unique expressions of intention, whether they are physical or physiological, of nonverbal children with severe disabilities.

Chapter 4 moves beyond issues of physical access and hones in on technologies that support functional communication, a key objective of interfacial technology. The authors focus on children who communicate differently due to difficulties related to either speaking or writing. These difficulties may be secondary to cerebral palsy, developmental or intellectual delays, or neuromuscular disease, among other conditions. The authors cover speech-generating devices, speech-recognition technology, note-taking technology, distance communication technology, whole-utterance-based communication, context-based vocabulary organization and online augmentative and alternative communication (AAC) training for clients and other stakeholders.

The clinical goal of assistive communication technologies is to enable children to communicate in a variety of everyday environments, including the home, school and community. The core chapter content is structured into four critical domains of influence, specifically, technologies that enable engagement, technologies that enable literacy, technologies that enable participation and finally technologies that enable support and training. The discussion of each domain is effectively introduced and embellished with interesting real-case vignettes. At the end of the chapter, the reader walks away with a deeper sense of (1) the dynamic nature of technology trends and innovations in the AAC field, (2) the philosophical shift in design and service delivery towards meaningful participation in *all* aspects of daily living, and (3) the recognition of children as competent social actors whose voices need to be heard.

The last chapter (Chapter 5) under the interfacial technologies umbrella is concerned with accessible graphical user and Web-based interfaces that mitigate sensitivity to motor and physical control difficulties, a timely topic for paediatric rehabilitation in the digital age. As the digital divide gradually dissolves and education becomes increasingly cybernated, it is only sensible to design Web and graphical interfaces that are accessible to as many potential users as possible. This chapter presents a pedagogical review of key considerations in accessible interface design in the context of Web-based surveys for adolescents with physical and sensory disabilities. Stimulating real-life examples that touch on practical and legal issues are provided throughout. The clinical impact of accessible interfaces is far reaching, with the potential to provide broadly accessible data collection tools for the evaluation of rehabilitation interventions, and the identification of user needs and priorities. Web-based data collection can be a powerful tool in paediatric rehabilitation where we are increasingly interested in soliciting the perspectives of children and youth directly rather than by proxy. Several valuable lessons are imparted to the reader. In designing Web-based surveys, international guidelines and standards as well as cognitive information processing and physical effort of the user need to be considered. Both usability and accessibility should be taken into account through extensive testing with target user groups.

Physical Compensatory Technologies

The second conceptual block in this book revolves around paediatric technologies that compensate for compromised or missing function (LoPresti, Mihailidis and Kirsch 2004). Chapter 6 addresses compensation for children who have difficulty maintaining a functional seated posture via an overview of seating principles and design considerations for specialised or adaptive seating systems. The paediatric populations requiring specialised or adaptive seating include those with cerebral palsy, neuromuscular disease and spinal disorders. Various technologies are mentioned, including seating systems that are planar, modular, custom-contoured, CAD-CAM designed, dynamic and shapeable. The primary rehabilitative goal of seating technology is to improve function by supporting the body in a functional posture. For example, appropriate seating may facilitate improved feeding and swallowing, respiration and distal hand movements. The chapter highlights the reality that effective adaptive seating for children with disabilities is a complex and evolving process, necessitating ongoing assessment of how seating supports function. Key areas for future research are identified as dynamic seating, that is, seating systems that accommodate rather than restrict natural movement, paediatric-only seating systems rather than scaled-down adult designs, improved monitoring of the tissue-support interface and the creation of paediatric anthropometric databases with 'seating-relevant' measures.

While Chapter 6 describes postural compensations, Chapter 7 discusses compensations for limb loss, that is, upper and lower extremity prostheses. In particular, Chapter 7 introduces the design, development, evaluation and application of technologies to decrease impairment associated with limb loss. A compendium of technologies is reviewed, including those common to lower and upper extremity prostheses (sockets and suspension), those unique to lower limbs (e.g., prosthetic feet, ankles and knees) and those exclusive to upper limbs (e.g., body-powered and electric prostheses). These technologies stand to benefit children and youth with limb differences, either congenital or acquired. The chapter also acquaints the readers with technologies to assist with prostheses fitting, training and outcome evaluation. Emerging technologies (e.g., neuroprostheses, intelligent prostheses, sensory feedback and modular component design) are also briefly introduced. The rehabilitative goals of prosthetic technologies are typically to mitigate the effects of limb loss and to allow individuals to achieve their functional goals. The authors adopt an engaging presentation style, whereby they trace a typical journey through paediatric rehabilitation from amputation surgery and prosthetics design, through to prosthesis fitting, training and outcome evaluation. While technological advances have allowed individuals with limb differences to achieve basic mobility and function more naturally and efficiently than in the past, the authors remark that there is still a long road ahead of research and development before prosthetic limbs rival their biological counterparts.

Multisensory, Interactive Machines and Environments

The final conceptual group of chapters is about machines and environments that provide stimulating and interactive platforms for therapy and research. In a critical narrative, Chapter 8 details contemporary global efforts in the area of robotics for autism research, diagnostics and therapeutics, highlighting the robots deployed, clinical goals and key findings. Generally, the habilitative goals of robots in the autism realm have been to enhance play and social interaction, to encourage children to break out of repetitive behaviours and to encourage verbal communication. Numerous robots are introduced in this chapter, spanning autonomous and remote-controlled machines, as well as object-like, humanoid and animal-like devices. The technology typically consists of machines outfitted with sensors to detect child interaction or presence and actuators to respond mechanically with motion, optically with lights or sonically with music. Many of the robots have significant on-board 'intelligence' to react appropriately to different interaction scenarios. The authors contend that robotics is a rapidly evolving discipline with tremendous potential as a platform for autism research, the habilitation of children with autism, and the development of therapies and diagnostic tools to complement existing behavioural instruments. The reader is cautioned, however, about the risk of robots becoming a technology that further socially isolates children with autism from their environments. The chapter closes with recommendations for conducting robot studies with children with autism and a discussion of challenges to the widespread adoption of robots in autism research and treatment.

Continuing on the theme of multisensory interaction, Chapter 9 introduces the reader to virtual reality (VR), that is, computer-generated environments that resemble real-world objects and events in terms of sight, sound and feel, as a tool for therapy, education and assessment of function. The clinical and educational goals are often to rehearse practical skills, to improve knowledge and achievement, to foster communication and creativity or to enhance physical functioning. Various clinical paediatric populations have been targeted with VR interventions. Children with attention deficit-hyperactivity disorder, autism spectrum disorder, intellectual developmental deficits and cerebral palsy are among those mentioned. The chapter begins with a pedagogical overview of the typical instrumentation, including computer technology, video capture devices, head-mounted displays, haptic and other sensors, actuators and immersive displays. The authors then present paediatric studies applying VR to achieve various educational goals and VR studies aimed at assessing and training specific clinical paediatric populations. By the end of the chapter, the reader becomes cognizant of the latitudinous application of VR as an educational and therapeutic tool for children, and of the potential for VR to enable clinicians to achieve therapeutic goals that would be difficult if not impossible to attain via conventional therapy. Despite encouraging evidence that in some instances

VR has surpassed traditional pen-and-paper or computer-based tools in its ability to engage children, the authors also call for controlled studies and careful scrutiny of current evidence.

LANDMARKS, NOT LANDSCAPE

Any work of this sort cannot possibly include a fair representation of all paediatric rehabilitation engineering-relevant research efforts around the world. As mentioned earlier, one should consider the works contained herein as a sampling of important landmarks in the paediatric rehabilitation engineering landscape. Due to a lack of intersection between book timelines and personal work agendas, other targeted authors were unable to contribute this time around. The editors would nonetheless like to acknowledge other important on-going research under the paediatric rehabilitation engineering umbrella, but not included in this book. These include, but are not limited to, paediatric functional electrical stimulation (Johnston et al. 2003), paediatric cognitive assistive technologies (Bodine and Scherer 2006), computer art therapy (Malchiodi 2000), computer-mediated sound therapy (Ellis 1995), and powered mobility for young children (Orpwood et al. 2005).

The editors hope that in reading this book or excerpts thereof, the reader will become intrigued by the endless possibilities offered by paediatric rehabilitation engineering. The fine work of the contributing authors herein exemplifies some of the important ways in which paediatric rehabilitation engineering is helping to aim the metaphorical arrows towards targets of achievement and success, and to draw back bow strings to ensure sufficient potential energy to go the distance. However, to most effectively launch arrows towards distant targets, one requires synergistic action between the archer, the bow and the arrow. In the same way, it is the harmonization of the expertise and energies of rehabilitation professionals, teachers, scientists, funders, policymakers, families, paediatric rehabilitation engineers and other stakeholders that will ensure that children are optimally supported as they embark on their journey from disability to possibility.

REFERENCES

Barker J. and S. Weller 2003. Never work with children? The geography of methodological issues in research with children. *Qualitative Research* 3(2):207–227.

Basil C. 1992. Social interaction and learned helplessness in severely disabled children. *Augmentative and Alternative Communication* 8(3):188–199.

Bates E. and F. Dick 2002. Language, gesture and the developing brain. *Developmental Psychobiology* 40:293–310.

Bodine C. and M. Scherer 2006. Technology for improving cognitive function. *Disability and Rehabilitation* 28(24):1567–1571.

Chau T. 2007. Intelligent systems in pediatric rehabilitation. *Assistive Technology* 19:17–20.

Clark A. and P. Moss 2001. *Listening to young children*, London: National Children's Bureau and Rowntree Foundation.

Colorado Consortium on Assistive Technology 2001. Assistive Technology for Infants, Toddlers, Children and Youth with Disabilities. http://www.cde.state.co.us (Accessed March 20, 2010).

Cooper R.A., H. Ohnabe and D.A. Hobson 2007. *An introduction to rehabilitation engineering.* New York: Taylor & Francis.

Copley J. and J. Ziviani 2004. Barriers to the use of assistive technology for children with multiple disabilities. *Occupational Therapy International* 11(4):229–243.

Einarsdóttir J. 2007. Research with children: Methodological and ethical challenges. *European Early Childhood Education Research Journal* 15(2):197–211.

Ellis P. 1995. Incidental music: A case study in the development of sound therapy. *British Journal of Music Education* 12:59–70.

Esptein I., B. Stevens, P. McKeever and S. Baruchel. 2006. Photo elicitation interview: Using photos to elicit children's perspectives. *International Journal of Qualitative Methods*, 5(3):Article 1.

Gibran K. 1923. *The Prophet.* New York: Alfred A. Knopf, Inc.

Hart R.A. 1997. *Children's participation.* London: Earthscan Publishers.

IEEE EMBS 2003. Designing a career in biomedical engineering. IEEE Engineering in Medicine and Biology Society. http://www.embs.org/docs/careerguide.pdf (Accessed March 20, 2010).

Johnston S.S. and J. Evans. 2005. Considering response efficiency as a strategy to prevent assistive technology abandonment. *Journal of Special Education Technology* 20(3):45–50.

Johnston T.E., R.R. Betz, B.T. Smith and M.J. Mulcahey. 2003. Implanted functional electrical stimulation: An alternative for standing and walking in pediatric spinal cord injury. *Spinal Cord* 41:144–152.

Judge S.L. 2000. Accessing and funding assistive technology for young children with disabilities. *Early Childhood Education Journal* 28(2):125–131.

Lewis T.L. and D. Maurer 2005. Multiple sensitive periods in human visual development: Evidence from visually deprived children. *Psychobiology* 46:163–183.

Lopresti E.F., A. Mihailidis and N. Kirsh 2004. Assistive technology for cognitive rehabilitation. *Neuropsychological rehabilitation* 14(1–2):5–39.

Malchiodi C. 2000. *Art therapy and computer technology: A virtual studio of possibilities.* London: Jessica Kingsley Publishers Ltd.

Newberger J. 1997. New brain development research – a wonderful opportunity to build public support for early childhood education. *Young Children* 52:4–9.

Orpwood R., S. Hasley, N. Evans and A. Harris. 2005. Development of a powered mobility vehicle for nursery-age children. In *Assistive technology from virtuality to reality*, A. Pruski and H. Knops, Eds., 540-543. Amsterdam: The Netherlands, IOS Press.

Vereijken B. 2005. Motor development. In *Cambridge encyclopedia in child development,* B. Hopkins, Ed., 217–226, Cambridge, MA: Cambridge University Press.

World Health Organization 2007. *International classification of functioning, disability and health: Children and youth version: ICF-CY.* Geneva: WHO Press.

Zentner M. and J.E. Bates 2007. Child temperament: An integrative review of concepts. *European Journal of Developmental Science* 2(1–2):7–37.

2 Microswitch-Based Programs for Children and Youth with Multiple Disabilities
An Overview of the Responses and Technology Adopted

*Giulio E. Lancioni, Nirbhay N. Singh, Mark F. O'Reilly,
Jeff Sigafoos, Doretta Oliva and Gabriella Basili*

CONTENTS

SUMMARY

Children and youth with profound and multiple disabilities are often unable to interact with their immediate surroundings and control relevant stimuli due to their limited response (motor) repertoire. A possible way to help them tackle their situation is the use of microswitch-based programs. To introduce a person with multiple disabilities to a microswitch-based program, one has to identify at least (1) a response that can be performed reliably and without excessive effort by the person, (2) a suitable microswitch to monitor the response reliably and allow the occurrence of such response to activate target stimulation, and (3) target stimulation that the person finds relevant and thus is motivated to reach. This chapter provides an overview of studies using microswitch-based programs for children and youth with multiple disabilities. The chapter is divided into four main sections, which are concerned with (1) an overview of studies aimed at establishing constructive responses and related microswitch technology, (2) an overview of studies aimed at promoting constructive responses and reducing problem behaviour/posture and related microswitch technology, (3) a discussion of the overall findings and their relevance in terms of educational/occupational impact as well as in terms of overall social appearance and quality of life, and (4) a conclusion section focusing on some relevant issues for future research in the area.

INTRODUCTION

Children and youth with profound and multiple disabilities are often unable to interact with their immediate surroundings and control relevant stimuli due to their limited response (motor) repertoire (Lancioni, O'Reilly and Basili 2001a,b; Lancioni et al. 2007a,b; Mechling 2006). This inability has far-reaching implications, making them look passive or inadequate, curtailing their opportunities of constructive engagement and impact, and harming their developmental prospects, their overall social appearance and, eventually, their quality of life (Lachapelle et al. 2005; Lancioni et al. 2001c,d, 2008a,b; Schalock et al. 2003). Their lack of constructive engagement with the outside world and the stimuli it produces can also be combined with forms of problem behaviour, such as eye poking and hand mouthing, or problem (inadequate) posture such as head tilting (Kurtz et al. 2003; Lancioni et al. 2009a; Matson et al. 2006; Richman 2008).

Intervention based on environmental enrichment and stimulation procedures handled by staff and parents would improve the child/youth's input level and might also reduce problem behaviours (e.g., Ringdahl et al. 1997), but could have two main drawbacks. First, enrichment/stimulation conditions could easily make the child/youth a recipient of external input rather than an active agent pursuing it purposefully. Second, those conditions may not encourage the development of any specific response scheme by the child/youth that could serve as a relevant developmental target and, at the same time, as an instrument to control stimulation in the surrounding context (Glickman et al. 1996).

A possible way to help children and youth with profound and multiple disabilities deal with their situations is the use of microswitch-based programs, that is, general occupation/recreation and rehabilitation programs relying on microswitch technology (Lancioni et al. 2001a, 2008b; Leatherby et al. 1992; Sullivan, Laverick and Lewis 1995; Sullivan and Lewis 1993). Microswitches are technical devices that a person with profound and multiple disabilities may use to control environmental events with simple responses (Crawford and Schuster 1993; Lancioni et al. 2001b, 2002a; Mechling 2006). For example, a pressure microswitch fixed to the headrest of a child's wheelchair and connected to a timing device and a light display may enable the child to activate such a display for brief periods of time (i.e., matching the intervals set in the timing device) through small head-movement responses. Similarly, a tilt microswitch fixed to a child's hand and connected to a timing device and a music player may enable the child to produce brief periods of musical stimulation through a small hand-movement response. An optic microswitch in front of the child's mouth and connected to a combination of massage vibrators may enable a child with pervasive motor disabilities to obtain brief periods of massage stimulation through simple mouth-opening responses. Also, optic sensors connected to the child/youth's legs or feet and to a music box may ensure that leg and foot responses are instrumental to bringing about brief intervals of preferred music. None of the first three cases mentioned above would have been able to access the stimulation through a direct manipulation of the stimulus source (i.e., light display, music player, or massage vibrators). The fourth case would not have been likely to find motivation for pre-ambulatory or ambulatory efforts based on the interest in the places he or she could reach or the activities he or she could eventually carry out (Lancioni et al. 2007f, 2008a).

To introduce a person with profound and multiple disabilities to a microswitch-based program, one has to identify a plausible response, that is, a response that can be performed reliably and without excessive effort by the person to successfully activate the microswitch available and produce the positive effect (Glickman et al. 1996; Lancioni et al. 2005h). The response selected for the program should also be adaptive (constructive), that is, it should be seen as beneficial for the person in terms of contact/interaction with the environment as well as physically and socially acceptable (Lancioni et al. 2001a,b,c; Mechling 2006; Sullivan et al. 1995). The program can continue with the use of the first (single) response introduced or can be extended with the addition of new responses that are expected to increase/strengthen as a consequence of the positive stimulation that their emission produces (Lancioni et al. 2001a; Sullivan and Lewis 1990, 1993). In some situations, the program can also be extended by adding to the adaptive response targeted for increase a problem behaviour or a problem/inadequate posture that should be reduced. For example, object manipulation and vocalization may be adaptive responses to be developed further and hand mouthing and head forward bending may represent problem behaviour and a problem/inadequate posture to be reduced (Lancioni et al. 2009a). To carry out a program directed at both (positive and negative) behavioural aspects, one has to resort to a microswitch cluster, that is, to a combination of microswitches that allow simultaneous monitoring of the adaptive response and the problem behaviour/posture and eventually ensure that the preferred stimulation for the adaptive responses occurs only when they are not accompanied by the problem behaviour/posture (cf. Lancioni et al. 2007c, 2008b,c).

There are no explicit guidelines as to the selection of the adaptive responses nor do specific rules exist whereby one can ensure that a program is going to be successful (Holburn, Nguyen and Vietze 2004; Lancioni et al. 2005h, 2008c). The most common views about the selection process converge on basic requirements such as the response (1) should already be present in the person's repertoire or very easy to shape through brief and simple prompting, (2) should not be too demanding in terms of performance cost/effort, and (3) should be discriminable for the person and feasible for the microswitch to detect reliably (Lancioni et al. 2001b, 2005h; Schlosser 2003; Sullivan et al. 1995). Moreover, the stimuli that the person is able to bring about through his or her response should be motivating (i.e., have a positive impact that can abundantly compensate for the overall cost of the response) (Kazdin 2001; Lancioni et al. 2001a, 2002a,c, 2004c; Langley 1990; Schlosser 2003). The combination of all of these elements should lead to a successful outcome. The person should increase the response emission presumably to increase the occurrence of the stimuli programmed for it, due to learning (awareness of) the association between the two events (Catania 2007; Kazdin 2001; Lancioni et al. 2001a, 2002c; Pear 2001).

The literature on microswitch programs has varied with regard to the types and numbers of responses adopted as well as with regard to microswitch systems used. These variations may be considered a reflection of (1) an increased effort to ensure a wider practical and developmental impact of these programs, and (2) an attempt to reach or serve a greater range of individuals than originally contemplated or deemed possible (i.e., including individuals with the most extensive developmental disabilities as well as individuals with relatively high developmental levels) (Lancioni et al. 2003b,c, 2004d, 2007a,b; Singh et al. 2003).

Examining the studies aimed at establishing one or more adaptive responses, the studies combining the goals of promoting constructive responses and reducing problem behaviour/posture, and the technology devised for the different types of studies may help one acquire a general picture of the reality in this area. In particular, it may help one to appreciate the opportunities currently available in this area and the new, potential options that may be worthwhile to investigate. The present chapter is an effort to provide this type of information. The chapter is divided into four main sections, which are concerned with (1) an overview of studies aimed at establishing adaptive responses and related microswitch technology, (2) an overview of studies aimed at promoting adaptive responses and reducing problem behaviour/posture and related microswitch technology, (3) a discussion of the overall findings and their relevance in terms of educational/occupational impact, social appearance and quality of life, and (4) a conclusion section focusing on some relevant issues for future research in the area. Figure 2.1 provides a general map of the first two sections as a general orientation for the reader.

STUDIES AIMED AT ESTABLISHING ADAPTIVE RESPONSES

For practical reasons, the studies aimed at establishing adaptive responses through microswitch-based programs were divided into five groups, according to the responses that they targeted (see Figure 2.1). The first group included a single, typical motor response, such as head turning and hand pushing, and generally relied on the use of

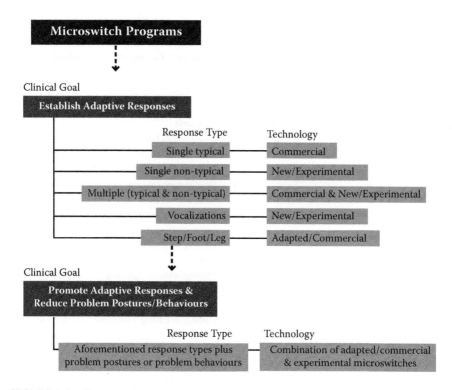

FIGURE 2.1   Conceptual roadmap of chapter content.

conventional, commercial microswitch devices. The second group included a single, non-typical response, which generally consisted of a detailed/small action, such as chin movements or vocalization, and relied on new/experimental microswitch devices. Such combinations of responses and devices were aimed at suiting persons with minimal motor behaviour. The third group included multiple responses, which could concern combinations of typical motor responses or combinations of these responses and non-typical ones. Those responses were targeted through conventional and new microswitches. The fourth group included multiple vocal responses and, specifically, combinations of vocal utterances, which were targeted with the use of adapted and new computer technology serving as multiple microswitch devices. The fifth group involved step responses (or foot/leg movements), which were targeted through optic (occasionally pressure) microswitches linked to the participants' legs or feet. These types of responses and microswitches were used together with special walker/support devices. Table 2.1 lists a number of studies considered to be representative of each of the groups mentioned. For every study listed, the table reports the number of participants and their ages (only participants up to 19 years of age are included in this review context), the response(s) used, and the outcome. The outcome is defined in terms of the number of participants with positive results, negative results, or partially positive results. Positive results refer to increased responding presumably due to the participants learning the link between responding and the preferred stimuli available for it (Lancioni et al. 2003a). Partially positive results refer to

TABLE 2.1
Studies Aimed at Establishing Adaptive Responses Grouped According to the Response(s) Targeted

Studies	Participants	Age	Response Types	Outcome
Single (Typical) Response				
Dattilo (1986)	3	6–10	Pushing with hand	3 Positive
McClure et al. (1986)	1	9	Pushing with both hands	1 Positive
Dattilo (1987)	1	7	Pushing with hand	1 Positive
Dewson and Whiteley (1987)	7	11–18	Head turning (pushing)	5 Positive 2 Negative
Sandler and McLain (1987)	5	6–8	Pushing with hand	5 Positive
Realon et al. (1988)	4	13–19	Pushing with hand, wrist or elbow	1 Positive 3 Negative
Realon et al. (1989)	8	—	Moving sideways (pushing with) hand	5 Positive 3 Negative
Sobsey and Reichle (1989)	6	6–16	Pushing with hand	6 Positive
Leatherby et al. (1992)[a]	5	7–13	Pushing or pulling with hand/ arm	3 Positive 2 Negative
Ivancic and Bailey (1996)	15	—	Pushing or pulling with hand or head turning (pushing)[b]	4 Positive 11 Negative
Lancioni et al. (2002c)	2	7, 14	Tapping with hand	2 Positive
Lancioni et al. (2003a)	3	9–15	Moving (pushing with) torso, tapping with one hand on other, or moving hand/knee	2 Positive 1 Partially positive
Lancioni et al. (2003b)	2	8, 9	Hand to forehead or on other hand	2 Positive
Singh et al. (2003)	1	14	Pushing with hand	1 Positive
Lancioni et al. (2004c)	1	7	Hand swaying	1 Positive
Mechling (2006)	3	5–19	Pushing with hand/arm or head turning (pushing)	3 Positive
Single (Non-Typical) Response				
Lancioni and Lems (2001)	2	4, 18	Vocalization	2 Positive
Lancioni et al. (2001c)	2	7, 10	Vocalization	2 Positive
Lancioni et al. (2004a)	1	18	Chin movements (as in chewing)	1 Positive
Lancioni et al. (2004b)	1	6	Chin movements (as in mouth opening)	1 Positive
Lancioni et al. (2004f)	1	17	Chin movements (as in chewing)	1 Positive
Lancioni et al. (2005a)	1	9	Repeated eye-blink pattern	1 Positive
Lancioni et al. (2006f)	2	10, 12	Eyelid upward movement	2 Positive
Lancioni et al. (2007a)	2	6, 14	Forehead skin movements	2 Positive
Lancioni et al. (2007b)	1	5	Hand-closure movements	1 Positive

TABLE 2.1 (CONTINUED)

Studies Aimed at Establishing Adaptive Responses Grouped According to the Response(s) Targeted

Studies	Participants	Age	Response Types	Outcome
Multiple (Typical and Non-Typical) Responses				
Crawford and Schuster (1993)	3	4	2 responses per participant: Pushing, pulling, or moving with hand, wrist or elbow	1 Positive 2 Partially positive
Sullivan et al. (1995)	1	3.5	2 responses: Head backward (pushing) and pushing with hand	1 Positive
Lancioni et al. (2001d)	2	10, 13	3 or 4 responses per participant: Vocalization, head turning, touching with hand, and raising foot	2 Positive
Lancioni et al. (2002a)	2	8, 12	3 responses per participant: Vocalization, head turning or backward (pushing), and pushing with hand	2 Positive
Lancioni et al. (2002b)	2	8, 13	3 responses per participant: Vocalization, head turning, tapping/stroking with fist or elbow, pushing with the back or hand	2 Positive
Lancioni et al. (2003c)	2	17, 19	4 responses per participant: Vocalization, raising head, pushing with left hand, with right hand or foot	2 Positive
Lancioni et al. (2004d)	2	7, 17	3 or 4 responses per participant: Vocalization, head forward, pushing with left hand, or with each hand	2 Positive
Lancioni et al. (2006a)	3	7–16	2 responses per participant: Vocalization and chin movements, knee movements and hand swaying, or mouth closing and hand opening	3 Positive
Lancioni et al. (2007g)	1	18	2 responses: Eye opening and mouth opening	1 Positive
Multiple (Vocal) Responses				
Lancioni et al. (2004b)	1	5	2 responses: Equivalents of a name and a falling-object sound	1 Positive
Lancioni et al. (2004e)	1	19	6 responses: Equivalents of words such as grandma, talc, cough, eyes, cat, and guitar	1 Positive

TABLE 2.1 (CONTINUED)
Studies Aimed at Establishing Adaptive Responses Grouped According to the Response(s) Targeted

Studies	Participants	Age	Response Types	Outcome
Lancioni et al. (2004g)	1	16	3 responses: These were syllable-like sounds	1 Positive
Lancioni et al. (2004i)	1	19	9 responses: Equivalents of words such as mama, pianoforte, song and singer's uncle's name, dance music and games	1 Positive
Lancioni et al. (2005e)	1	18	7 responses: Equivalents of myself, pets, a caregiver's name, papa, popular songs, friends and funny stories	1 Positive
Step Responses or Foot/Leg Movements				
Lancioni et al. (2005f)	1	13	Step responses for supported locomotion	1 Positive
Lancioni et al. (2005g)	1	11	Step responses for supported locomotion	1 Positive
Lancioni et al. (2007d)	2	7, 9	Step responses for supported locomotion	2 Positive
Lancioni et al. (2007f)	2	8, 10	Pre-ambulatory foot/leg movements	2 Positive
Lancioni et al. (2008a)	2	3, 12	Step responses for supported locomotion	2 Positive

Note: (–) Information is missing.
[a] The data refer to Study 1.
[b] No details are provided.

the situation in which a participant succeeds only in part of the program (i.e., failing to increase some of the targeted responses or exhibiting response decline during the post-intervention period).

Studies Targeting a Single (Typical) Response

Table 2.1 provides a list of 16 studies targeting a single, typical response (Dattilo 1986, 1987; Dewson and Whiteley 1987; Ivancic and Bailey 1996; Lancioni et al. 2002c, 2003a,b, 2004c; Leatherby et al. 1992; McClure et al. 1986; Mechling 2006; Realon, Favell, and Dayvault 1988; Realon, Favell and Phillips 1989; Sobsey and Reichle 1989; Sandler and McLain 1987; Singh et al. 2003). Although the response adopted could vary considerably across studies, the most common examples consisted of head turning and hand pushing. The microswitches adopted for them generally consisted of pressure devices or similar kinds of instruments. Other forms of responses varied from tapping with the hand on a tabletop to moving the hands downward or bringing one hand onto the other (with the use of vibration-sensitive devices or tilt/mercury and optic microswitches that were activated by movement rather than pressure; see Lancioni et al. 2002c, 2003a,b).

For example, McClure et al. (1986) taught an 8-year-old boy to push with both hands on pressure microswitches mounted approximately 40 cm apart on his wheelchair's board. This response allowed him to obtain brief periods of preferred stimuli such as vibration and music. The boy, who had profound intellectual disability and visual impairment, acquired high levels of responding (suggesting that his responses were largely influenced by the contingent occurrence of preferred stimuli) and engaged in such responding successfully during different periods of the day.

Leatherby et al. (1992) worked with five children, who were between 7 and 13 years of age. The response selected for the activation of the microswitches involved pushing, pulling or moving aside with the hand. Microswitch activation (produced by the hand movements selected as responses) turned on a preferred toy for a 3-s interval. One of the five children did not produce any meaningful responding and thus was excluded from the study. Of the remaining four children, three increased their level of responding during the intervention as opposed to the baseline (i.e., when no toys were available for their responding) or a non-contingent stimulation phase (i.e., when toys were presented independently of their responding).

Ivancic and Bailey (1996) worked with 15 persons, 10 of whom were known as having a long history of learning failure due to their complex situation. The responses targeted by the authors were seemingly simple movements of the hand and head, such as pushing/pulling or turning. The microswitches were apparently pressure devices or simple variations thereof. The intervention phases included the use of more preferred or less preferred stimuli on the target responses, across groups of sessions of 10 min. The results showed that the use of highly preferred stimuli was effective in increasing the frequency of the target responses for four of the seven participants for whom highly preferred stimuli had been identified. The use of non-highly preferred stimuli was consistently ineffective.

Lancioni et al. (2002c) taught two girls of 7 and 14 years of age to use hand-tapping responses to access preferred stimuli. Hand tapping on the tabletop was considered more plausible for the participants (as it required lower performance efforts and motor coordination) than pushing on a specific microswitch placed on the table. The hand-tapping responses were monitored through a vibration microswitch. During the intervention phase, the participants' production of those responses, and consequent activation of the vibration microswitch, led to the occurrence of preferred stimuli for 7 s. The results showed that both girls had a very consistent increase in responding during the intervention as opposed to the baseline phase (i.e., when no stimuli were available for their response efforts).

Lancioni et al. (2003b) taught two children of 8 and 9 years of age to activate optic microswitches with hand movements such as bringing the left hand almost in contact with the forehead and bringing the right hand almost in contact with the back of the left hand. The reason for (the hypothesised advantage in) using these responses, which were already present in the children's repertoire, was that they did not require a precise/forceful physical action such as that needed for pushing on specific pressure devices. During the intervention period, the responses triggered preferred stimuli for 7 s. Both children showed an increase in responding during intervention as opposed to baseline.

Mechling (2006) included three participants of 5 to 19 years of age. They activated a pressure microswitch either with head or with arm/hand movements. The intervention (comparison of conditions) comprised nine sessions of 9 min each. Every session consisted of three 3-min intervention periods, which involved the three stimulus conditions compared. A stimulus condition was activated for 10 s after microswitch activation. The stimulus conditions concerned adapted toys and devices (i.e., three new objects per participant, such as a train moving, a blowing whistle and flashing lights), commercial cause-and-effect software (i.e., three programs per participant, such as *Teach Me to Talk: Animals,* which involved sound, music and animation), and instructor-created video programs (i.e., three recordings of different events/ activities per participant, such as group singing, which presented preferred persons, sounds and occupations). Once the comparison had been completed, each participant received three sessions with the most effective condition only. During the comparison phase, each participant showed a higher frequency of microswitch activations with the instructor-created video programs. The mean frequencies of activations with this condition ranged between 5 and 9 for the three participants. The mean frequencies for the intervention periods with adapted toys and devices ranged between 1 and 3, while the mean frequencies for the periods with commercial cause-and-effect software were low for two participants and approximately 6 for the third. During the best condition only, the participants' mean frequencies of microswitch activations were between 6 and 7.

STUDIES TARGETING A SINGLE (NON-TYPICAL) RESPONSE

Table 2.1 provides a list of nine studies targeting a single, non-typical response for microswitch activation (Lancioni and Lems 2001; Lancioni et al. 2001c, 2004a,b,f, 2005a, 2006f, 2007a,b). The non-typical responses targeted in these studies included vocalization (i.e., a brief sound emission), chin movements (mouth opening), eye-lid movements, forehead skin movements and small hand-closure movements. The search for non-typical, novel responses and matching/suitable microswitches originated from two considerations. First, some of the failures reported with the use of typical responses may have been due to the excessive effort that the performance of such responses required of the participants with very extensive motor impairment (Ivancic and Bailey 1996; Lancioni et al. 2007c). Second, a number of those individuals may not even qualify for microswitch-aided programs given their extremely limited behavioural repertoire and the consequent absence of responses suitable for the microswitches commercially available (cf. Lancioni et al. 2001c, 2004f, 2007b,g; Leatherby et al. 1992).

For example, Lancioni and Lems (2001) worked with two participants of 4 and 18 years of age, who had pervasive multiple disabilities that made it impossible for them to manage motor responses such as those reported in the first group of studies. Both participants, however, presented spontaneous vocal responses, which were viewed as a potential resource to develop through a new (specifically built) microswitch. The new microswitch consisted of a battery-powered, sound-detecting device connected to a throat microphone (insensitive to environmental noise), which was held at the participants' larynx with a simple neckband. Data showed that prior to the intervention, the participants had mean frequencies of vocal responses between 1 and 2 per minute. During the intervention, the response rates more than doubled for both participants, indicating clear performance (and sensory input) changes for them.

Lancioni et al. (2004b) conducted a program with a 6-year-old boy, who usually sat in a reclined position with his body largely static. The response that seemed most plausible for him to perform (and it was already present in his repertoire) was chin movements, as in mouth opening. The microswitch for this response involved (1) a small box with a position sensor, which was attached to the side of a hat that the boy was to wear, and (2) a light band that connected the position sensor to the other side of the hat, passing under the boy's chin. When a downward chin movement pulled the position sensor, the microswitch was activated and consequently preferred environmental stimuli were delivered. The boy's response frequency increased more than twofold during the intervention phases compared to the baseline periods. An alternative microswitch technology for this response was later developed (Lancioni et al. 2006e) to intervene with an 8-year-old boy, who disliked things touching his face. The microswitch for this boy consisted of an optic sensor held under his chin. The microswitch activated as its distance from the chin decreased (i.e., in relation to the boy's mouth opening). The results were satisfactory with the boy showing a large response increase during the intervention periods.

Lancioni et al. (2005a) reported an intervention with a 9-year-old boy, who presented with profound developmental and physical disabilities and minimal motor behaviour. The most reliable response for him seemed to be eye blinking. A specific response pattern (i.e., two blinks occurring within a 2-s interval) was identified as distinct from the common blinking behaviour. The microswitch for the response included (1) an optic sensor mounted on an eyeglass frame that the boy wore during the sessions, and (2) an electronic unit that emitted a signal when a response (two blinks within a 2-s interval) was detected. Data showed that the response rates increased largely during the intervention periods (i.e., when responding allowed the participant to access preferred stimuli).

Lancioni et al. (2006f) worked with two children of 10 and 12 years of age using upward eyelid movements as the response through which they could produce environmental changes (i.e., causing brief periods of preferred stimulation). The microswitch technology involved optic sensors mounted on eyeglasses such as those reported in the study by Lancioni et al. (2005a). However, the functioning of the technology was modified in order to suit the response selected for the two participants. This consisted of raising one eyelid or both eyelids markedly as it occurs when looking at something that is high up. In this study, the optic sensor was not to detect the blinks as in the Lancioni et al. (2005a) study, but rather the transition from the eyelid (which it normally pointed at) to the eye (which it would point at in the case of a looking-up response). Both participants showed extensive response increases during the intervention periods (i.e., when the response was instrumental to obtain preferred stimuli). The increases were maintained at a 2-month post-intervention check.

Lancioni et al. (2007a) explored the possibility of using small upward or downward movements of the forehead skin as the response for two children of approximately 6 and 14 years of age. The microswitch consisted of an optic sensor (barcode reader) with an electronic regulation unit, and a small tag with horizontal bars (kept on the participants' foreheads). The optic sensor was held in front of the tag and small movements of this (following upward or downward movements of the forehead skin) activated the microswitch system and caused brief periods of preferred stimulation. Both participants showed a clear response increase during the first intervention period. Such an increase was replicated during a second intervention phase and successfully retained at a 1.5-month post-intervention check.

Lancioni et al. (2007b) reported the use of small hand-closure movements as the response with a girl of slightly more than 5 years of age. The response consisted of the girl's fingers touching or pressing on a microswitch fixed to the palm of her hand. The microswitch involved a two-membrane thin pad. The outer membrane (i.e., the one facing the girl's fingers) was a touch-sensitive sensor and was activated by simple contact with any of her fingers. The inner membrane was activated if the girl applied pressure of approximately 20 g. This second membrane allowed microswitch activation to occur even if the girl's fingers remained in contact with the outer membrane. In such cases, the girl was not required to remove her fingers from contact to activate the microswitch, but rather to intensify such contact (triggering the inner membrane) to access preferred environmental stimulation. The girl showed a gradual but highly consistent response increase during the first intervention phase, which was replicated during the second intervention phase and successfully maintained at a 1-month post-intervention check.

STUDIES TARGETING MULTIPLE (TYPICAL AND NON-TYPICAL) RESPONSES

Table 2.1 provides a list of nine studies involving the use of multiple responses with multiple microswitches to allow the participants to access different sets of stimuli (Crawford and Schuster 1993; Lancioni et al. 2001d, 2002a,b, 2003c, 2004d, 2006a, 2007g; Sullivan et al. 1995). For example, Crawford and Schuster (1993) involved three children of 4 years of age. Each child was taught to use two responses, which involved pushing, pulling or moving aside with the hand, wrist or elbow. The performance of a response, with the help of a prompt from the research assistant or independently, led to the activation of a preferred toy for 5 to 7 s. Two of the children showed successful acquisition (i.e., independent performance) of only one of the two responses targeted during the intervention. Data for the third child showed successful acquisition of the response taught during the intervention and of the second response available, which apparently required no teaching.

Sullivan et al. (1995) worked with a girl, whose age was 3.5 years. The responses selected for the girl consisted of a head backward (pushing) movement and pushing with the hand. The two microswitches (pressure devices) were simultaneously available and the activation of either of them through the aforementioned responses led to the occurrence of preferred stimuli. Data indicated that both responses were increasing in relation to the availability of the stimuli.

Lancioni et al. (2002b) conducted a study with two participants, who were 8 and 13 years of age. For each participant, three responses were targeted. Those responses were vocalization, head-sideways and elbow-stroking motions for the first participant, and fist tapping, back pushing and a hand-to-shoulder motion for the second participant. The responses were taught individually and each of them led to a specific set of preferred stimuli throughout the intervention. Once the intervention had covered all responses, the participants could use any of them at any time. This response freedom allowed them continuous access to (with the opportunity of choosing among) all three sets of preferred stimuli. The results showed that both participants had an increased use of all three responses. Their performance was largely maintained over post-intervention checks covering 4 or 6 months.

Lancioni et al. (2006a) worked with three participants whose ages ranged between 7 and 16 years. Each participant was taught two simple responses. The responses consisted of vocalization and repeated chin movements, light knee movement and gentle swaying of a grid suspended above the participant's face, and mouth closing and hand opening. The microswitches for vocalization and chin movements were the same as those previously described for these responses (Lancioni and Lems 2001). The microswitches for mouth closing and hand opening were variations of the microswitch used for chin movements. The microswitches used for knee movement and grid swaying were combinations of tilt devices. Each participant was taught the responses individually. Subsequently, the microswitches for the two responses were simultaneously available and the participant could choose between the two. The last period of the study was aimed at assessing whether the participants' preference for one response or the other was due to a choice between the stimuli available for the responses or simply to the response per se. The results indicated that all three participants succeeded in acquiring the responses selected for them and showed clear response choices. These choices seemed to be largely due to the stimuli available for one response or the other at least for two of the participants. For the third participant, the level of simplicity of the responses seemed also to play a role. In other words, one of the responses seemed simpler for the participant than the other and this aspect had an impact on the overall choice rates.

Lancioni et al. (2007g) reported a study with an 18-year-old participant. The participant had previously been involved in a program with multiple responses and multiple microswitches. However, the previous responses (hand pushing and head turning) were no longer present in his repertoire due to a deterioration of his general motor condition. The new responses used to replace the old ones were eye and mouth opening. The microswitch technology for these responses included two optic sensors mounted on an eyeglasses' frame. The first optic sensor was in front of the participant's left eye and it was triggered when the eye was opened. The second optic sensor was held through a light wire in front of the participant's mouth and was triggered when the mouth was opened. The two responses were instrumental to access two different sets of preferred stimuli. The results showed that the participant was successful in replacing the old (hand and head) responses that were no longer feasible for him with the new eye- and mouth-opening responses. These responses

were successfully combined (after their individual teaching) and were retained satisfactorily at the 2-month post-intervention check.

STUDIES TARGETING MULTIPLE (VOCAL) RESPONSES

Table 2.1 provides a list of five studies using multiple vocal responses (Lancioni et al.
2004b,e,g,i, 2005e). These studies originated from the notion that (1) a number of persons with multiple disabilities may be able to produce different vocal utterances, and
(2) such utterances could become relevant responses/instruments through which the
persons can bring about environmental changes and specifically produce periods of
preferred stimulation. To make the responses powerful instruments as just mentioned,
a computer system was recently developed. The system works as a combination of
microswitches, which discriminate among the participants' utterances and ensure
that different utterances can cause different/appropriate environmental effects.

For example, Lancioni et al. (2004g) conducted a study with two participants with
multiple disabilities, who presented some vocal behaviour. One was 16 years old (in
the age range covered in this chapter), while the other was 20 years old (outside the
range covered here). The vocal behaviour consisted of one-syllable utterances for the
younger participant and word-like utterances for the older participant. Totals of three
and nine utterances were available for the two participants, respectively. The software program for the discrimination of the first participant's utterances was based
on locally recurrent neural networks and time sequences of cepstral parameters. The
software used for the discrimination of the second participant's utterances involved
the combination of a commercially available speech recognition program and an
experimental control program developed specifically for the study. Both participants
increased the frequencies of their utterances drastically during the intervention (i.e.,
when their utterances allowed them to access specific, positive environmental stimuli). The system's percentages of correct utterance discrimination were more than 70
for the two participants.

Lancioni et al. (2004i) extended the work in this area with two additional participants with multiple disabilities. One of them was within the age range of this chapter
(19 years old), while the other was outside the range (23 years old). For each of
these participants, nine word-like utterances were used as specific responses, which
allowed access to different stimulation events. The computer system employed for
them combined a commercially available speech recognition program and a special
control program like the one described previously. Data showed that both participants increased the frequencies of their utterances during the intervention. The system's percentages of correct utterance discrimination were greater than or equal to
80 for the two participants.

STUDIES TARGETING STEP RESPONSES OR BASIC FOOT/LEG MOVEMENTS

Table 2.1 lists five studies reporting the use of support/walker devices and microswitches with contingent stimulation for children with multiple disabilities, that is,
intellectual, motor and, often, sensory disabilities (Lancioni et al. 2005f,g, 2007d,f,
2008a). Their level of intellectual disability was estimated to be in the severe to

profound range. These studies, except the one by Lancioni et al. (2007f), were aimed at promoting stepping responses (locomotion) with six children. The study by Lancioni et al. (2007f) targeted pre-ambulatory leg-foot movements with two children. The walker/support device ensured upright posture and provided sufficient body-weight lifting through a saddle or harness and a fitting frame. These conditions were aimed at ensuring that the child could produce step responses (or other leg-foot movements) without excessive effort. The microswitches monitored the occurrence of the target responses and allowed the responses to cause brief periods of preferred stimulation. Preferred stimulation was considered of critical importance to motivate the children to perform independent responses and enjoy the experience (Lancioni et al. 2007d; Miltenberger 2004).

For example, Lancioni et al. (2007d) used the aforementioned approach with two children of 7 and 9 years of age. The children were reported to be in the profound intellectual disability range but could stand and take some steps with support. One of them presented with spastic tetraparesis and visual impairment while the other had low muscle tone and visual impairment. Both children received several 5-min sessions per day. The design of the study involved an ABAB sequence (in which A represented baseline phases and B represented intervention phases) and a 1-month post-intervention check. The B (intervention) phases, contrary to the A (baseline) phases, included brief stimulation events for the step responses, which were detected through optic microswitches attached to their shoes. The results showed that both children had a clear increase in the frequencies of step responses during the intervention phases and retained this increase at the post-intervention check. During those periods, the children also showed an increase in indices of happiness, such as smiles.

Lancioni et al. (2007f) used the same approach to enhance pre-ambulatory responses with two children of 8 and 10 years of age. The procedural conditions were similar to those of the study summarised previously (Lancioni et al. 2007d), while the responses targeted were foot-leg movements. These movements, which were detected through optic or pressure microswitches, involved the child's foot touching the floor after any minimal lifting of it (i.e., in a way that resembled a side, forward, or backward step). Both children showed relatively low levels of responses during the baseline phases and rises in response levels during the intervention phases.

STUDIES AIMED AT PROMOTING ADAPTIVE RESPONSES AND REDUCING PROBLEM BEHAVIOUR/POSTURE

Table 2.2 presents a list of 10 studies that assessed the impact of microswitch clusters, that is, combinations of microswitches used simultaneously for promoting adaptive responses and reducing problem behaviour/posture (Lancioni et al. 2004h, 2005b,c,d, 2006c, 2007c,e,h, 2008c,d). Six of those studies involved the reduction of problem postures such as leg flexing and head forward tilting and four involved the reduction of problem behaviours such as hand mouthing and eye poking. The use of microswitch clusters is based on the notion that educational intervention with persons with profound and multiple disabilities needs to reduce the problem behaviour/posture as part of the effort to promote constructive responding in order to have

TABLE 2.2

Studies Aimed at Establishing Adaptive Responses and Reducing Problem Behaviour/Posture

Studies	Participants	Age	Response Types	Outcome
Adaptive Responses and Problem Posture				
Lancioni et al. (2004h)	3	6–12	Adaptive responses: Touching, manipulating objects or lifting a foot Problem posture: Leg flexed, and head forward tilting or backward stretching	3 Positive
Lancioni et al. (2005b)	1	7	Adaptive responses: Pushing on a small sensitive board Problem posture: Head forward tilting	1 Positive
Lancioni et al. (2005c)	2	6, 8	Adaptive responses: Pushing on a small sensitive board or lifting arm and hand Problem posture: Head forward tilting	2 Positive
Lancioni et al. (2005d)	3	7–9	Adaptive responses: Lifting a foot, touching an object on a leg, and vocalization Problem posture: Head forward tilting	3 Positive
Lancioni et al. (2007c)[a]	4	8–10	Adaptive responses: Touching an object on a leg, pushing an object in front, lifting arm and hand, and vocalization Posture: Head forward tilting	2 Positive 2 Partially positive
Lancioni et al. (2008d)	3	8–17	Adaptive responses: Lifting a foot or stroking a table area or the other hand Problem posture: Head forward tilting	3 Positive
Adaptive Responses and Problem Behaviour				
Lancioni et al. (2006c)	1	12	Adaptive responses: Head and foot movements Problem behaviour: Hand mouthing	1 Positive
Lancioni et al. (2007e)	1	13	Adaptive responses: Foot movements Problem behaviours: Hand mouthing and eye poking	1 Positive
Lancioni et al. (2007h)	2	8, 12	Adaptive responses: Manipulation of objects Problem behaviours: Hand or object mouthing	2 Positive
Lancioni et al. (2008c)	1	12	Adaptive responses: Manipulation of objects Problem behaviour: Hand mouthing	1 Positive

[a] The data refer to Study I.

positive developmental/clinical implications (Lancioni et al. 2004, 2005d, 2008c). Programs based on microswitch clusters allow one to (1) concurrently monitor adaptive responses and problem behaviour/posture, and (2) deliver preferred stimuli automatically for adaptive responses occurring in the absence of the problem behaviour/ posture (Lancioni et al. 2006).

STUDIES DEALING WITH PROBLEM POSTURE

In one of the initial studies in this area, Lancioni et al. (2004h) studied three children with multiple disabilities between 6 and 12 years of age. The adaptive response for the three children consisted of touching, manipulating an object/microswitch or lifting a foot (i.e., removing it from a pressure microswitch), which allowed them access to brief periods of preferred environmental stimulation. The target problem posture was (1) a flexed (rather than extended) leg for one of the participants who was standing with support during the sessions and (2) head forward tilting or backward stretching for the other two participants who were sitting during the sessions. Initially, the participants were able to access preferred stimulation each time they performed the adaptive response. Subsequently, the adaptive response led to preferred stimulation only if it occurred in the absence of the problem posture, which was detected through pressure or tilt microswitches. All three participants showed a vast increase in their adaptive responses and a significant decrease in the problem posture. Essentially, most of the adaptive responses were performed with the leg extended (one participant) and the head upward (the other two participants).

Lancioni et al. (2007c) carried out a long-term assessment with four children who had been involved in a program aimed at promoting two adaptive responses while reducing head forward tilting. The program had been carried out according to the procedures summarised for the study mentioned previously (Lancioni et al. 2004h). That is, the emphasis of the intervention was first on promoting the adaptive responses by allowing them to produce preferred stimulation. Then, the adaptive responses were made to turn on preferred stimulation only if they occurred in the absence of the problem posture. The results had shown large increases in the frequencies of the adaptive responses, which mostly occurred in the absence of head tilting. The data of the long-term assessment indicated that two of the children maintained the head upright for nearly the entire stimulation period, while the other two children did not maintain the correct posture through the stimulation period. In an attempt to modify the situation of the latter children, a program revision was carried out for them. In essence, adaptive responses occurring in the absence of head tilting continued to turn on the preferred stimulation. This stimulation, however, lasted the 8 s scheduled only if the child maintained upright head position through that period. Otherwise, it was interrupted. The outcome of this program revision was largely satisfactory with both children. That is, they acquired the ability to maintain the head upright for most of the stimulation time and the session duration.

Lancioni et al. (2008d) attempted to replicate the results of the aforementioned program revision with three new participants of approximately 8 to 17 years of age with multiple disabilities. The adaptive response consisted of foot lifting or hand stroking. The problem posture was head forward tilting. Initially, the participants were provided with 9 s of preferred stimulation for each adaptive response they performed. Subsequently, only the adaptive responses that occurred in the absence of the problem posture were allowed to turn on the stimulation. This lasted the scheduled 9-s period if the participant kept the head upward throughout. Yet, it would be interrupted if the problem posture reappeared. The results indicated that all three participants increased the overall frequency of adaptive responses and the frequency of those responses with the head upright. The upright head position was maintained through most of the scheduled stimulation periods as well as most of the session time. An expert validation assessment of this program with physiotherapist trainees and professionals supported its practical relevance and indicated that such a program could be conceived as a useful complement to formal motor rehabilitation procedures.

STUDIES DEALING WITH PROBLEM BEHAVIOUR

Lancioni et al. (2007e) carried out a program to deal with problem behaviours with a 13-year-old boy, who was diagnosed with profound mental retardation, motor impairment and minimal residual vision. The boy did not possess recognizable adaptive responses to control environmental stimulation and engaged in problem behaviours such as hand mouthing and eye poking, which were deemed to occur independent of social contingencies. The boy was initially taught an adaptive foot-movement response, which activated a special microswitch and turned on preferred stimuli for 8 s. Subsequently, foot responses produced preferred stimuli only if they occurred in the absence of hand mouthing and eye poking. Moreover, the stimuli were on for the 8-s period scheduled only if the problem behaviours did not appear during that time. Occurrence of any problem behaviour led to stimulus interruption. Data showed that the boy (1) increased his adaptive responding, (2) learned to perform this responding largely free from problem behaviour and refrained from that behaviour for most of the session time, and (3) maintained this positive performance through the 3-month post-intervention check.

Lancioni et al. (2008c) worked with a girl of 12 years of age, who presented with spastic tetraparesis, minimal residual vision and reportedly profound intellectual disability. The girl had only minimal interest in the objects presented in front of her and tended to engage in hand mouthing. The intervention program was directed at promoting object contact/manipulation and reducing hand mouthing. The adaptive response was detected by optic microswitches, which were arranged inside a box containing vibrating devices. The problem behaviour was detected through optic microswitches on the girl's shirt across her chest. When the girl brought one or both hands into the box and touched the objects/devices available, these were turned on to provide preferred vibratory stimulation combined with music or voices for 8 s. The stimulation (1) started only if the girl did not simultaneously engage in hand mouthing and (2) continued for the scheduled 8 s provided that the girl did not engage in hand mouthing during that period. If she did, the stimulation would immediately stop. The results were highly encouraging. The girl exhibited a large increase in the number of adaptive responses free of the problem behaviour. The mean session time without hand mouthing was approximately 2.5 min at the beginning of the program. It increased to approximately 7 min by the end of the program.

DISCUSSION

OUTCOME OF THE STUDIES

Most of the studies reported in Table 2.1 and Table 2.2 had a positive outcome, that is, clear increases in adaptive responses or increases in adaptive responding and declines in problem behaviour/posture. Most of the exceptions (i.e., negative or partially positive results) were reported in the studies using a single (typical) response. Some doubts were also raised by the long-term data obtained with the first version of the clusters when the scheduled stimulation was provided in its entirety regardless of the lasting absence or reappearance of the problem posture.

In view of all of the results with the single (typical) responses, several considerations can be formulated. First, one could argue that some of the studies reporting failures did apparently set up a program without a clearly recognised collection of highly preferred stimuli to use contingent on the responses being taught (e.g., Dewson and Whiteley 1987; Ivancic and Bailey 1996; Realon et al. 1988, 1989). In some situations, it was clearly reported that no high-preference stimuli existed for the participants (e.g., Ivancic and Bailey 1996). This lack of preferred stimuli (absence of motivating/reinforcing events), together with a very low level of functioning of the participants, can definitely be considered an extremely serious problem in a program in which learning is the objective being pursued (Crawford and Schuster 1993; Kazdin 2001).

Second, it is easily conceivable that participants with a very limited level of functioning are much more at risk of failure when the response requirement is harder (i.e., when the response is not yet in the person's repertoire or it requires a fairly high level of effort to be performed). In these cases, the only chances of learning success are tied to three conditions, that is, (1) adequate physical skills for the independent performance of the response, (2) very powerful stimuli contingent on the response (i.e., highly effective reinforcing events) so that the positive value of the stimuli by far exceeds the efforts required for performing the response, and (3) carefully programmed and sufficiently protracted teaching time (Kazdin 2001; Lancioni et al. 2001a; Saunders et al. 2003). Apparently, these conditions were not always available in the studies that reported failures (e.g., Dewson and Whiteley 1987; Ivancic and Bailey 1996; Realon et al. 1988).

Third, with regard to the notion of careful programming, Saunders et al. (2001, 2003) have suggested that adopting a momentary functioning of the microswitches might be more useful than resorting to their combination with timers. In the first case, the microswitch ensures the activation of preferred stimuli throughout the duration of the response. In the second case, the stimuli are activated for a specific period of time, generally a few seconds, consequent to the response (irrespective of its duration). While these authors have reported encouraging data in support of their view, they also found failures or partial success with momentary functioning of the microswitches (Saunders et al. 2001, 2003). The idea that a person may not easily associate response and stimulation when a timer is used with the microswitch (i.e., because new response emissions during the stimulation do not cause new effects) may be inaccurate and questionable. In fact, the chances that the person produces a new response emission during the stimulation following his or her previous response is limited due to the brevity of the stimulation periods typically used (e.g., 7 s). Moreover, any new response instance occurring during the stimulation period would be paired with an on-going positive event rather than meeting with neglect (Kazdin 2001; Miltenberger 2004).

Fourth, selecting a suitable response may entail different things for different people. For some people, one may successfully select fairly simple (typical) movements that do not need to be particularly precise spatially, do not involve any remarkable physical effort, and can provide obvious feedback (e.g., swaying a grid above one's face with small hand movements). For others, one may need to resort to less conventional forms of behaviour such as vocalizations, eyelid movements, or chin movements as plausible responses (Lancioni et al. 2001c, 2004b, 2005a,i).

In view of the unsatisfactory data reported in some applications of the microswitch clusters, at least two points may be underlined. The first point concerns the fact that maintaining an appropriate posture (e.g., head upright) and avoiding an inappropriate posture (e.g., head forward tilting) may be quite difficult for some participants and thus it may be possible only for brief periods at a time or only when very high motivation is ensured. Initiatives to facilitate the new posture (e.g., via a less stringent posture request or more favourable positioning) could be beneficial in those cases (Lancioni et al. 2007c, 2008d). The second point concerns the need to use the reinforcing stimulation correctly. Allowing the stimulation to continue even if the problem posture reappears amounts to reinforcing rather than discouraging such behaviour (Kazdin 2001; Lancioni et al. 2008d). On the contrary, interrupting the stimulation whenever the problem posture reappears may help the person to discriminate between appropriate and inappropriate posture (amounting to a form of *response cost* for the problem posture) (Kazdin 2001; Miltenberger 2004).

The positive outcome obtained in the studies using a single, non-typical response may underline the possibility of successfully serving participants with minimal motor behaviour and limited response opportunities. In these cases (like in any other case), a satisfactory outcome would depend on the respect of a number of basic conditions regarding the response per se, the microswitch, and the stimuli. For example, one should (1) select a response that is already in the participant's repertoire and is not too difficult for him or her to perform, (2) use a microswitch that is suitable to the response and the participant's situation, and (3) ensure the availability of stimuli that are highly motivating for the participant. New research with regard to non-typical responses would be highly desirable to determine the generality of the data collected thus far and extend the assessment to other types of responses and microswitches to open new intervention opportunities that were not previously available or conceivable (Barlow, Nock, and Hersen 2009; Kennedy 2005).

The studies using multiple responses have mostly reported successful results, with participants increasing the level of response engagement, improving self-determination, and enriching positive environmental stimulation (cf. Algozzine et al. 2001; Felce and Perry 1995; Schalock et al. 2003). A positive view may also be taken about the studies involving multiple vocal responses. In spite of the encouraging picture emerging from this latter group, the results should be interpreted with caution. In fact, only a small number of participants were included in these studies and the availability of differentiated vocal responses can be expected only in a minority of participants with multiple disabilities (Barlow et al. 2009; Kazdin 2001; Lancioni et al. 2004i, 2005e).

The studies involving support/walker devices with microswitches and contingent stimulation have illustrated the possibility of using this intervention package in a very functional way for special groups of participants, that is, (1) those with a relevant level of motor performance potentially usable for supported ambulation and (2) those with basic foot/leg movements that may be profitably exercised (cf. Lancioni et al. 2007d,f). The possibility of following step responses or simple foot/leg movements with preferred (reinforcing) stimulation is expected to compensate for the response efforts (i.e., compete with their cost) and motivate the children to increase the response frequency on an independent basis. Such a situation of great motivation through preferred stimulation may also be favourable for improving the children's general mood (i.e., increasing indices of happiness) with important implications for their social, emotional and practical outlook (Dillon and Carr 2007; Lancioni et al. 2007d,f).

IMPLICATIONS OF THE STUDIES AND PRACTICAL PERSPECTIVES

The results of the studies using microswitch-based programs represent a substantial body of evidence that clarifies (and emphasises) the relevance of this approach and also suggests possible ways of expanding and improving it. In an appraisal of past/present solutions and a search for innovations, the first consideration concerns the use of single, non-typical responses. The studies adopting those responses have provided a new level of evidence about the possibility of helping persons with very minimal motor behaviour. These persons could seldom be considered for intervention programs involving typical motor responses and traditional microswitches (Lancioni et al. 2004b,f, 2005a, 2007a,b,g). The possibility of offering these individuals a chance to be active and to effectively and independently pursue environmental stimulation according to their own preferences can be considered highly relevant, both technically and in terms of the individual's own quality of life (Browder et al. 2001; Karvonen et al. 2004; Lachapelle et al. 2005). With regard to the latter aspect, the possibility of being constructively engaged and determining one's own level of stimulation may be considered a critically positive achievement with beneficial effects in terms of social image and, possibly, personal satisfaction (Felce and Perry 1995; Petry, Maes and Vlaskamp 2005; Wehmeyer and Schwartz 1998; Zekovic and Renwick 2003).

From a technical standpoint, one can underline the importance of having isolated and successfully targeted small responses and having developed viable interfaces (microswitch devices) to connect the responses identified to the outside world. The non-typical responses thus far used in the studies include vocalization (i.e., a brief sound emission), chin movements (mouth opening), eyelid movements, small hand-closure movements, and forehead skin movements. The eyelid movements have involved four different types of responses, that is, single eye blink, double eye blink, eye opening, and upward looking, which were reported to successfully suit the conditions of different participants. Similarly, the chin-movement response has been modified in terms of the number and amplitude of movements for different participants.

The aforementioned response variations and their successful applications can be taken as an indication of the wide range of opportunities that may be available by adapting the response requirement and technology to the individual characteristics of the participants. One could also identify additional response variations as supplementary practical solutions. For example, one could target full/protracted eyelid closures as specific responses for participants for whom such behaviours may be much more likely than double blinks or upward looking. Such closures could be detected with simple adaptations of the optic-microswitch technology used for the other eyelid responses. One could identify simple lip movements (e.g., closing the lips or pulling them slightly apart) for participants for whom those movements do not lead to reliable chin responses (Lancioni et al. 2007g). In these cases, optic sensors could be adapted to detect the target movements (i.e., the light changes caused by them) and allow the participants to control environmental events through those movements. One could also decide to target small hand-opening movements for participants who tend to have their hands closed (i.e., with the fingers against the palm of the hand). One solution could involve the use of the same microswitch now employed for the hand-closure responses, but the microswitch would be activated when the person decreases the applied pressure or lifts the fingers off the microswitch.

The second consideration concerns the possibilities of extending the performance (learning) opportunities of persons who present a more favourable condition than those involved in the previous group of studies. Having the opportunity to use multiple responses through multiple microswitches allows a person to increase the range of his or her engagement and the variety of sensory input (preferred stimulation) obtainable. Different responses are generally related to different sets of stimuli, and this condition is useful to limit the risks of saturation. Besides enjoying the variation of stimuli, the person may also satisfy his or her possible preferences for some of them by selecting the response leading to them more often than the other responses (Cannella, O'Reilly and Lancioni 2005; Lancioni et al. 2006b,d; Stafford et al. 2002). This choice situation may constitute a guarantee of high personal fulfilment and strong/lasting engagement motivation (Hoch et al. 2002; Kazdin 2001; Lancioni et al. 2003c, 2006a).

The strong motivation to be active and the possibility of choosing among a variety of stimuli may eventually promote positive mood expressions such as indices of happiness (Dillon and Carr 2007; Favell, Realon and Sutton 1996; Green and Reid 1999; Lancioni et al. 2002b; Ross and Oliver 2003). This condition may be considered highly desirable for the participant, with positive implications on his or her quality of life (Crocker 2000; Dillon and Carr 2007; Szymanski 2000). It may also provide extra encouragement to parents and staff, motivate them to continue with these programs, and convince them of the usefulness of their efforts (Clarke et al. 2002; Lancioni et al. 2002a, 2006a; Sullivan et al. 1995).

While the aforementioned points underline the great potential of programs involving multiple responses with multiple microswitches, a general concern may arise from the view that these programs do not pay direct attention to a person's hypothetical/possible desires for contact with the caregiver. Such a concern might be considered more realistic when the program includes participants who are used to and apparently enjoy social contact and caregivers who are able to integrate the provision of social contact within their daily work schedule. In such a situation, microswitches whereby the participant can obtain different environmental stimuli would need to be supplemented with a Voice Output Communication Aid (VOCA), that is, a device that the participant can activate to ask for caregiver's contact (cf. Lancioni et al. 2008b; Schlosser 2003; Schlosser and Sigafoos 2006). Combining a VOCA, for the request of caregiver attention or mediation, with regular microswitches that allow direct access to environmental stimuli, may be conceived as a fairly simple and practical strategy (cf. Lenker and Paquet 2004; Parette, Huer and Hourcade 2003). The possibility for a participant to ask for caregiver attention/mediation parallel to his or her independent engagement could justify longer periods of engagement and thus provide a more viable occupational condition. Obviously, the evidence available is still minimal and new research seems necessary to include other participants and assess the level of generality of the available data.

The third consideration concerns the potential usability and practical implications of microswitch clusters. With regard to the use of microswitch clusters, one may argue that it represents the most constructive and positive way to help persons with severe/profound intellectual and multiple disabilities progress in their development. In fact, the use of microswitch clusters integrates the intervention for positive and negative aspects of the person's performance within the same program, relying on a technology that may be considered reasonably accessible in terms of both complexity and cost. Within such programs, it is critical to establish an independent and constructive response by which the participant obtains preferred stimulation that can compete favourably with (1) the possible effects of the problem behaviour that needs to be reduced or (2) the efforts required by the correct posture that needs to be consolidated. The importance of such a careful program arrangement may not only be decisive in the short term (i.e., to ensure the initial learning process) but also in the long term (i.e., to ensure the maintenance of the learning effects) (cf. Lancioni et al. 2008c,d). The examples considered in this chapter were concerned with specific forms of problem behaviour and inadequate posture (e.g., hand mouthing and head forward tilting). Other applications may also be conceived and some indeed have already been addressed, albeit in a preliminary way. For example, new applications may deal with the goal of helping participants with cerebral palsy and other developmental disabilities perform small/basic responses (of practical or physical utility) without triggering dystonic/spastic reactions (Lancioni et al. 2009b).

The fourth consideration concerns the usability and practical value of microswitch technology combined with support/walker devices for promoting step responses and assisted locomotion for participants with multiple disabilities. The most common/traditional intervention approach employed for fostering locomotion with these participants has relied on the neuro-developmental method (Bar-Haim et al. 2006; Begnoche and Pitetti 2007; Day et al. 2004; Ketelaar et al. 2001). The neuro-developmental method emphasises the importance of inhibiting abnormal movements and facilitating postural adjustments through therapist-directed practice (Cherng et al. 2007; Ketelaar et al. 2001). Current views within this intervention area, however, emphasise an active (child-centred), task-specific practice as the basis for improving the targeted motor function. According to these views, the way to improve a child's locomotor behaviour is to allow the child to successfully practice such behaviour (Begnoche and Pitetti 2007). The most popular approach developed in line with this new perspective of behaviour practice concerns the use of treadmills generally combined with partial body weight support (Begnoche and Pitetti 2007; Day et al. 2004). The use of microswitch technology combined with support/walker devices may represent a second approach with seemingly high potential. In fact, the support/walker devices contain supporting features ensuring adequate posture and partial weight lifting while the microswitches monitor the child's stepping responses and provide motivation (reinforcement) for those responses through the automatic delivery of brief periods of preferred, contingent stimulation (Lancioni et al. 2007d, 2008a).

CONCLUSION

A variety of studies have used microswitch programs to allow children and youth with profound and multiple disabilities to interact with the surrounding world and control environmental stimulation with simple responses. Studies have varied widely. The first level of differentiation between studies was based on their clinical goals: whether the studies were exclusively aimed at establishing adaptive responses or combined the dual goals of promoting adaptive responses and reducing problem behaviour/posture. The studies aimed at establishing constructive responses were then divided into five groups, according to the responses that they targeted. The first group included a single, typical motor response, such as head turning and hand pushing, and generally relied on the use of conventional, commercial microswitch devices. The second group included a single, non-typical response, which generally consisted of a detailed/small action, such as chin movements, eyelid movements or vocalization, and relied on new/experimental microswitch devices. The third group included multiple responses, which encompassed combinations of typical motor responses or combinations of these responses with non-typical ones. The fourth group included multiple vocal responses, which were targeted with the use of adapted and new computer technology. The fifth group involved step responses (or foot/leg movements), which were targeted through optic (occasionally pressure) microswitches linked to the participants' legs or feet.

The studies combining dual goals were divided into two groups. The first group targeted adaptive responses such as touching or manipulating an object/microswitch and problem postures such as a flexed (rather than extended) leg or head forward tilting (Lancioni et al. 2004h). The second group targeted adaptive responses including foot, head and hand movements and problem behaviours such as hand mouthing and eye poking (Lancioni et al. 2007e).

The discussion of the outcomes was combined with an analysis of the importance of selecting suitable responses for the participants and ensuring that the responses would produce interesting (preferred) effects so that their cost would be amply compensated by their benefits (Miltenberger 2004). Efforts to find suitable responses for persons with multiple disabilities and minimal motor behaviour led to the identification of the non-typical responses (e.g., chin movements, eyelid movements and forehead skin movements).

The positive implications of using multiple responses were examined with particular emphasis on the benefits one may derive from extending the level of engagement and the opportunities of choice among environmental stimuli (or simply among responses). With regard to this aspect of multiple responses and choice, comments were also made as to the possibility (desirability) of combining microswitches and VOCA to guarantee the participants an opportunity of social contact in addition to the direct access to various environmental stimuli.

The use of microswitch clusters was indicated as the most constructive and positive way to help persons with severe/profound intellectual and multiple disabilities progress in their development. In fact, such an approach integrates the intervention for positive and negative aspects of the person's performance within the same program arrangement using a technology package that may be considered reasonably accessible in terms of both complexity and cost (Lancioni et al. 2008c).

The combination of microswitches and support/walker devices was considered to be a particularly useful approach for helping children with profound and multiple disabilities develop foot/leg movements and practice supported step responses leading to basic locomotion. With regard to locomotion, this combination approach was seen as (1) a supplement to the use of treadmill training, which in turn is becoming a strong alternative to the traditional neuro-developmental method, and (2) a great opportunity to achieve developmental goals with positive client involvement in terms of motivation and mood (Lancioni et al. 2007d).

In view of the data and the discussion reported previously, three issues of high practical relevance may be identified for immediate research work in this area. First, finding additional non-typical responses and corresponding microswitches would be essential for helping other persons who have minimal chances of active and constructive engagement with their environment. The range of non-typical responses investigated thus far is relatively narrow. Other responses, such as eyebrow movements, lip separation or closing, and tongue protrusion/withdrawal could also be examined. Obviously, any attempt to examine other responses requires the introduction of suitable microswitches. Some of these microswitches may need to be designed and realised entirely for the purpose of these new investigations.

Second, the actual applicability of microswitch clusters for participants with problem behaviour/posture would need to be determined. One approach to this challenge would be to carry out intervention programs with participants who show problem behaviours or inadequate postures other than those targeted in the studies reviewed. Results indicating a beneficial impact of microswitch clusters would open up new directions/opportunities in terms of intervention and underline a constructive approach in tackling problematic aspects in the participant's performance (i.e., an approach that seeks the reduction of the problematic aspects as part of an effort directed at strengthening adaptive responses).

Third, finding ways of coordinating the use of walkers with microswitches and contingent stimulation, and treadmill programs within practical rehabilitation situations may also be of great relevance. For example, children could start with a treadmill program that helps them develop basic stepping (walking) responses. Subsequently, they could rely on the use of a walker with microswitches and contingent stimulation to enhance their self-determination and independent locomotor behaviour (cf. Begnoche and Pitetti 2007; Katelaar et al. 2001; Provost et al. 2003).

REFERENCES

Algozzine, B., D. Browder, M. Karvonen, D.W. Test, and W.M. Wood. 2001. Effects of interventions to promote self-determination for individuals with disabilities. *Review of Educational Research* 71:219–277.

Bar-Haim, S., N. Harries, M. Belokopytov, A. Frank, L. Copeliovitch, J. Kaplanski, and E. Lahat. 2006. A comparison of efficacy of Adeli suit and neurodevelopmental treatments in children with cerebral palsy. *Developmental Medicine and Child Neurology* 48:325–330.

Barlow, D.H., M. Nock, and M. Hersen. 2009 *Single-case experimental designs*. (3rd ed.) New York: Allyn & Bacon.

Begnoche, D., and K.H. Pitetti. 2007. Effects of traditional treatment and partial body weight treadmill training on the motor skills of children with spastic cerebral palsy: A pilot study. *Pediatric Physical Therapy* 19:11–19.

Browder, D.M., W.M. Wood, D.W. Test, M. Karvonen, and B. Algozzine. 2001. Reviewing resources on self-determination: A map for teachers. *Remedial and Special Education* 22:233–244.

Cannella, H.I., M.F. O'Reilly, and G.E. Lancioni. 2005. Choice and preference assessment research with people with severe to profound developmental disabilities: A review of the literature. *Research in Developmental Disabilities* 26:1–15.

Catania, A. C. 2007. *Learning* (4th Interim ed.). New York: Sloan Publishing.

Cherng, R.J., C.F. Liu, T.W Lau, and R.B. Hong. 2007. Effect of treadmill training with body weight support on gait and gross motor function in children with spastic cerebral palsy. *American Journal of Physical Medicine and Rehabilitation* 86:548–555.

Clarke, S., J. Worcester, G. Dunlap, M. Murray, and K. Bradley-Klug. 2002. Using multiple measures to evaluate positive behavior support: A case example. *Journal of Positive Behavior Interventions* 4:131–145.

Crawford, M.R., and J.W. Schuster. 1993. Using microswitches to teach toy use. *Journal of Developmental and Physical Disabilities* 5:349–368.

Crocker, A.C. 2000. Introduction: The happiness in all our lives. *American Journal on Mental Retardation* 105:319–325.

Dattilo, J. 1986. Computerized assessment of preferences for severely handicapped individuals. *Journal of Applied Behavior Analysis* 19:445–448.

Dattilo, J. 1987. Computerized assessment of leisure preferences: A replication. *Education and Training in Mental Retardation* 22:128–133.

Day, J.A., E.J. Fox, J. Lowe, H.B. Swales, and A.L. Behrman. 2004. Locomotor training with partial body weight support on a treadmill in a nonambulatory child with spastic tetraplegic cerebral palsy: A case report. *Pediatric Physical Therapy* 16:106–113.

Dewson, M.R.J., and J.H. Whiteley. 1987. Sensory reinforcement of head turning with nonambulatory, profoundly mentally retarded persons. *Research in Developmental Disabilities* 8:413–426.

Dillon, C.M., and J.E. Carr. 2007. Assessing indices of happiness and unhappiness in individuals with developmental disabilities: A review. *Behavioral Interventions* 22:229–244.

Favell, J.E., R.E. Realon, and K.A. Sutton. 1996. Measuring and increasing the happiness of people with profound mental retardation and physical handicaps. *Behavioral Interventions* 11:47–58.

Felce, D., and J. Perry. 1995. Quality of life: Its definition and measurement. *Research in Developmental Disabilities* 16:51–74.

Glickman, L., J. Deitz, D. Anson, and K. Stewart. 1996. The effect of switch control site on computer skills of infants and toddlers. *American Journal of Occupational Therapy* 50:545–553.

Green, C.W., and D.H. Reid. 1999. A behavioral approach to identifying sources of happiness and unhappiness among individuals with profound multiple disabilities. *Behavior Modification* 23:280–293.

Hoch, H., J.J. McComas, L. Johnson, N. Faranda, and S.L. Guenther. 2002. The effects of magnitude and quality of reinforcement on choice responding during play activities. *Journal of Applied Behavior Analysis* 35:171–181.

Holburn, S., D. Nguyen, and P.M. Vietze. 2004. Computer-assisted learning for adults with profound multiple disabilities. *Behavioral Interventions* 19:25–37.

Karvonen, M., D.W. Test, W.M. Wood, D. Browder, and B. Algozzine. 2004. Putting self-determination into practice. *Exceptional Children* 71:23–41.

Kazdin, A. E. 2001. *Behavior modification in applied settings* (6th ed.). New York: Wadsworth.

Kennedy, K. 2005. *Single case designs for educational research*. New York: Allyn & Bacon.

Ketelaar, M., A. Vermeer, H. Hart, E. van Petegem-van Beek, and P.J. Helders. 2001. Effects of a functional therapy program on motor abilities of children with cerebral palsy. *Physical Therapy* 81:1534–1545.

Kurtz, P.F., M.D. Chin, J.M. Huete, R.S.F. Tarbox, J.T. O'Connor, T.R. Paclawskyj, and K.S Rush. 2003. Functional analysis and treatment of self-injurious behavior in young children: A summary of 30 cases. *Journal of Applied Behavior Analysis* 36:205–219.

Ivancic, M.T., and J.S. Bailey. 1996. Current limits to reinforcement identification for some persons with profound multiple disabilities. *Research in Developmental Disabilities* 17:77–92.

Lachapelle, Y., M.L. Wehmeyer, M.C. Haelewyck, Y. Courbois, K.D. Keith, R. Schalock, M.A. Verdugo, and P.N. Walsh. 2005. The relationship between quality of life and self-determination: An international study. *Journal of Intellectual Disability Research* 49:740–744.

Lancioni, G.E., C. De Pace, N.N. Singh, M.F. O'Reilly, J. Sigafoos, and R. Didden. 2008a. Promoting step responses of children with multiple disabilities through a walker device and microswitches with contingent stimuli. *Perceptual and Motor Skills* 107:114–118.

Lancioni, G.E., and S. Lems. 2001. Using a microswitch for vocalization responses with persons with multiple disabilities. *Disability and Rehabilitation* 23:745–748.

Lancioni, G.E., M.F. O'Reilly, and G. Basili. 2001a. An overview of technological resources used in rehabilitation research with people with severe/profound and multiple disabilities. *Disability and Rehabilitation* 23:501–508.

Lancioni, G.E., M.F. O'Reilly, and G. Basili. 2001b. Use of microswitches and speech output systems with people with severe/profound intellectual or multiple disabilities: A literature review. *Research in Developmental Disabilities* 22:21–40.

Lancioni, G.E., M.F. O'Reilly, D. Oliva, and M.M. Coppa. 2001c. A microswitch for vocalization responses to foster environmental control in children with multiple disabilities. *Journal of Intellectual Disability Research* 45:271–275.

Lancioni, G.E., M.F. O'Reilly, D. Oliva, and M.M. Coppa. 2001d. Using multiple microswitches to promote different responses in children with multiple disabilities. *Research in Developmental Disabilities* 22:309–318.

Lancioni, G.E., M.F. O'Reilly, D. Oliva, N.N. Singh, and M.M. Coppa. 2002a. Multiple microswitches for multiple responses with children with profound disabilities. *Cognitive Behaviour Therapy* 31:81–87.

Lancioni, G.E., M.F. O'Reilly, J. Sigafoos, N.N. Singh, D. Oliva, and G. Basili. 2004a. Enabling a person with multiple disabilities and minimal motor behaviour to control environmental stimulation with chin movements. *Disability and Rehabilitation* 26:1291–1294.

Lancioni, G.E., M.F. O'Reilly, N.N. Singh, D. Oliva, S. Baccani, L. Severini, and J. Groeneweg. 2006a. Micro-switch programmes for students with multiple disabilities and minimal motor behaviour: Assessing response acquisition and choice. *Pediatric Rehabilitation* 9:137–143.

Lancioni, G.E., M.F. O'Reilly, N.N. Singh, D. Oliva, M.M. Coppa, and G. Montironi. 2005a. A new microswitch to enable a boy with minimal motor behavior to control environmental stimulation with eye blinks. *Behavioral Interventions* 20:147–153.

Lancioni, G.E., M.F. O'Reilly, N.N. Singh, D. Oliva, and J. Groeneweg. 2003a. Using microswitches with persons who have multiple disabilities: Evaluation of three cases. *Perceptual and Motor Skills* 97:909–916.

Lancioni, G.E., M.F. O'Reilly, N.N. Singh, D. Oliva, G. Piazzolla, P. Pirani, and J. Groeneweg. 2002b. Evaluating the use of multiple microswitches and responses for children with multiple disabilities. *Journal of Intellectual Disability Research* 46:346–351.

Lancioni, G.E., M.F. O'Reilly, N.N. Singh, D. Oliva, L. Scalini, C.M. Vigo, and J. Groeneweg. 2005b. Further evaluation of microswitch clusters to enhance hand response and head control in persons with multiple disabilities. *Perceptual Motor Skills* 100:689–694.

Lancioni, G.E., M.F. O'Reilly, N.N. Singh, D. Oliva, L. Scalini, C.M. Vigo, and J. Groeneweg. 2005c. Microswitch clusters to enable hand responses and appropriate head position in two children with multiple disabilities. *Pediatric Rehabilitation* 8:59–62.

Lancioni, G.E., M.F. O'Reilly, N.N. Singh, D. Oliva, L. Scalini, C.M. Vigo, and J. Groeneweg. 2005d. Microswitch clusters to enhance adaptive responses and head control: A programme extension for three children with multiple disabilities. *Disability and Rehabilitation* 27:637–641.

Lancioni, G.E., M.F. O'Reilly, N.N. Singh, J. Sigafoos, R. Didden, D. Oliva, and G. Montironi. 2007a. Persons with multiple disabilities and minimal motor behavior using small forehead movements and new microswitch technology to control environmental stimuli. *Perceptual and Motor Skills* 104:870–878.

Lancioni, G.E., M.F. O'Reilly, N.N. Singh, J. Sigafoos, R. Didden, D. Oliva, G. Montironi, and M.L. La Martire. 2007b. Small hand-closure movements used as a response through microswitch technology by persons with multiple disabilities and minimal motor behavior. *Perceptual and Motor Skills* 104:1027–1034.

Lancioni, G.E., M.F. O'Reilly, N.N. Singh, J. Sigafoos, R. Didden, D. Oliva, and L. Severini. 2006b. A microswitch-based program to enable students with multiple disabilities to choose among environmental stimuli. *Journal of Visual Impairment and Blindness* 100:488–493.

Lancioni, G.E., M.F. O'Reilly, N.N. Singh, J. Sigafoos, D. Oliva, S. Baccani, A. Bosco, and F. Stasolla. 2004b. Technological aids to promote basic developmental achievements by children with multiple disabilities: Evaluation of two cases. *Cognitive Processing* 5:232–238.

Lancioni, G.E., M.F. O'Reilly, N.N. Singh, J. Sigafoos, D. Oliva, S. Baccani, and J. Groeneweg. 2006c. Microswitch clusters promote adaptive responses and reduce finger mouthing in a boy with multiple disabilities. *Behavior Modification* 30:892–900.

Lancioni, G.E., M.F. O'Reilly, N.N. Singh, J. Sigafoos, D. Oliva, G. Montironi, M. Savino, and A. Bosco. 2005e. Extending the evaluation of a computer system used as microswitch for word utterances of persons with multiple disabilities. *Journal of Intellectual Disability Research* 49:639–646.

Lancioni, G.E., M.F. O'Reilly, N.N. Singh, J. Sigafoos, D. Oliva, and L. Severini. 2006d. Enabling persons with multiple disabilities to choose among environmental stimuli and request stimulus repetitions through microswitch and computer technology. *Perceptual and Motor Skills* 103:354–362.

Lancioni, G.E., M.F. O'Reilly, N.N. Singh, J. Sigafoos, D. Oliva, and L. Severini. 2008b. Enabling two persons with multiple disabilities to access environmental stimuli and ask for social contact through microswitches and a VOCA. *Research in Developmental Disabilities* 29:21–28.

Lancioni, G.E., M.F. O'Reilly, N.N. Singh, J. Sigafoos, A. Tota, M. Antonucci, and D. Oliva. 2006e. Children with multiple disabilities and minimal motor behavior using chin movements to operate microswitches to obtain environmental stimulation. *Research in Developmental Disabilities* 27:290–298.

Lancioni, G.E., M.F. O'Reilly, N.N. Singh, F. Stasolla, F. Manfredi, and D. Oliva. 2004c. Adapting a grid into a microswitch to suit simple hand movements of a child with profound multiple disabilities. *Perceptual and Motor Skills* 99:724–728.

Lancioni, G.E., N.N. Singh, M.F. O'Reilly, F. Campodonico, D. Oliva, and C.M. Vigo. 2005f. Promoting walker-assisted step responses by an adolescent with multiple disabilities through automatically delivered stimulation. *Journal of Visual Impairment and Blindness* 99:109–113.

Lancioni, G.E., N.N. Singh, M.F. O'Reilly, F. Campodonico, G. Piazzolla, L. Scalini, and D. Oliva. 2005g. Impact of favorite stimuli automatically delivered on step responses of persons with multiple disabilities during their use of walker devices. *Research in Developmental Disabilities* 26:71–76.

Lancioni, G.E., N.N. Singh, M.F. O'Reilly, and D. Oliva. 2002c. Using a hand-tap response with a vibration microswitch with students with multiple disabilities. *Behavioural and Cognitive Psychotherapy* 30:237–241.

Lancioni, G.E., N.N. Singh, M.F. O'Reilly, and D. Oliva. 2003b. Evaluating optic microswitches with students with profound multiple disabilities. *Journal of Visual Impairment and Blindness* 97:492–495.

Lancioni, G.E., N.N. Singh, M.F. O'Reilly, and D. Oliva. 2003c. Extending microswitch-based programs for people with multiple disabilities: Use of words and choice opportunities. *Research in Developmental Disabilities* 24:139–148.

Lancioni, G.E., N.N. Singh, M.F. O'Reilly, and D. Oliva. 2004d. A microswitch program including words and choice opportunities for students with multiple disabilities. *Perceptual and Motor Skills* 98:214–222.

Lancioni, G.E., N.N. Singh, M.F. O'Reilly, and D. Oliva. 2005h. Microswitch programs for persons with multiple disabilities: An overview of the responses adopted for microswitch activation. *Cognitive Processing* 6:177–188.

Lancioni, G.E., N.N. Singh, M.F. O'Reilly, D. Oliva, and J. Groeneweg. 2005i. Enabling a girl with multiple disabilities to control her favorite stimuli through vocalization and a dual-microphone microswitch. *Journal of Visual Impairment and Blindness* 99:179–182.

Lancioni, G.E., N.N. Singh, M.F. O'Reilly, D. Oliva, and G. Montironi. 2004e. A computer system serving as a microswitch for vocal utterances of persons with multiple disabilities: Two case evaluations. *Journal of Visual Impairment and Blindness* 98:116–120.

Lancioni, G.E., N.N. Singh, M.F. O'Reilly, D. Oliva, G. Montironi, and S. Chierchie. 2004f. Assessing a new response-microswitch combination with a boy with minimal motor behavior. *Perceptual and Motor Skills* 98:459–462.

Lancioni, G.E., N.N. Singh, M.F. O'Reilly, D. Oliva, G. Montironi, F. Piazza, F. Ciavattini, and F. Bettarelli. 2004g. Using computer systems as microswitches for vocal utterances of persons with multiple disabilities. *Research in Developmental Disabilities* 25:183–192.

Lancioni, G.E., N.N. Singh, M.F. O'Reilly, D. Oliva, L. Scalini, C.M. Vigo, and J. Groeneweg. 2004h. Microswitch clusters to support responding and appropriate posture of students with multiple disabilities: Three case evaluations. *Disability and Rehabilitation* 26:501–505.

Lancioni, G.E., N.N. Singh, M.F. O'Reilly, and J. Sigafoos. 2009a. An overview of behavioral strategies for reducing hand-related stereotypes of persons with severe to profound intellectual and multiple disabilities. *Research in Developmental Disabilities* 30:20–43.

Lancioni, G.E., N.N. Singh, M.F. O'Reilly, J. Sigafoos, R. Didden, and D. Oliva. 2009b. Two boys with multiple disabilities increasing adaptive responding and curbing dystonic/spastic behavior via a microswitch-based program. *Research in Developmental Disabilities* 30:378–385.

Lancioni, G.E., N.N. Singh, M.F. O'Reilly, J. Sigafoos, R. Didden, D. Oliva, and E. Cingolani. 2008c. A girl with multiple disabilities increases object manipulation and reduces hand mouthing through a microswitch-based program. *Clinical Case Studies* 7:238–249.

Lancioni, G.E., N.N. Singh, M.F. O'Reilly, J. Sigafoos, R. Didden, D. Oliva, and L. Severini. 2007c. Fostering adaptive responses and head control in students with multiple disabilities through a microswitch-based program: Follow-up assessment and program revision. *Research in Developmental Disabilities* 28:187–196.

Lancioni, G.E., N.N. Singh, M.F. O'Reilly, J. Sigafoos, D. Oliva, A. Costantini, S. Gatto, V. Marinelli, and A. Putzolu. 2006f. An optic microswitch for an eyelid response to foster environmental control in children with minimal motor behaviour. *Pediatric Rehabilitation* 9:53–56.

Lancioni, G.E., N.N. Singh, M.F. O'Reilly, J. Sigafoos, D. Oliva, M. Gatti, F. Manfredi, G. Megna, M.L. La Martire, A. Tota, A. Smaldone, and J. Groeneweg. 2008d. A microswitch-cluster program to foster adaptive responses and head control in students with multiple disabilities: Replication and validation assessment. *Research in Developmental Disabilities* 29:373–384.

Lancioni, G.E., N.N. Singh, M.F. O'Reilly, J. Sigafoos, D. Oliva, and G. Montironi. 2004i. Evaluating a computer system used as a microswitch for word utterances of persons with multiple disabilities. *Disability and Rehabilitation* 26:1286–1290.

Lancioni, G.E., N.N. Singh, M.F. O'Reilly, J. Sigafoos, D. Oliva, G. Piazzolla, S. Pidala, A. Smaldone, and F. Manfredi. 2007d. Automatically delivered stimulation for walker-assisted step responses: Measuring its effects in persons with multiple disabilities. *Journal of Developmental and Physical Disabilities* 19:1–13.

Lancioni, G.E., N.N. Singh, M.F. O'Reilly, J. Sigafoos, D. Oliva, S. Pidala, G. Piazzolla, and A. Bosco. 2007e. Promoting adaptive foot movements and reducing hand mouthing and eye poking in a boy with multiple disabilities through microswitch technology. *Cognitive Behaviour Therapy* 36:85–90.

Lancioni, G.E., N.N. Singh, M.F. O'Reilly, J. Sigafoos, D. Oliva, L. Scalini, F. Castagnaro, and M. Di Bari. 2007f. Promoting foot-leg movements in children with multiple disabilities through the use of support devices and technology for regulating contingent stimulation. *Cognitive Processing* 8:279–283.

Lancioni, G.E., N.N. Singh, M.F. O'Reilly, J. Sigafoos, D. Oliva, L. Severini, and J. Groeneweg. 2007g. Eye- and mouth-opening movements replacing head and hand responses in a microswitch program for an adolescent with deteriorating motor condition. *Perceptual and Motor Skills* 105:107–114.

Lancioni, G.E., N.N. Singh, M.F. O'Reilly, J. Sigafoos, D. Oliva, L. Severini, A. Smaldone, and M. Tamma. 2007h. Microswitch technology to promote adaptive responses and reduce mouthing in two children with multiple disabilities. *Journal of Visual Impairment and Blindness* 101:628–636.

Langley, M.B. 1990. A developmental approach to the use of toys for facilitation of environmental control. *Physical and Occupational Therapy in Pediatrics* 10:69–91.

Leatherby, J.K., D.L. Gast, M. Wolery, and B.C. Collins. 1992. Assessment of reinforcer preference in multi-handicapped students. *Journal of Developmental and Physical Disabilities* 4:15–36.

Lenker, J.A., and V.L. Paquet. 2004. A new conceptual model for assistive technology outcomes research and practice. *Assistive Technology* 16:1–10.

Matson, J.L., N.F. Minshawi, M.L. Gonzalez, and S.B. Mayville. 2006. The relationship of comorbid problem behaviors to social skills in persons with profound mental retardation. *Behavior Modification* 30:496–506.

McClure, J.T., R.A. Moss, J.W. McPeters, and M.A. Kirkpatrick. 1986. Reduction of hand mouthing by a boy with profound mental retardation. *Mental Retardation* 24:219–222.

Mechling, L.C. 2006. Comparison of the effects of three approaches on the frequency of stimulus activation, via a single switch, by students with profound intellectual disabilities. *The Journal of Special Education* 40:94–102.

Miltenberger, R.G. 2004. *Behavior modification: Principles and procedures* (3rd ed.). New York: Wadsworth.

Parette, P., M.B. Huer, and J.J. Hourcade. 2003. Using assistive technology: Focus groups with families across cultures. *Education and Training in Developmental Disabilities* 38:429–440.

Pear, J. 2001. *The science of learning*. New York: Psychology Press.

Petry, K., B. Maes, and C. Vlaskamp. 2005. Domains of quality of life of people with profound multiple disabilities: The perspective of parents and direct support staff. *Journal of Applied Research in Intellectual Disabilities* 18:35–46.

Provost, B., K. Dieruf, P.A. Burtner, J.P. Phillips, A. Bernitsky-Beddingfield, K.J. Sullivan, C.A. Bowen, and L. Toser. 2007. Endurance and gait in children with cerebral palsy after intensive body weight-supported treadmill training. *Pediatric Physical Therapy* 19:2–10.

Realon, R.E., J.E. Favell, and K.A. Dayvault. 1988. Evaluating the use of adapted leisure materials on the engagement of persons who are profoundly multiply handicapped. *Education and Training in Mental Retardation* 23:228–237.

Realon, R.E., J.E. Favell, and J.F. Phillips. 1989. Adapted leisure material vs. standard leisure material: Evaluating several aspects of programming for persons who are profoundly handicapped. *Education and Training in Mental Retardation* 24:168–177.

Richman, D.M. 2008. Early intervention and prevention of self-injurious behaviour exhibited by young children with developmental disabilities. *Journal of Intellectual Disability Research* 52:3–17.

Ringdahl, J.E., T.R. Vollmer, B.E. Marcus, and H.S. Roane. 1997. An analogue evaluation of environmental enrichment: The role of stimulus preference. *Journal of Applied Behavior Analysis* 30:203–216.

Ross, E., and C. Oliver. 2003. The assessment of mood in adults who have severe or profound mental retardation. *Clinical Psychology Review* 23:225–245.

Sandler, A.G., and S.C. McLain. 1987. Sensory reinforcement: Effects of response-contingent vestibular stimulation on multiply handicapped children. *American Journal of Mental Deficiency* 91:373–378.

Saunders, M.D., K.A. Questad, T.L. Kedziorski, B.C. Boase, E.A. Patterson, and T.B. Cullinan. 2001. Unprompted mechanical switch use in individuals with severe multiple disabilities: An evaluation of the effects of body positions. *Journal of Developmental and Physical Disabilities* 13:27–39.

Saunders, M.D., G.R. Timler, T.B. Cullinan, S. Pilkey, K.A. Questad, and R.R. Saunders. 2003. Evidence of contingency awareness in people with profound multiple impairments: Response duration versus response rate indicators. *Research in Developmental Disabilities* 24:231–245.

Schalock, R., I. Brown, R. Brown, R.A. Cummins, D. Felce, L. Matikka, K.D. Keith, and T. Parmenter. 2003. Conceptualization, measurement, and application of quality of life for persons with intellectual disabilities: Reports of an international panel of experts. *Mental Retardation* 40:457–470.

Schlosser, R.W. 2003. Roles of speech output in augmentative and alternative communication: Narrative review. *Augmentative and Alternative Communication* 19:5–27.

Schlosser, R.W., and J. Sigafoos. 2006. Augmentative and alternative communication interventions for persons with developmental disabilities: Narrative review of comparative single-subject experimental studies. *Research in Developmental Disabilities* 27:1–29.

Singh, N. N., G.E. Lancioni, M.F. O'Reilly, E.J. Molina, A.D. Adkins, and D. Oliva. 2003. Self-determination during mealtimes through microswitch choice-making by an individual with complex multiple disabilities and profound mental retardation. *Journal of Positive Behavior Interventions* 5:209–215.

Sobsey, D., and J. Reichle. 1989. Components of reinforcement for attention signal switch activation. *Mental Retardation and Learning Disability Bulletin* 17:46–60.

Stafford, A.M., P.M. Alberto, L.D. Fredrick, L.J. Heflin, and K.W. Heller. 2002. Preference variability and the instruction of choice making with students with severe intellectual disabilities. *Education and Training in Mental Retardation and Developmental Disabilities* 37:70–88.

Sullivan, M.W., D.H. Laverick, and M. Lewis. 1995. Fostering environmental control in a young child with Rett syndrome: A case study. *Journal of Autism and Developmental Disorders* 25:215–221.

Sullivan, M.W., and M. Lewis. 1990. Contingency intervention: A program portrait. *Journal of Early Intervention* 14:367–375.

Sullivan, M.W., and M. Lewis. 1993. Contingency, means-end skills and the use of technology in infant intervention. *Infants and Young Children* 5:58–77.

Szymanski, L.S. 2000. Happiness as a treatment goal. *American Journal on Mental Retardation* 105:352–362.

Wehmeyer, M.L., and M. Schwartz. 1998. The relationship between self-determination, quality of life, and life satisfaction for adults with mental retardation. *Education and Training in Mental Retardation and Developmental Disabilities* 33:3–12.

Zekovic, B., and R. Renwick. 2003. Quality of life for children and adolescents with developmental disabilities: Review of conceptual and methodological issues relevant to public policy. *Disability and Society* 18:19–34.

3 Access Technologies for Children and Youth with Severe Motor Disabilities

Natasha Alves, Stefanie Blain, Tiago Falk,
Brian Leung, Negar Memarian and Tom Chau

CONTENTS

INTRODUCTION

An access solution translates a user's functional intent, be it manifested as a physical movement, facial gesture, physiological change or combinations thereof, into a functional activity (Tai, Blain and Chau 2008). An access technology constitutes the technological front end of an access solution and encompasses two main elements: (1) an access pathway, that is, the actual sensors or input devices that transduce an expression of intent into an electrical signal, and (2) a signal processing unit, which filters and classifies the transduced signal, generating some command signal for interfacing to an augmentative and alternative communication aid, a computer or an environmental control unit.

Many children and youth have no access to communication, the environment or a computer; they possess limited functional movements or speech as a result of motor neuron diseases (e.g., Noda et al. 1990), severe cerebral palsy (Clarke and Wilkinson 2007), ventral pontine stroke (Juneja et al. 2009; Bruno et al. 2009), posterior fossa lesions (Miller et al. 2010) or acquired brain injuries (Morgan and Vogel 2008). Although this population is growing globally and life expectancy has been extended significantly by improved complex care, medications, nutritional supplements and artificial ventilation, their quality of life remains minimal. It is believed that many of these individuals have capable minds, but are locked inside a non-functional body. Today, the majority of this population does not have any assistive technology to facilitate access to communication, environment or computer. For many, off-the-shelf input devices such as button switches are often highly unreliable due to issues such as poor motor coordination, involuntary or inconsistent movements, and muscle weakness, fatigue and spasticity.

In this chapter, we introduce five novel access solutions, each one motivated by at least one paediatric client with severe physical disabilities who did not have any physical access or functional speech. The presentation of the solutions is loosely arranged by the anatomic location of interest. The first two solutions, namely, the facial infrared thermography and multi-camera tongue detection, involve activity around the mouth. Still associated with the oropharyngeal region, the third solution invokes vocal cord vibrations as an access pathway. Moving away from the mouth, mechanomyographic access is described in the next section as a means of harnessing eyebrow and thumb movements. Finally, moving to the fingers and removing the requirement for extant physical movement, the last solution exploits the electrical activity of the skin along with other peripheral autonomic signals as a composite access channel. Figure 3.1 summarises the sequence in which the solutions will be introduced.

Each access solution will constitute a section of the chapter, with all sections generally adhering to a uniform format. Specifically, each section begins with the clinical and technical rationale for considering the proposed access pathway, followed by a brief description of one of the key clients motivating the research and development. The technical components of the solution, the clinical testing procedures and the ensuing empirical data are presented next. Each section closes with a discussion of the merits and limitations of the access solution.

INFRARED THERMOGRAPHY-BASED ACCESS

Motivation

Infrared thermography refers to the measurement of the radiation in the infrared range of the electromagnetic spectrum, that is, between wavelengths of 0.8 μm and 1.0 mm (Jones 1998) emitted by the surface of an object. Infrared cameras use specialised lenses manufactured from materials such as germanium to focus thermal radiation onto a focal plane array of infrared detectors (Balcerak and Lupo 2002). Cameras with the capability of producing digital output yield an image that is a spatial two-dimensional (2-D) map of the three-dimensional (3-D) temperature distribution of the object (Jones and Plassmann 2002).

Infrared thermography potentially can be used in the development of new access solutions. Recently, Nhan and Chau (2009) examined the baseline characteristics of facial skin temperature, as measured by dynamic infrared thermal imaging, to gauge its potential as an emotion detector for non-verbal individuals with severe motor impairments. This study showed that emotional thermoregulation manifests as detectable changes in facial skin temperature. While a skin temperature-based emotion detector can be a valuable access pathway for individuals without any voluntary physical ability (e.g., patients with locked-in syndrome), infrared thermal imaging

Access Technologies

Infrared Thermography-Based Access Solution

A case study describing the design and development of a non-invasive and non-contact switch that detects voluntary mouth opening and closing via infrared thermal imaging

Motivation, client profile, infrared thermal switch development and evaluation, merits and limitations

Multiple Camera Tongue Switch

A case study documenting the development of a non-contact tongue switch for a child with severe spastic quadriplegic cerebral palsy

Motivation, client profile, multiple cameras and image processing, switch evaluation, merits and limitations

Vocal Cord Vibration Detection

A case study describing the development of a periodic vocal-cord vibration switch that overcomes three major limitations of existing speech-based technologies

Motivation, client profile, switch development and evaluation, merits and limitations

Mechanomyography-Based Access

Case studies describing the use of remnant muscle activity, measured by muscle sounds, to control a switch

Motivation for muscle sounds, client profiles – forehead and forearm muscle activity, mechanomyography access development, evaluation, merits and limitations

Electrodermal Activity and Other Peripheral Physiological Signals

Potential use of electrodermal activity and other signals from the peripheral autonomic nervous system to control a switch, illustrated by a case study with an individual with severe spastic quadriplegia

Physiological background of electrodermal activity, fingertip temperature, and cardiorespiratory signals, client profile, access pathway development, switch evaluation, merits and limitations

FIGURE 3.1 Roadmap of chapter.

can also be utilised to develop access solutions that can be voluntarily controlled by the patients. Memarian, Venetsanopolous and Chau (2009) proposed an access solution that generates a binary control signal when activated by a user's voluntary mouth opening, exploiting the fact that the temperature inside the human mouth is generally higher than that of the surroundings. A relatively constant temperature is always maintained within the human body (Jones 1998), and therefore localised temperature changes due to mouth opening and closing can serve as a switch. A simple binary switch can open many doors to a person with severe motor disabilities (Blain, McKeever and Chau 2010). For example, he or she can use it to select characters from a scanning keyboard, or control his or her wheelchair. In this section, the process of developing the thermal switch and its application to a young adult with severe motor impairment is discussed.

CLIENT PROFILE

David (pseudonym) is a 26-year-old male with severe spastic quadriplegic cerebral palsy. While he is not a paediatric client per se, he has been a long-term client of a paediatric rehabilitation hospital where he still receives seating services. His case mirrors that of many younger clients who exhibit the same challenges faced in seeking access pathways. David's family first noticed signs of physical disability subsequent to a high fever and febrile seizure during infancy. David is not able to move his limbs or upper body voluntarily. However, he has adequate control of his jaw and can open and close his mouth quite reliably. David's most comfortable position is a semi-supine position in his wheelchair with his head facing either left or right (Figure 3.2). He rarely maintains a forward-looking head posture. While he can change his direction of gaze with effort, he usually relies on the assistance of a third party for repositioning. David has very little involuntary body or head movement and can maintain a stationary position for extended periods of time. David

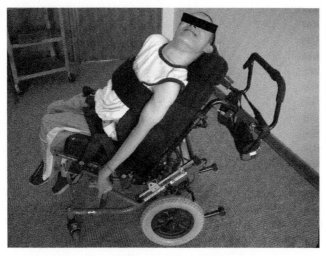

FIGURE 3.2   (See color insert following page 240.) Client's typical posture in his wheelchair.

lives with his family and his primary caregiver is his mother. He has some vocalizations that can be interpreted by his mother. He can also smile, blink and take food orally. Despite his physical disability, David is cognitively intact, follows instructions promptly and can focus on a task willingly. He is literate and has attended a year of college.

INFRARED THERMOGRAPHY ACCESS SOLUTION

Figure 3.3 shows a schematic of our automated algorithm for detecting mouth opening activity from the thermal video data. The system consists of three main modules, namely face segmentation, motion and intensity analyses, and filtering of non-mouth objects. Face segmentation isolates the client's face from other objects that may appear in the video frame. Since the activity of interest, that is, mouth opening, is a facial gesture, the first step is to accurately localise the client's face. Opening and closing the mouth involve jaw motion. Furthermore, the human mouth is typically warmer than the surrounding facial regions outside the mouth, suggesting that the thermal signature of an open mouth is different from that of a closed mouth. Therefore, the second module of the algorithm scans the client's face to pinpoint facial regions that are both sufficiently warm *and* moving as candidate mouth openings. This module usually results in multiple objects as open mouth candidates. Some of the non-mouth regions that are commonly selected as open mouth candidates are the chin and forehead. These objects are also warm and moving and are therefore retained subsequent to motion and thermal intensity filtering. For example, according to the literature, the forehead is the warmest part of the human body with a temperature (34.5°C) close to that inside the mouth (Moriyamashi et al. 1996). Therefore, motion of the forehead may result in a false positive. To eliminate these non-mouth objects, we employ morphological and anthropometric filters. Objects that do not satisfy the expected size, shape and location of an open mouth within the face are thus filtered out. The reader

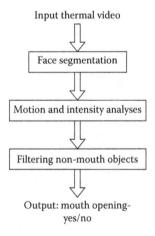

FIGURE 3.3 Components of the mouth detection algorithm for the proposed access solution.

is referred to Memarian, Venetsanopolous and Chau (2009) for technical details of the algorithm.

Upon detection of a mouth open-close sequence, a mouse click/space bar press was generated using a module latching relay by DLP Design Inc. and a Swifty USB switch interface by Origin Instruments™.

TESTING PROTOCOL

David participated in two rounds of experiments with the thermal switch. The first round verified the functionality of the aforementioned video processing algorithm. In the second round, David used the thermal switch to perform interactive tasks with the computer. The instrumentation and testing protocol for each round are discussed briefly in the following subsections.

Algorithm Functionality Verification

A THERMAL-EYE 2000B infrared thermal video camera by L-3 Communications with thermal sensitivity ≤ 100 mK (GotoInfrared 2007) was connected via an NTSC to USB TV convertor (Dazzle Multimedia). Videos were recorded as 240 × 320 AVI files (30 frames per second) and processed offline in MATLAB and Simulink (version R2007b).

David was comfortably seated in his wheelchair within a laboratory environment. The thermal camera was positioned anterior and lateral to him at a 45° angle (Figure 3.4). This camera location was chosen over the often-used frontal view, keeping in mind the target application as an access switch where the user's field of view ought to be unobstructed. David was cued to open his mouth, hold it ajar for 1-s and finally close his mouth. He was given an auditory prompt upon every open and close action. The end of each mouth closing was followed by a 3-s rest before the onset of the next mouth opening. David was cued to open and close his mouth 15 times.

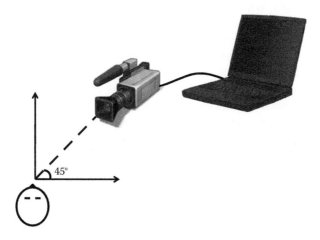

FIGURE 3.4   Thermal switch instrumentation setup.

Testing the Usability of the Thermal Switch

In the second round, thermal videos of David were processed in real-time, providing him a binary switch triggered by mouth opening. David used this switch to inter-act with the computer (e.g., play games, type). Thermal video was acquired by a ThermaCam SC640 infrared thermal video camera by FLIR with thermal sensitivity ≤ 60 mK (FLIR Systems 2005) and sent to a laptop computer via a firewire cable. Videos were recorded as 640 × 480 MP4 files (30 frames per second) and processed online in Simulink (version R2008a). Client posture and position with respect to the infrared thermal camera was the same as round 1.

David used the thermal switch to complete interactive tests. First, to give David some familiarity with the real-time thermal switch, he played two single switch games, that is, Cheat7 from OneSwitch.org.uk (Becker 2005) and Transport Snap from BBC (BBC 2009). The former was a targeting game, while the latter was an object match-ing game. He was then tested with a standard scan switch test using the Compass Assessment Software (version 1.2; Koester Performance Research 2007). In the scan switch test, David was prompted with an audiovisual cue, namely the phrase 'press the switch' displayed in a yellow square on the computer screen and accompanied by an engaging sound. Each cue lasted for 10-s and was punctuated by a pause of random duration, between 1 and 4-s long. David responded to this prompt by opening his mouth. Basically, he opened and closed his mouth each time he wanted to gener-ate a switch press (Figure 3.5). The software provided audiovisual feedback to him. It rewarded David with positive phrases such as 'Good job!' or 'Well done!' for correct activations and informed him of the instances where he missed with phrases such as 'Sorry.' The test was repeated three times, through which David was cued a total of 48 times (8 times in trial one, 20 times in trial two, and 20 times in trial three).

RESULTS

The computerised mouth detection algorithm resulted in 60% sensitivity and 99% specificity in round 1. While the very high specificity figure verified the algorithm's capacity to filter out non-mouth objects (false positives), the sensitivity was rather low compared to results previously achieved from testing the algorithm with able-bodied participants (Memarian et al. 2009). This was mainly due to frequent invol-untary head rotation away from the camera and suboptimal camera placement as a consequence of his awkward posture. David was asked to maintain a constant head position, so that his mouth movement stayed within the camera's field of view. However, because of involuntary spastic head rotation, his face turned away from the thermal camera's field of view during several instances of mouth opening. In such circumstances, a third party was needed to either turn David's head back to face the camera or to move his wheelchair such that his face was captured by the camera. Also, David's awkward position in his wheelchair forced us to position the thermal camera at an angle and distance from him that was not consistent with the settings used in pervious able-bodied tests.

The algorithm parameters were fine-tuned from rounds 1 to 2 to enhance the system's performance and speed. Table 3.1 shows the results of the round 2 scan

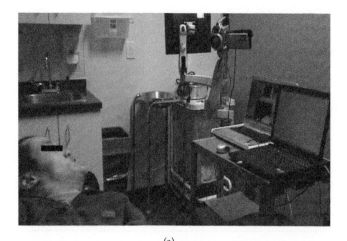

(a)

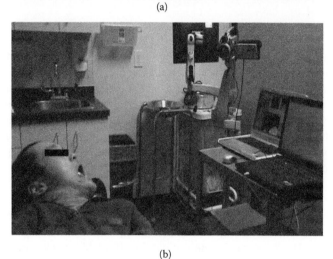

(b)

FIGURE 3.5   (See color insert following page 240.) Client responding to audiovisual cues generated by the Compass Assessment Software (Koester Performance Research 2007): (a) client in rest state, (b) client making a switch press by opening his mouth.

switch test with Compass Assessment Software. System sensitivity improved substantially from the round 1 level. Also, the sensitivity increased from trial one to trial three. Response time was measured from the moment of prompt presentation to the instance of switch activation. The last column of Table 3.1 indicates David's average response time for each trial.

Discussion

Merits

For a client who can exercise voluntary control over mouth open and close motions, possible access technologies include sip and puff devices, electromyography (EMG)

TABLE 3.1

Results of Scan Switch Test with Compass Assessment Software

Trial No.	Number of Cues	Hits (TP)	False Alarms (FP)	Misses (FN)	Sensitivity $\left(\dfrac{TP}{TP+FN}\right)$	Specificity $\left(\dfrac{TN}{TN+FP}\right)$	Average Response Time [s]
1	8	6	0	2	75%	100%	5.77
2	20	18	0	2	90%	100%	2.1
3	20	19	0	1	95%	100%	3.45

Source: Koester Performance Research 2007. *Compass Assessment Software* [online]. http://www. kpronline.com/products.html (accessed February 2009).
TP: true positives, *FP*: false positives, *FN*: false negatives, *TN*: true negatives.

and computer vision. Compared to EMG and sip and puff, the proposed thermography-based access solution is both non-invasive and non-contact, that is, it does not require the attachment of any sensors or external objects to the user. The thermography solution is more hygienic and safe as the risk of infection, ingestion of small parts, or physical injury from switch or mounting hardware is mitigated. Unlike visible light computer vision-based access solutions, infrared thermography is not dependent on lighting or colour conditions, and thus can be used both night and day, indoor and outdoor.

Limitations and Future Directions

Despite these encouraging early findings, thermal imaging does have its limitations. Infrared thermal cameras are generally more expensive than conventional (visible light) cameras. However, recent innovations in affordable, pocket-sized, portable thermal cameras (e.g., SPi Infrared 2008) have brought down the costs of thermal imaging. Thermal image quality is susceptible to fluctuations in ambient temperature, humidity and regional air circulation (Jones 1998). A robust thermographic access solution may need to dynamically compensate for changes in these contextual factors. A final limitation of thermal imaging is the relatively low resolution of infrared cameras and the inherent difficulty in distinguishing fine facial features. These issues may be mitigated by fusing thermal videos with simultaneously recorded visible spectrum imagery (Wang and Sung 2007).

Several improvements can be made to enhance detection performance when faced with a challenging posture or spastic head movements. The algorithm can be dynamically updated to track and focus on the region of interest (i.e., the participant's face) more accurately. Multiple cameras can be invoked, each capturing the participant's facial region from a different angle, thereby minimizing the chance of the participant's mouth leaving the camera's field of view. Finally, the user can undergo training. The results in Table 3.1 suggest a potential positive effect of client training on overall performance.

TONGUE-BASED ACCESS VIA MULTIPLE CAMERAS

MOTIVATION

Children with severe cerebral palsy may use a facial gesture as a pathway for single switch access. The premise is that these children may already be using one or more facial expressions to indicate preference to their caregivers. Thus, a facial movement involved in creating one of these facial expressions may be used to drive a single switch output.

Facial gestures can be captured and processed via video in order to implement a non-contact access technology. The user produces the expected facial gesture toward a video camera placed at some distance in front of the user. The signal processing component of the access technology performs real-time video processing to detect the facial gestures. The BlinkLink and Eyebrow Clicker (Grauman et al. 2003) are two example systems that use a single video camera to capture and process eye blinks and eyebrow raises, respectively, for single switch access.

We developed a multiple camera tongue switch for a child with severe spastic quadriplegic cerebral palsy. This access technology consisted of three webcams simultaneously capturing the child's tongue protrusions from distinct perspectives. The system conducted real-time colour video processing on the three video streams to detect instances of tongue protrusion, and each detected instance caused an activation of the single switch output. The multiple cameras relieved the child from having to aim his face in one specific direction — a difficult targeting problem due to spasticity in his neck muscles.

CLIENT PROFILE

Jason (pseudonym) is a 7-year-old boy. He has spastic quadriplegic cerebral palsy with severity conforming to level 5 on the Gross Motor Function Classification Scale (Palisano et al. 1997). In particular, he has no independent mobility and sits in a manual wheelchair while in the community. His four limbs and head are affected by sporadic yet frequent bouts of spasticity. At times, the spastic muscle activity will persist for extended periods (e.g., more than 30-s), which renders him stuck to a pose. Due to this lack of adequate voluntary control of his limb and head movements, he is unable to achieve consistency in targeting mechanical switches located proximal to his body.

Jason can comprehend verbal instructions and react to verbal inquiries. He is considered non-verbal but can voluntarily articulate one-word responses to indicate preference or YES/NO decisions.

An initial assessment identified tongue protrusion as a potential pathway for single switch access. Jason has voluntary control of his facial movements; he can smile and express displeasure. He struggles at performing voluntary eye blinks with consistency and has even greater difficulty with voluntary eyebrow movements. He has adequate control of his lips, although the quality of control diminishes in the presence of head and neck spasticity. Jason can produce voluntary tongue protrusions with consistency. During spasticity, he would be too distracted by discomfort to attempt tongue protrusions. However, Jason rarely produces involuntary tongue protrusions. Tongue protrusion was thus selected for single switch access because Jason could modulate this facial gesture most reliably.

Jason did not have an access technology prior to the multiple camera tongue switch. Instead, he relied on caregiver-mediated access, that is, a caregiver physically issued commands on his behalf. His past history of switch-fitting attempts included an assortment of wheelchair-mounted mechanical switches, sip-and-puff switches, and voice-activated switches. Jason's parents were interested in a non-contact solution because of the child's difficulty with targeting mechanical switches and concerns about his head and arms violently colliding with wheelchair-mounted devices during bouts of involuntary movement.

DEVELOPMENT AND TESTING OF THE MULTIPLE CAMERA TONGUE SWITCH

The multiple camera tongue switch is a software solution deployed using off-the-shelf hardware, which consists of three webcams and a laptop computer. Jason was provided with an implementation consisting of three Logitech Quickcam Pro 5000 webcams and a laptop computer equipped with an Intel Core 2 Duo 1.5 GHz processor and 1 GB of memory. Each webcam streamed RGB24 video into the laptop computer at a resolution of 320×240 pixels and a frame rate of 15 Hz. The software implemented the tongue switch algorithm and a user interface for the caregiver to set up the tongue switch. Single switch output could be configured to be either a keyboard/mouse event sent via software or an electrical pulse delivered via hardware (e.g., toggling one of the RS-232 serial port signals).

The tongue switch algorithm treated the three webcams as independent input sources. Each video stream had its own instance of a single camera algorithm that performed colour video processing to detect tongue protrusions. Then, a fusion algorithm periodically sampled the results of all three single camera algorithm instances to produce a final single switch output. The three video streams were independent input sources because each single camera algorithm instance was not aware of the other two instances. This further implies the webcams may be freely placed at setup-time and repositioned during run-time without compromising correct system behaviour. Hence, the multiple camera tongue switch is functionally equivalent to three single camera tongue switches simultaneously observing the user from three distinct perspectives.

The three webcams were placed in front of the user. The centre camera was directly in front of the user as in a single camera system. The two peripheral cameras were placed to the left and right of the centre camera and toed-in toward the user. Figure 3.6 shows an example setup with the three webcams in a linear arrangement, which is suitable for deployment on a tabletop. Alternatively, for deployment on a wheelchair tray, the three webcams can be positioned along an arc such that they are equidistant to the user.

Figure 3.7 summarises the single camera algorithm. Face localization finds the user's face and tracks it in subsequent frames. It consists of segmentation of skin-coloured objects on the YCg′Cr′ luma-colour-difference space (de Dios 2007) followed by colour tracking using the CAMSHIFT algorithm (Bradski 1998). For

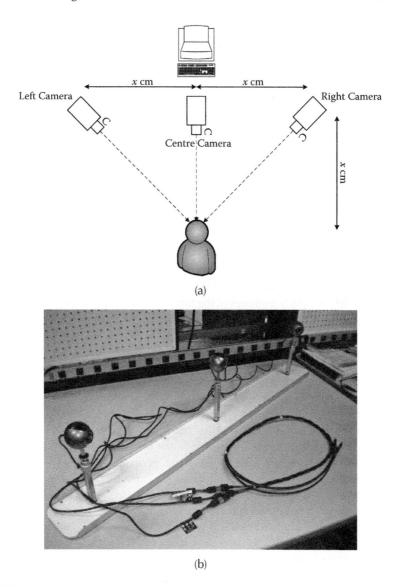

(a)

(b)

FIGURE 3.6 Example deployment of the multiple camera tongue switch. (a) The diagram shows the positioning of the three cameras as a linear array in front of the user (Reprinted with permission from Leung, B., and T. Chau. 2010. A multiple camera tongue switch for a child with severe spastic quadriplegic cerebral palsy. *Disability and Rehabilitation: Assistive Technology* 5(1):58–68.) (b) The picture shows the linear array on a mounting platform.

mouth localization, the algorithm computes a feature map on the face region of interest that accentuates saturated red pixels. The premise is that skin tone is typically not saturated and that the lips and tongue associate with most of the saturated red pixels. The tongue switch module determines the single camera single switch output by detecting influxes of saturated red pixels in the mouth region of interest, which

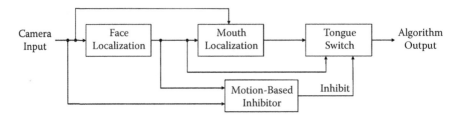

FIGURE 3.7 Block representation of the single camera algorithm (Reprinted with permission from Leung, B., and T. Chau. 2010. A multiple camera tongue switch for a child with severe spastic quadriplegic cerebral palsy. *Disability and Rehabilitation: Assistive Technology* 5(1):58–68.)

corresponds to tongue protrusions. The module also computes a frontal face view measure that determines whether the camera perceives a frontal view of the user's face. The camera does not have a frontal view of the face if the mouth region of interest is near the left or right boundaries of the face region of interest. The motion-based inhibitor temporarily disables algorithm output whenever it measures large amounts of motion from motion history images (Davis 2001) of the face region of interest, which is usually a consequence of spastic head movements.

The fusion algorithm of the multiple camera tongue switch follows the best camera paradigm. At any given time, the fusion algorithm decides on switch activation using data coming from the camera that has the best frontal view of the user's face, that is, the camera with the largest frontal face view measure. For further details of the tongue protrusion algorithm, see Leung and Chau (2010).

Jason participated in an experiment that tested the performance of the multiple camera tongue switch and the added value of the peripheral cameras in facilitating his single switch access. During each of five experiment sessions on separate days, Jason worked through several iterations of a picture matching game with 2 min of rest in-between iterations. A single iteration of the picture matching game consisted of a target picture and 20 choice pictures presented one-by-one on screen. Using the multiple camera tongue switch to drive the picture matching game, Jason was asked to identify instances where the choice and target pictures matched. Concurrently, a human observer recorded the choices for which Jason protruded his tongue. This record was used to verify (1) whether single switch activations were caused by tongue protrusion and (2) whether switch inaction was caused by the absence of the protruded tongue. Finally, we simulated the performance of a single camera system by deriving the tongue switch output using only data from the centre camera.

The performance of the multiple camera tongue switch was quantified in terms of sensitivity and specificity to intentional tongue protrusions. These performance measures were calculated from the counts of true positive instances n_{TP} (switch activation with tongue protrusion), false negative instances n_{FN} (switch inaction despite tongue protrusion), true negative instances n_{TN} (switch inaction in the absence of tongue protrusion), and false positive instances n_{FP} (switch activation without tongue protrusion).

TABLE 3.2

Performance of the Multiple Camera Tongue Switch to the Emulated Single Camera Setup

	Sensitivity		Specificity		True +ve Activations	
	Multiple	Centre-Only	Multiple	Centre-Only	Centre	Peripheral
Session 1	83 ± 17	37 ± 34	91 ± 11	93 ± 16	5	13
Session 2	78 ± 26	26 ± 23	77 ± 11	98 ± 3	3	13
Session 3	87 ± 22	77 ± 25	76 ± 10	86 ± 11	15	2
Session 4	91 ± 18	63 ± 40	73 ± 9	84 ± 11	19	14
Session 5	69 ± 24	27 ± 30	85 ± 9	91 ± 7	3	11

RESULTS

Table 3.2 summarises the experimental results. Over the five sessions, the multiple camera tongue switch performed with an average sensitivity of 82% and an average specificity of 80%. This is remarkable for a child who had not been using an access technology regularly. Moreover, the sensitivity for the centre-camera-only detection (column 2) reduced significantly in sessions 1, 2, and 5, where switch activations came primarily from the peripheral cameras. This result demonstrates that the peripheral cameras provided enhanced detection and that the centre-camera-only system missed intentional tongue protrusions when Jason's head was turned to the left or right.

DISCUSSION

The multiple camera tongue switch comes with significant clinical benefits. Most importantly, it is a hygienic solution that minimises the risk of skin rashes and infections because there is no physical contact between the user and the tongue switch. Second, the multiple camera tongue switch is financially affordable given that its components are exclusively off-the-shelf items. Finally, a caregiver with minimal training can deploy the multiple camera tongue switch; as aforementioned, correct system behaviour does not depend on exact placement of the three cameras.

However, clinicians must exercise caution when prescribing tongue protrusion for single switch access. In many cultures and social settings, protruding one's tongue toward another person is an offensive gesture. Second, the amount of tongue protrusions necessary for single switch access far exceeds the amount of protrusions one would otherwise produce. This raises concerns about potential long-term deterioration of oral and vocalization functions. Finally, the child should feel physically and mentally comfortable with tongue protrusions as his or her access pathway. At times, this can be difficult to ascertain from a non-verbal child.

A future development of the multiple camera tongue switch will be to move the implementation onto FPGA or microcontroller platforms. Such development will result in improved portability and lower energy consumption, making the tongue switch applicable in a greater number of settings. In the next section, we move away from the mouth, down to the pharyngeal region.

VOCAL FOLD VIBRATION-BASED ACCESS

MOTIVATION

It is known that, worldwide, approximately 1 in 100 individuals have complex communications needs and cannot rely on speech for daily communication (Beukelman and Mirenda 2005). As examples, in North America, of the 3.7% Canadian children aged 5 to 14 years with a disability, 44.8% possess speech production impairments (Statistics Canada 2007); in the United States, an estimated 5% of all children entering first grade have moderate to severe speech disorders (Data Resource Center 2005/2006). Moreover, a majority of these individuals, as a result of, for example, degenerative neuromotor diseases, cerebral palsy, or brain injuries, have multiple disabilities and hence also possess no functional movements. These limitations preclude the use of augmentative and alternative communication (AAC) devices with existing mechanical switches (Lancioni et al. 2001) or speech recognition technologies (Noyes and Frankish 1992; Havstam et al. 2003). One emergent alternative access pathway exploits non-verbal vocalizations for AAC device activation (Lancioni et al. 2005; Lancioni and Lems 2001).

Speech production disorders can be associated with poor respiratory control, laryngeal dysfunction, or oral-facial muscular weakness. Studies suggest, however, that voluntary non-verbal vocalizations can be developed in individuals with multiple and severe disabilities (Lancioni and Lems 2001; Yorkston et al. 1999). Commonly, vocalizations are captured with a close-talking microphone or a throat microphone (Lancioni et al. 2005). Close-talking microphones, although more robust than airborne microphones, are still sensitive to environment noise and the speech output from the user's speech-generating devices (Harada et al. 2009). In order to reduce false activations, sound-based systems are equipped with a 'sensitivity' dial that, when set to low, allows for increased robustness against environment noise. The major drawback is that loud vocalizations have to be produced for accurate switch activation, thus leading to premature fatigue (Chang and Karnell 2004). To guard against environmental effects, throat microphones have been employed (Lancioni and Lems 2001). With throat microphones, however, false activations may occur due to user-generated artefacts such as coughs, throat clearings, heavy breathing, congested airways, or involuntary spastic head movements (Lancioni et al. 2005). To overcome such limitations, periodic vocal cord vibration detection has been proposed as an alternative access pathway (Falk et al. 2009).

CLIENT PROFILE

Experiments with the vocal cord vibration detection system were conducted with three clients diagnosed with cerebral palsy. For the remainder of this section, we will use the pseudonyms Edmond, Oswald and Samuel. Edmond is almost 6 years old and, due to dystonia, has strong spasticity and involuntary movements that prohibit computer access. Edmond had been previously prescribed a jellybean switch for right foot, left elbow or chin control. The chin control was shown to be more consistent and accurate, but involuntary movements and emotion-bound muscle hypertonicity cause its use to be overly fatiguing.

Oswald is 11 years and 7 months old and has spastic quadriplegia with dystonia. Strong spasticity has limited Oswald's ability to use any mechanical switches to access a computer effectively. He had been previously prescribed with a commercial speech-based system called Words+,* which was quickly abandoned due to the excessive effort required for switch activation. Subsequently, touch-sensitive switches were tested and activated by tongue, cheek, lips, nose or chin. The chin switch was shown to be the most successful but still resulted in premature fatigue and was not very reliable.

Samuel is 19 years old and has severe hypotonia and mitochondrial myopathy. Samuel's motor abilities are restricted to very minimal arm and hand control and little to no head movement. Samuel has had a long history of switch trials, which include bite, foot (i.e., a mechanical button switch activated by leg extension), thumb, and sound-based switches. The bite and foot switches were abandoned due to excessive fatigue. The thumb switch measured muscle vibrations that occurred during muscle activity, and was found to work well for activities that did not require timed responses such as online shooting video games. For timed responses, such as using a virtual on-screen keyboard for school-related activities, Samuel currently uses the Words+ sound switch to detect the vocalization /ah/ with a miniature close-talking microphone held near his mouth by a clip on his headband. Samuel has shown disinterest in the current Words+ solution due to the excessive effort required for switch activation and the numerous false activations caused by environmental noise in his classroom.

ACCESS PATHWAY DEVELOPMENT AND METHODS OF TESTING

Non-verbal vocalizations are produced by forced air from the lungs as it passes between the vocal folds, causing the vocal cords to vibrate. Inherently, by measuring vocal cord vibrations, AAC access becomes insensitive to environment noise, as illustrated by the block diagram in Figure 3.8. Moreover, it is known that certain vocalizations (e.g., vowels) and hums cause *periodic* vibrations of the vocal cords (Titze 1994). User-generated artefacts such as coughs, swallows and throat clearing, on the other hand, cause *aperiodic* vibrations. Periodic vocal cord vibrations can be non-invasively detected by means of a dual-axis accelerometer placed on the anterior surface of the throat with a neckband and aligned to the anterior-posterior (AP) and superior-inferior (SI) anatomical axes. Figure 3.9 depicts 40-ms excerpts of an accelerometer signal, measured in the AP direction, during instances of vowel production (top subplot) and cough (bottom subplot). As observed, vocalizations exhibit strong periodic behaviour whereas coughs and other user-generated artefacts are aperiodic.

Periodicity in vocal cord vibrations can be detected by means of the normalised cross-correlation function, which exhibits values close to unity for highly periodic signals. The reader is referred to Falk et al. (2009) for more details regarding the normalised cross-correlation function and the signal processing strategies involved in periodicity detection. A real-time prototype was built using a PIC microcontroller. The implemented system along with the accelerometer and custom-made neckband are depicted in Figure 3.8. Figure 3.9, in turn, shows a client using the prototype to access a virtual on-screen keyboard.

---

* Words+ Infrared/Sound/Touch (IST) Switch. URL: http://www.words-plus.com

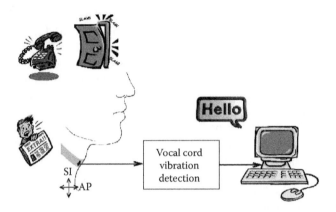

FIGURE 3.8 (See color insert following page 240) Block diagram of the vocal cord vibration detection system. Insensitivity to environment noise and user-generated artefacts such as coughs are two major advantages of the system over existing speech-based solutions.

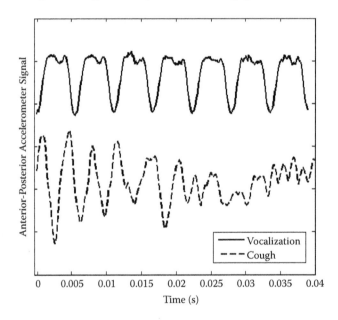

FIGURE 3.9 Short 40-millisecond segments of anterior-posterior accelerometer signals captured during a vocalization (top plot) and a cough (bottom plot).

To test the throat vibration switch, three client-specific tests were used. For Edmond, school-related tasks were performed such as turning pages of electronic storybooks, playing songs, and engaging in different cause-and-effect activities during two 30-min periods spread over a 2-week period. For Oswald, environmental control tasks were performed via an environmental control unit for two 15-min periods. The first session focused on non-verbal vocalizations and the second session focused on hums. Representative tasks included turning on/off the radio, TV, and

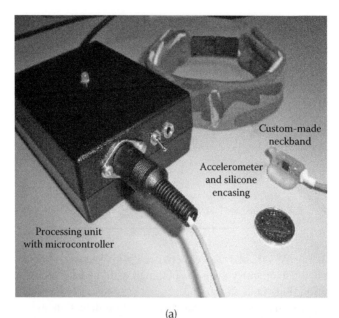

(a)

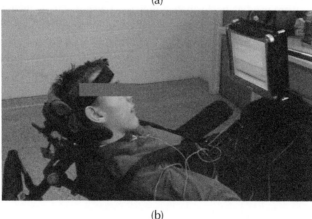

(b)

FIGURE 3.10 View of (a) hardware prototype along with the accelerometer with a silicone encasing and a custom-made neckband, (Reprinted with permission from Falk, T.H., Chan, J., Duez, P., Teachman, G., and Chau, T. 2010. Augmentative communication based on realtime vocal cord vibration detection. *IEEE Trans. Neural Systems and Rehabilitation Engineering* Digital Object Identifier: 10.1109/TNSRE.2009.2039593. © 2010 IEEE), and (b) (See color insert following page 240.) An adolescent participant with cerebral palsy using the system to access a virtual on-screen keyboard.

lights, volume control, and channel surfing. Lastly, Samuel was asked to perform a sentence writing task using the WiViK* virtual on-screen keyboard. The sentence included all letters of the alphabet and tests were conducted in eight sessions (four in the morning and four in the afternoon) over a 2-week period. Since Samuel was

---

* WiViK, URL: http://www.wivik.com

TABLE 3.3
Five-Point Rating Scale for User-Perceived Exertion

Rating	Description
1	Nothing at all, not tired
2	A little, not tired
3	Moderate, a little tired
4	A lot, tired
5	Too much, very tired

Question asked was, 'How much effort was required and how tired do you feel?'

proficient in using WiViK and was experienced with Words+, a comparative task was also conducted to quantify the gains obtained with the new vocal cord vibration detection solution (Falk et al. 2009).

To test the performance of the vocal cord vibration detection switch, sensitivity and specificity were used as performance metrics. False positives included detected coughs, while false negatives were undetected volitional vocalizations. For the writing task performed by Samuel, additional measures were also used; more specifically, the average time taken to complete the task and the change in perceived exertion before and after the completion of the task. In order to measure user-perceived exertion, a modified five-point Borg scale (Borg 1982) was used, as shown in Table 3.3. The participant was asked to rate how much effort was required to complete the task and how tired he felt before and after the task. During each session, the participant was asked to rest between tasks such that pre-task exertion levels remained the same for the two switches. Manual scanning of the five rating levels was performed and the participant indicated his choice with a single tongue click (i.e., his conventional method for a "yes" response).

RESULTS

For Edmond, sensitivity values of 96.75% and 99.25% were observed during the first and second 30-min sessions, respectively. For Oswald, sensitivity values of 99.3% and 100% were observed for the sessions using non-verbal vocalizations and hums, respectively. For both individuals, a specificity of 100% was attained, indicating that false positives were not present. Table 3.4 further reports specificity and sensitivity values for Samuel using either the Words+ or the vocal cord vibration detection solutions. As can be seen, no significant changes in sensitivity were observed between the morning and afternoon sessions for the vocal cord vibration detection system. For the Words+ switch, on the other hand, a significant decrease in performance was obtained in the afternoon ($p < 0.005$, with a paired t-test), mostly due to the fact that Samuel is known to fatigue as the day progresses. This is further corroborated by the task time and perceived exertion metrics also reported in the table. In the afternoon,

TABLE 3.4

Performance Comparison between the Vocal Cord Vibration-Based System and Words+ for the Sentence Writing Task Performed by Samuel

	Words+		Vocal Cord Vibration	
	Morning	Afternoon	Morning	Afternoon
Sensitivity (%)	84.0	65.2	91.4	96.6
Specificity (%)	100.0	99.8	100.0	100.0
Task time (s)	371.6 ± 90.9	783.3 ± 91.4	324.7 ± 47.0	379.6 ± 70.8
Perceived exertion	1.75	2.00	0.50	0.50

Task time is reported as average time ± standard deviation.

Samuel was able to perform the writing task with the vocal cord vibration switch roughly twice as fast as with the Words+ switch. In terms of perceived exertion, represented by the average difference between post- and pre-task perceived exertion levels, Samuel consistently reported significantly lower ($p < 0.005$, t-test) fatigue levels with the vocal cord vibration detection switch.

DISCUSSION

Merits

Using periodic vocal cord vibration detection as an alternative access pathway overcomes three major limitations of existing speech-based technologies: (1) sensitivity to environment noise, (2) sensitivity to user-generated artefacts, and (3) user fatigue. The improvements obtained across these three categories are likely to contribute positively to AAC outcomes (Lund and Light 2007). Additionally, the use of hums for switch activation has important clinical and social advantages. Clinically, hums are less strenuous on the vocal folds relative to voiced vocalizations and reduce the risk of vocal fold strain during prolonged periods of usage. Socially, soft hums are less disruptive to individuals in the surrounding environment such as peers in a classroom setting. Moreover, the use of an accelerometer placed non-invasively on the anterior region of the neck offers the advantage that vocal cord vibrations can be detected even in the presence of strong spastic head movements, which are known to encumber microphone-dependent speech-based solutions (Lancioni et al. 2005).

Limitations and Future Directions

A majority of the individuals who are candidates for using the vocal cord vibration switch possess severe dysarthria. Produced vocalizations are seldom intelligible and are mono-pitched and of reduced loudness (Langley and Lombardino 1991), thus prohibiting the use of existing speech recognition technologies (Havstam et al. 2003). Notwithstanding, it is common to witness such individuals using their vocalizations to communicate with familiar partners (Smith 1994). As described previously, placement and use of a neckband can allow for increased robustness against spastic head movements. The other side of the coin, however, is that false switch activations may occur if the individual attempts to communicate with a partner in parallel to performing a task. This was observed a few times with Oswald during pilot experiments when he requested that his mother "move" his legs into a more comfortable position in his wheelchair. To overcome this limitation, a disable function triggered by an external device, can be incorporated. Users who have an additional, yet not as reliable, access pathway may choose to disable vocal cord vibration detection by accessing a separate switch. In the case of Oswald, it was found that he could disable vocal cord vibration detection by using a separate chin switch.

Moreover, the vocal cord vibration detection system currently operates as a binary switch. Studies have shown, however, that some phonatory control can be attained with able-bodied children (Patel and Brayton 2008) and with adults with cerebral palsy and severe dysarthria (Patel 2002). Voluntary control of the frequency of vibrations (commonly termed pitch or fundamental frequency) of produced hums and vocalizations can allow for the development of tertiary or possibly quaternary switches (Patel 2002). Further experiments are being conducted to determine if such volitional control is possible with *children* with cerebral palsy.

MECHANOMYOGRAPHY-BASED ACCESS SOLUTION

MOTIVATION

While individuals with profound physical disabilities may not have sufficient strength or range of physical movement to reliably manipulate a mechanical switch, often the individual still possesses some voluntary muscle control. The muscle or muscle group that an individual can voluntarily control could serve as an access site. In its simplest form, the user may be able to contract and relax the muscle at will, and can thus generate ON/OFF commands to the user-interface. The primary advantage of using muscle activity as an access pathway is that explicit physical movement is not required. In principle, the user should be able to actuate a switch by low-force muscle twitches that can be repeated with minimal fatigue.

When the muscle is the access site, the access pathway is a signal that represents the activity of the muscle under consideration. Surface electromyogram (EMG) electrodes are most commonly used for monitoring muscle activity for the purpose of controlling external devices. Surface EMG signals represent the electrical activity of the underlying active muscle fibres. Applications of EMG as an access pathway for individuals with disabilities have included EMG switches controlled by a viable muscle of the hand, foot, cheek or forehead (Gryfe et al. 1996; Kennedy and Adams 2003).

In addition to electrical activity, a contracting muscle also generates mechanical activity. When a muscle contracts, its fibres shorten, resulting in an increase in fibre diameter. The dimensional changes produce pressure waves that are manifested as low-frequency vibrations on the surface of the overlying skin (Orizio et al. 1999). Further, there is a gross lateral movement of the muscle at the initiation of a contraction and smaller subsequent lateral oscillations at the resonant frequency of the muscle (Barry and Cole 1990; Orizio 1993). These mechanical vibrations have been measured by microphones (Watakabe et al. 2001), piezoelectric contact sensors

(Barry 1991; Watakabe et al. 1998), accelerometers (Barry 1992), and laser distance sensors (Orizio et al. 1999) on the surface of the skin. The superficial measurement of these vibrations is known as the mechanomyogram (MMG). It is suggested that MMG reflects the intrinsic mechanical activity of muscle contraction (Orizio 1993). MMG has been applied in the evaluation of muscle myopathies (Barry, Gordon and Hinton 1990; Ng et al. 2006), the monitoring of muscle pain (Madeleine and Arendt-Nielsen 2005), and the study of muscle fatigue (Madeleine et al. 2002; Shinohara and Sogaard 2006). Investigational studies have also employed MMG as a control signal in upper limb prostheses (Barry et al. 1986; Silva, Heim and Chau 2005).

MMG has several attributes that make it a promising access pathway. The signal reflects force output in both normal and diseased muscles (Barry et al. 1990). Further, an MMG signal is detectable even at low contraction levels due to asynchronous firing of active motor units (Madeleine et al. 2001). This activity burst may be useful in detecting low-force contractions of atrophied muscles. MMG provides a good estimation of inflection points in motor-unit recruitment (Akataki, Mita and Watakabe 2004), which may be useful when monitoring voluntary activations within spasticity. Unlike EMG, MMG is not affected by skin impedance changes. It has also been suggested that the MMG signal propagates along the longitudinal axis of the muscle fibre, and may be less critical to transducer position relative to the muscle belly (Orizio 1993).

CLIENT PROFILE

To exemplify MMG as a binary access pathway, we focus on two clients: John (pseudonym), 9, diagnosed with dystonic quadriplegic cerebral palsy, and Jane (pseudonym), 19, diagnosed with spastic quadriplegic cerebral palsy.

John's method of communication was limited speech and partner-assisted auditory and visual scanning. He needed a switch for computer access and, eventually, a high-tech communication device. He had previously tried mechanical head switches, an infrared hand switch, and a voice-activated switch. Initial assessments by his clinical team indicated that these switches were impractical access alternatives. John had limited muscle strength, confounding involuntary arm and head movements, and was unable to generate loud vocalizations. His bouts of involuntary head movements made positioning the head switch cumbersome. Although he could voluntarily clench his fist, spastic involuntary clenching was frequent, making the infrared hand switch unreliable. John could vocalise a soft 'ya' to activate a voice switch. However, he found this mode of access very fatiguing. Moreover, due to his violent head movements, the microphone was placed distal to his mouth and thus highly susceptible to false activations in the presence of ambient sounds. We identified eyebrow movement (i.e., raising and lowering) as a motion that John could repeatedly execute with minimal physical effort.

Jane used a mechanical head switch and a Dynavox for communication. Her occupational therapist indicated that the head switch needed to be repositioned frequently. Jane has voluntary control of small thumb movements. While her clinical team attempted to harness this movement with infrared switches and bend-sensitive sensors, the movement was too small to generate reliable activations.

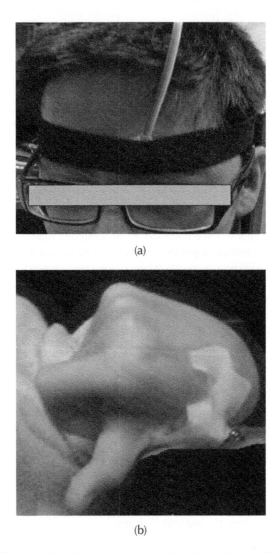

(a)

(b)

FIGURE 3.11   Sensor position for monitoring muscle activity: (a) frontalis muscle (b) brevis muscle.

Access Pathway Development and Methods for Testing

Muscle Site Selection

The frontalis muscles of the forehead appeared to be a candidate access site to monitor John's eyebrow movement. Muscle activity was recorded by an MMG sensor attached to his forehead by an extensible head band, as shown in Figure 3.11a. In attempting to detect Jane's thumb movements, we initially recorded muscle activity from the flexor pollicis longus muscle of her forearm. However, since the activity could not be isolated from other involuntary forearm muscle activations, we

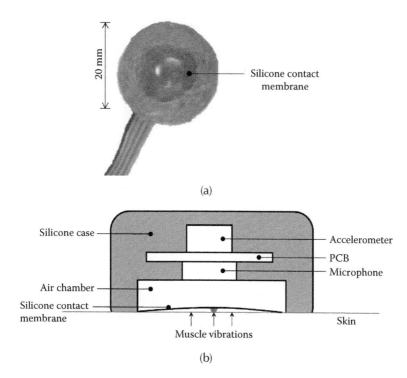

FIGURE 3.12   (a) MMG sensor. (b) Schematic diagram of the MMG sensor

determined that her abductor pollicis brevis muscle would generate cleaner signals. The MMG sensor was fastened with cloth tape, as shown in Figure 3.11b.

Mechanomyogram Measurement

The MMG signal is measured by a sensor comprised of a microphone-accelerometer pair enclosed in a silicon casing, as shown in Figure 3.12(a) (Silva and Chau 2003). As depicted in Figure 3.12(b), the microphone measures muscle vibrations via a silicone contact membrane and an air chamber. The microphone measures muscle vibrations via a silicone contact membrane and an air chamber. Since the microphone signal is affected by motion artefact, the sensor also contains an accelerometer that allows for separation of movement from muscle contractions (Silva and Chau 2005). This sensor pair is particularly useful when measuring MMG for access, since artefact-like involuntary spastic movement or body spasms are often encountered. Figure 3.13 is an example of recordings from the forearm of an individual with quadriplegia due to spinal cord injury who was able to produce small, low-force thumb and wrist flexions. As seen in the magnified microphone signal, the MMG signal is markedly different during rest and contraction. However, the signal is much noisier when the individual experiences body spasms. This movement artefact is detected by the accelerometer and can be used to determine when to suspend control of the access device.

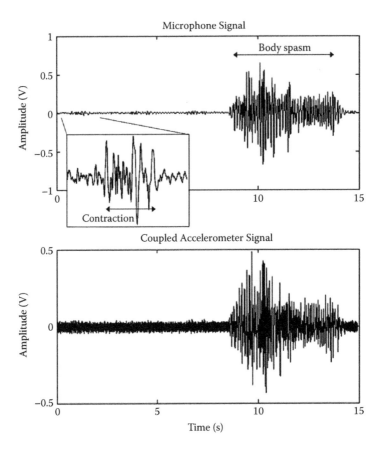

FIGURE 3.13 Signals from the microphone and accelerometer in the presence of movement artefact.

Data Collection and Offline Analysis

Once a reliable muscle site was determined for each client, MMG data were acquired and digitised at 1 kHz (NI USB-6210, National Instruments). The data were recorded over multiple sessions, during which the participants were cued to repeatedly contract and relax their target muscle.

The recorded data were analyzed in MATLAB for signal features that could detect the onset of muscle activity during a contraction. The data were spliced into 200-ms segments. Two potential features were identified: the root mean square (RMS) value of the microphone signal (John) and the percentage change in variance (Jane). Muscle activation was detected if the feature value exceeded a predefined threshold for at least two successive signal segments. A post-processing algorithm was developed to perform switch de-bouncing and allow a single activation per contraction.

Algorithm Modification and Verification

The detection algorithm was programmed in LabView to perform real-time acquisition (NI USB-6210), data processing, and switch activation. This software allowed us to modify the choice of features, response delay and activation threshold, in an online manner while obtaining immediate feedback about the algorithm's performance. The software provided the user with auditory feedback when a muscle contraction was detected. In addition, the program asserted the DTR pin of the computer's serial port. The serial port was interfaced to a conventional 1/8-in. mono-plug to generate a conventional switch output. John experimented with using the switch output for computer access (with a Swifty USB interface), and Jane used the switch to operate her Dynavox. Through trial and error, optimal parameter settings, such as sensitivity and response delay, were determined for each client.

Hardware Implementation

A custom hardware implementation of the proposed MMG switch was developed. Signals from the MMG sensor were filtered (5 to 50 Hz), digitised (1 kHz) and processed by a microcontroller (MSPF2013, Texas Instruments) programmed with each client's personal detection algorithm. A 5-kΩ potentiometer allowed the user to control the threshold for activity detection. When muscle activity was detected, the processor generated a signal that triggered a binary switch. The implementation allowed the user to toggle between a conventional switch interface and a pre-selected keystroke for use as a computer interface. An LED provided the user with feedback of detected activations. The system is depicted in Figure 3.14.

Performance Testing

The detection algorithm was tested offline to estimate switch performance metrics such as the number of correctly detected muscle contractions (true positives, TP),

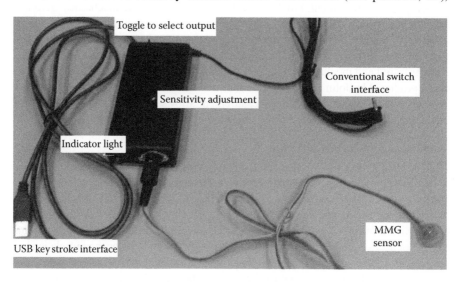

FIGURE 3.14   Hardware implementation of the MMG switch.

TABLE 3.5

Results of the Detection Algorithm (Offline Analysis)

Client	Test Duration	Cues	True Positives	False Positives	False Negatives
John	3 min	68	53	15	9
Jane	2 min	48	36	12	6
Jane	3 min	59	50	9	10

the number of muscle contractions missed by the detection algorithm (false negatives, FN), the number of contractions detected when the client was resting or did not intend to contract their muscle (false positives, FP), and the number of correctly identified resting periods (true negatives, TN).

MMG data were continuously recorded while the participants were cued to contract and relax their muscles. Since muscle contraction was accompanied by a small movement, the observation of a movement was considered the gold standard to which the detection algorithm's output was compared. The client was cued to contract the target muscle. The number of correctly identified contractions and false detections were recorded, and are shown in Table 3.5.

Discussion

Merits

The primary advantage of the MMG-driven switch is that it obviates the need for explicit physical movement. Further, because we are measuring mechanical activity, the switch is robust to skin impedance changes due to perspiration. The switch is sensitive to low-force muscle contractions, and thus requires minimal effort by the user, making it an attractive solution for extended use. Alignment issues, which affect infrared and mechanical switches that can potentially harness the small movements produced by John and Jane, are circumvented because the sensor is secured to the muscle site. The accelerometer measurement allows us to suspend control of the switch during periods of head or limb movement.

Limitations and Future Direction

While sensitivity to small muscle contractions serves as an advantage, the device may sometimes be overly sensitive and generate false activations, such as when the user blinks or smiles. This may be overcome in the future by changing the detection algorithm to recognise a specific pattern of muscle activation. The switch's sensitivity to small activations also makes it difficult for the user to control, particularly when the user is not accustomed to inhibiting the activation of the muscle, or the muscle is also used for other purposes, such as facial expressions. Although the trade-off between sensitivity and specificity may be adjusted by tuning the switch's threshold, arriving at an optimal setting may be difficult given the participants' dynamic motor characteristics.

Switch usability could be considerably improved if the system was designed to be robust to movement. In its current implementation, the switch is turned off when movement is detected. However, this implementation may not be suitable for users who need to control the switch during prolonged periods of continuous involuntary movement. To this end, a source separation method, such as the one proposed by Silva and Chau (2005), would need to be implemented.

ELECTRODERMAL ACTIVITY AND OTHER PERIPHERAL AUTONOMIC PHYSIOLOGICAL SIGNALS

MOTIVATION

All activities that can possibly be executed by the human body are commanded and coordinated by the central nervous system. The controls issued by the brain and spinal cord are in turn transmitted by the two branches of the peripheral nervous system: the sensory-somatic nervous system and the autonomic nervous system (Figure 3.15).

Over half a million people worldwide are affected by conditions that cause deterioration of the mechanisms that enable somatic muscle control, such as cerebral palsy, amyotrophic lateral sclerosis (ALS), brainstem stroke, and spinal cord injury (Barnett et al. 1992). While these conditions cause changes in the sensory-somatic nervous system, the functions of the autonomic nervous system often remain intact. The peripheral autonomic nervous system and the functions that it controls are therefore candidate access pathways for individuals affected by such conditions. By learning to exert voluntary control of these signals, an individual with severe physical disabilities may gain the ability to express his or her functional intent and the means of interacting with his or her environment.

Overview of the Peripheral Autonomic Nervous System

The autonomic nervous system is comprised of the sensory and motor neurons that connect the central nervous system with internal organs, including the heart, the

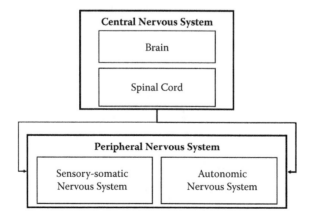

FIGURE 3.15 Organization of the central and peripheral nervous sytems of the human body.

lungs, the viscera and the exocrine and endocrine glands. Its primary function is to coordinate the internal environment and maintain homeostasis. The autonomic nervous system is subdivided into two further sections: the sympathetic nervous system, which coordinates the responses associated with 'fight or flight', and the parasympathetic nervous system, which returns the body to homeostatic balance after being stimulated by the sympathetic system. Together, these branches exert antagonistic control on the internal functions of the body, including, but not limited to: heart rate, respiration rate, pupil dilation/contraction, secretion of digestive enzymes, secretion of hormones, electrodermal activity, vasodilation and vasocontraction of blood vessels, and contraction of the smooth muscles. This section focuses specifically on four signals of the peripheral autonomic nervous system and their potential to be used as an access pathway: electrodermal activity, fingertip temperature, respiration patterns and cardiovascular patterns.

Electrodermal Activity

Electrodermal activity (EDA), often called galvanic skin resistance (GSR), is a measure of the electrical conductance of the skin. The skin's conductance changes as a result of cholinergic stimulation of the sweat glands, causing them to release ion-rich sweat, thus increasing the overall conductance of the skin. These changes can be generated spontaneously, reflexively or voluntarily by a variety of internal or externally applied arousal stimuli (Vetrugno et al. 2003), and have been used in decades of research as one of the most popular and convenient measures of arousal of the autonomic nervous system (Boucsein 1992). Electrodermal activity consists of two components: a slowly evolving baseline component, known as the electrodermal level (EDL), and a phasic component, known as the electrodermal reaction (EDR) (Figure 3.16). While EDL changes are indicative of homeostatic and thermoregulatory processes, electrodermal reactions are increases in electrodermal activity of more than 0.05 µS within a 10-s window, and are indicative of ANS activation (Hot et al. 1999). A variety of arousal stimuli can induce an EDR, including startling and threatening stimuli, emotional or affective processes, memory recall, orientation to a novel stimulus and attention orientation (Blain, Chau and Mihailidis 2008).

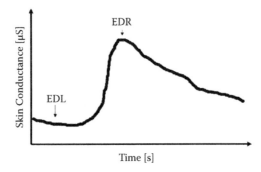

FIGURE 3.16 Electrodermal levels (EDL), indicative of thermoregulatory sweat gland activity, and electrodermal reactions (EDR), indicative of sympathetic sweat gland activity.

It has been used as a measure of arousal, attention and orientation in fields such as psychology, emotion recognition and psychophysiology.

Fingertip Temperature

The circulatory system branches into a complex network of cutaneous microcirculation when the blood reaches the hands, especially around the fingertips. Among the fingertip cutaneous vascular structures are ateriovenous anatomoses (AVAs), which are densely innervated by sympathetic nerve fibres, and consequently react to stimulation of the ANS (Hales 1985). The direction of their response is dependent on the overall temperature of the body; when fingertip temperature is above $33 \pm 2°C$, sympathetic stimulation induces vasoconstriction, and below this temperature, the same stimuli induces vasodilation (Elam and Wallin 1987). Changes in microcirculation manifest after a latency period of approximately 15-s, and have been recorded in response to arousal stimuli such as forced arithmetic, deep inspirations, sudden noises and pain, and are an established indicator of the state of an individual's ANS (Elam and Wallin 1987; Kistler, Mariauzouls and von Berlepsch 1998; Krogstad et al. 1995)

Cardiorespiratory Signals

The cardiovascular and respiratory systems are dually innervated by both branches of the autonomic nervous system; stimulation from the sympathetic branch causes increased functioning in both systems and stimulation from the parasympathetic branch reverses this behaviour. In both systems, it is difficult to trace a change in function back to its source, but for different reasons; the heart's responses to stimuli of a specific valence are highly stimulus dependent, whereas the respiratory musculature is innervated by both autonomic and somatic mechanisms, rendering the separation of involuntary reaction from voluntary control very challenging. Nevertheless, both heart and respiration rates have shown significant changes in response to sympathetic stimuli, including emotion and attention orientation (Blain, Chau and Mihailidis 2008).

Peripheral Autonomic Signals as an Access Pathway

Thus far, the reported responses of the four autonomic signals of interest have all been involuntary reactions to sympathetic arousing stimuli. The ability for an individual to control his or her autonomic signals has been widely debated for several decades (Miller 1969; Birbaumer 2006). To date, voluntary control of peripheral ANS signals has been used in fields such as biofeedback, polygraphy and mental imagery. While issues such as the slow rate of response, metabolic noise and pathological change must be addressed, evidence gathered from these fields suggests that peripheral ANS signals can be brought under voluntary control and that they may constitute a viable access pathway for individuals with severe and multiple disabilities (Blain, Chau and Mihailidis 2008). The remainder of this section focuses on a case study of a 15-year-old boy with severe disabilities for whom an access pathway comprised of signals from the autonomic nervous system is being developed.

CLIENT PROFILE

Reed is a 15-year-old boy who was born with severe spastic quadriplegic cerebral palsy, global developmental delay and visual impairment secondary to birth asphyxia. His medical history includes infantile seizures, on-going respiratory and swallowing difficulties, gastroesophageal reflux, frequent bouts of bronchiolitis and pneumonia. Reed is dependent on trained caregivers for all activities of daily living and is fed non-orally via a G-tube. He presents with marked or fluctuating increased tone throughout his extremities, and reduced or fluctuating tone in his neck and trunk. Reed's personalised equipment includes bilateral wrist splints and ankle-foot orthoses and a Tilt-in-Space manual wheelchair. Reed has been involved in speech-language pathology services for the past 9 years. Augmentative and alternative communication strategies and devices that were attempted in the past included a BIGmack communicator via an external switch mounted above his left arm to convey a pre-recorded message, a paper board with Mayer-Johnson Picture Communication Symbols (PCS) where selection was indicated by eye gaze, auditory scanning supplemented with printed pictures where selection was via a wheelchair-mounted Buddy Button, and various switch-activated software programs controlled by a custom chin switch. To date, none of these have been successfully used for environmental control or communication, largely due to issues of fatigue and involuntary movement.

ACCESS PATHWAY DEVELOPMENT

Due to Reed's extremely limited physical vocabulary and the lack of success with conventional augmentative and alternative communication devices, he was selected as a potential candidate for an access pathway based on peripheral autonomic nervous system signals. In order for this to be a viable pathway, we had to determine whether Reed was physiologically labile; in other words, whether the signals of his peripheral ANS responded to external stimuli. An access pathway was envisioned for Reed that he would control by changing the patterns of his peripheral ANS signals via a simple mental activity: thinking of things that he liked, and thinking of things that he did not like. Consequently, the initial step in access pathway development was to determine whether the patterns of the four physiological signals of interest changed upon presentation of different objects of preference.

As a result of not having a reliable access pathway, Reed was unable to express his own preferences. Instead, the proxy report of his primary caregiver, his mother, was used as a de facto standard to identify 10 objects that she believed would evoke an emotional response — five associated with a positive emotion, and five associated with a negative emotion. These objects were presented to him for 1-min each, over five different sessions, such that each object was presented five separate times. Reed's electrodermal activity, fingertip temperature, heart rate and respiration rate were recorded with a ProComp Infiniti data acquisition system from Thought Technology. Each of the signals was then independently analyzed offline to determine whether significant changes away from their baseline states had occurred, and whether Reed's physiological lability was sufficient to pursue peripheral physiological signals as an access pathway.

RESULTS

Reed's frequent bouts of respiratory and swallowing difficulty manifested as frequent occurrences of high amplitude, high frequency noise in both the respiratory and blood volume pulse signals, as depicted in Figure 3.17. These changes occluded many of the cardiorespiratory responses to the stimuli that we were expecting to see; as a result, these two signals were excluded from consideration as access pathways.

Examining the patterns of Reed's electrodermal activity, it was clear that he demonstrated electrodermal lability. He presented clear electrodermal reactions in response to both positive and negative stimuli, as illustrated in Figure 3.18. Clear changes in temperature were not as easy to discriminate; this fact, combined with the significantly longer latency of temperature responding, led to the selection of electrodermal activity as the physiological signal with the highest potential as a viable access pathway.

On average, electrodermal reactions were not present in baseline (resting) recordings, and appeared in response to both objects that his mother believed that he liked, such as his Tyrannosaurus Rex toy, and objects that his mother believed he disliked, such as his toothbrush. These reactions demonstrated that Reed was conscious of and responded to his external environment, and that he had the potential to be trained to voluntarily control his electrodermal activity to interact with his environment.

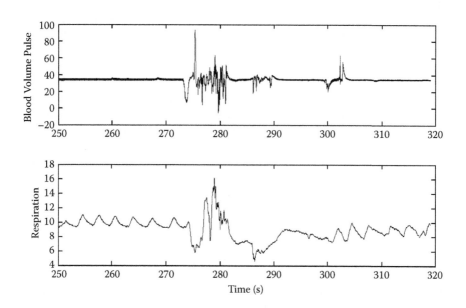

FIGURE 3.17 Examples of cardiorespiratory noise that occurs in Reed's physiological signals.

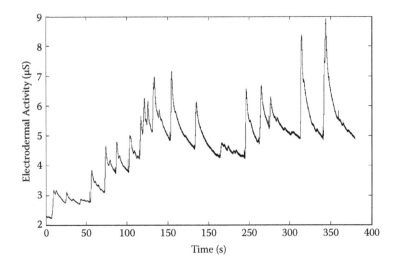

FIGURE 3.18   Electrodermal reactions generated by Reed as a result of watching one of his favourite videos.

DISCUSSION

Merits

Peripheral physiological signals are easily recorded by readily available commercial equipment. This equipment is relatively inexpensive, and is often operable by non-experts, facilitating its use by caregivers and family members. For experts wishing to analyze the signals beyond the basic outputs of such systems, reactions in the peripheral autonomic nervous systems are amenable to single-trial analysis, as changes in these signals often manifest as discrete events, such as an electrodermal reaction, or a large breath. Unlike many brain-computer interface paradigms that require the repetition of one trial many times before a conclusion can be drawn based on the average pattern, reactions in the peripheral physiological signals can be detected on a single-trial basis, making this access pathway amenable to real-time control. The signals can be recorded non-invasively, often requiring no more than a few sensors on the fingers, and one around the chest cavity to record respiration. Every individual has a response to stress that is predominantly manifested in one mode of his or her autonomic nervous system; recording the multitude of peripheral physiological signals allows algorithms to be developed that cater the access pathway to the response patterns of a particular individual, enabling a more accurate and sensitive pathway to be developed.

Limitations

There are three predominant limitations to using peripheral physiological signals as an access pathway: speed, metabolic noise and pathological change. Peripheral ANS changes manifest after a physiological process has occurred in the body; the mechanisms of these processes may take anywhere from 1- to 5-s (e.g., EDA) to 15-s (e.g., fingertip temperature) to occur (Boucsein 1992; Elam and Wallin 1987). Compared to signals in the central nervous system that change on the order of milliseconds, these changes may seem slow indeed (Birbaumer 2006). However, the benefits of a speedy access pathway may be offset by other factors, such as invasiveness, cost, inconvenience and system complexity. For individuals for whom speed is not the dominant priority, peripheral ANS signals may be an appealing alternative due to their non-invasive, affordable and convenient measurement.

Metabolic noise also presents difficulties in using these signals as an access pathway. While physiological signals can change as a result of external and internal stressors, they often also change in response to internal bodily processes, in the effort to maintain homeostasis. Separating out these metabolic changes from those that are deliberately generated remains challenging. Finally, the etiologies of some conditions of individuals in the target population often cause changes in the functioning of the peripheral autonomic nervous system. For example, individuals with complete spinal cord injury can no longer sweat below the level of injury, thereby rendering their EDA signal uninformative. These changes must be addressed and taken into consideration when developing an access pathway using these signals for a particular individual.

Future Directions

While electrodermal activity and other peripheral autonomic nervous system signals have demonstrated promise in being voluntarily controlled by able-bodied individuals, individuals within the target population have yet to demonstrate this ability. Programs need to be developed to train an individual with severe disabilities to become aware of these naturally involuntary signals, and to train these individuals to bring them under voluntary control. Furthermore, most of the work that has been accomplished in this area has examined individual peripheral ANS signals outside the context of the other signals. Evidence suggests that there is a strong relationship between many of the peripheral ANS signals; for example, when an individual is at rest, inhalation causes heart rate acceleration and exhalation causes heart rate deceleration (Lacey and Lacey 1980). These relationships between signals may contain a great deal of information, and further work must be conducted to exploit the maximum possible information from this unique access pathway.

CONCLUDING REMARKS

This chapter has introduced a number of emerging and investigational access technologies for non-verbal children and youth with severe disabilities. For those who retain voluntary mouth opening and closing or tongue protrusion amid involuntary head movements, infrared facial thermography or multiple camera computer vision systems, respectively, may be viable access technologies. Likewise, for children and youth who can create barely audible vocalizations but not functional speech, the vocal cord vibration technology described herein may provide an access possibility. Voluntary twitching of small or atrophied muscles may be detected using mechanomyography even if anti-gravity movement is not possible. Finally, when an individual with a capable mind has no controllable physical movements or vocalizations, signals of the autonomic nervous system might be considered as potential cues to a child's preferences. With growing numbers of children and youth presenting with complex and multiple disabilities, continued clinical-driven engineering research into novel access technologies is warranted.

REFERENCES

Akataki, K., K. Mita, and M. Watakabe. 2004. Electromyographic and mechanomyographic estimation of motor unit activation strategy in voluntary force production. *Electromyography and Clinical Neurophysiology* 44(8):489–496.

Balcerak, R., and J. Lupo. 2002. Advances in infrared sensor technology and systems. *24th Annual IEEE Engineering in Medicine and Biology Society Conference*, 2:1124–1125, October 23–26, 2002, Houston, TX. IEEE Press New York: NY.

Barnett, H.J.M., J.P. Mohr, B.M. Stein et al. 1992. Stroke: *Patho-physiology, diagnosis & management*. Edinburgh: Churchill Livingstone.

Barry, D.T. 1991. Muscle sounds from evoked twitches in the hand. *Archives of Physical Medicine and Rehabilitation* 72(8):573–575.

Barry, D.T. 1992. Vibrations and sounds from evoked muscle twitches. *Electromyography and Clinical Neurophysiology* 32(1-2):35–40.

Barry, D.T., and N.M. Cole. 1990. Muscle sounds are emitted at the resonant frequencies of skeletal muscle. *IEEE Transactions on Bio-Medical Engineering* 37(5):525–531.

Barry, D.T., K.E. Gordon, and G.G. Hinton. 1990. Acoustic and surface EMG diagnosis of pediatric muscle disease. *Muscle & Nerve* 13(4):286–290.

Barry, D.T., J.A. Leonard, A.J. Gitter Jr., and R.D. Ball. 1986. Acoustic myography as a control signal for an externally powered prosthesis. *Archives of Physical Medicine and Rehabilitation* 67(4):267–269.

BBC. Cbeebies Something Special Games. *Transport Snap* [online]. BBC. http://www.bbc.co.uk/cbeebies/somethingspecial/games/transportsnap (accessed February 2009).

Becker, P. 2005. *Cheat7* [online]. OneSwitch.org.uk. http://www.oneswitch.org.uk/2/sd-shoot-em-ups.htm (accessed February 2009).

Beukelman, D., and P. Mirenda. 2005. *Augmentative and alternative communication: Supporting children and adults with complex communication needs*, 3rd ed. Baltimore, MD: Paul H. Brookes Publishing.

Birbaumer, N. 2006. Breaking the silence: Brain-computer interfaces (BCI) for communication and motor control. *Psychophysiology* 43(6):517–532.

Blain, S., T. Chau, and A. Mihailidis. 2008. Peripheral autonomic signals as access pathways for individuals with severe disabilities: A literature appraisal. *The Open Rehabilitation Journal* 1:27–37.

Blain, S., P. McKeever, and T. Chau. 2010. Bedside computer access for an individual with severe and multiple disabilities: A case study. *Disability and Rehabilitation: Assistive Technology* 5(5):359–369.

Borg, G. 1982. Psychophysical bases of perceived exertion. *Medicine and Science in Sports and Exercise* 14(5):377–381.

Boucsein, W. 1992. *Electrodermal activity*. New York: Plenum Press.

Bradski, G.R. 1998. Computer vision face tracking for use in a perceptual user interface. *Intel Technology Journal* 2(12):1–15.

Bruno, M.A., C. Schnakers, F. Damas, F. Pellas, I. Lutte, J. Bernheim, S. Majerus, G. Moonen, S. Goldman, and S. Laureys 2009. Locked-in syndrome in children: Report of five cases and review of the literature. *Pediatric Neurology* 41(4):237–246.

Chang, A., and M. Karnell. 2004. Perceived phonatory effort and phonation threshold pressure across a prolonged voice loading task: A study of vocal fatigue. *Journal of Voice* 18(4):454–466.

Clarke M., and R. Wilkinson. 2007. Interaction between children with cerebral palsy and their peers. 1. Organizing and understanding VOCA use. *Augmentative and Alternative Communication* 23(4):336–348.

Data Resource Center. 2005/2006. Child and adolescent health measurement initiative. National survey of children with special health care needs. http://cshcndata.org/Content/Default.aspx (accessed June 2009).

Davis, J.W. 2001. Hierarchical motion history images for recognizing human motion. In: *Proceedings of the IEEE Workshop on Detection and Recognition of Events in Video*, 39–46. Conference paper, Vancouver, BC, Canada July 8, 2001 New York: IEEE Press.

de Dios, J.J. 2007. Skin colour and feature-based segmentation for face localization. *Optical Engineering* 46(3):037007-1–037007-6.

Elam, M., and B.G Wallin. 1987. Skin blood flow responses to mental stress in man depend on body temperature. *Acta Physiologica Scandinavica* 129:489–497.

Falk, T.H., Chan, J., Duez, P., Teachman, G., and Chau, T. 2010. Augmentative communication based on realtime vocal cord vibration detection. *IEEE Transactions Neural Systems and Rehabilitation Engineering* 18(2):159–163.

FLIR Systems. 2005. ThermaCAM SC640 [online]. FLIR Systems Inc. http://www.flirthermography.com/cameras/camera/1101/ (accessed January 2009).

GotoInfrared. 2007. L-3 Communications: Thermal-Eye 2000B/300D [online]. GotoInfrared. http://gotoinfrared.com/L3.htm (accessed April 23, 2009).

Grauman, K., M. Betke, J. Lombardi, J. Gips, and G. Bradski. 2003. Communication via eye blinks and eyebrow raises: Video-based human-computer interfaces. *Universal Access in the Information Society* 2(4):359–373.

Gryfe, P., I. Kurtz, M. Gutmann, and G. Laiken. 1996. Freedom through a single switch: Coping and communicating with artificial ventilation. *Journal of the Neurological Sciences* 139:132–133.

Hales, J.R.S. 1985. Skin arteriovenous anatomoses: Their control and role in thermoregulation. In Johansen, K., Burggen, W. editors. *Cardiovascular shunts*: *Phylogenetic, ontogenetic and clinical aspects*. Copenhagen, Denmark: Munksgaard. pp. 433–451.

Harada, S., J. Wobbrock, J. Landay, J. Malkin, and J. Bilmes. 2009. Longitudinal study of people learning to use continuous voice-based cursor control. In: *Proc. Conf. Human Factors in Computing Systems* 347–356.

Havstam, C., M. Buchholz, and L. Hartelius. 2003. Speech recognition and dysarthria: A single subject study of two individuals with profound impairment of speech and motor control. *Logopedics Phoniatrics Vocology* 28:81–90.

Hot, P., J. Naveteur, P. Leconte et al. 1999. Diurnal variations of tonic electrodermal activity. *International Journal of Psychophysiology* 33(3):223–230.

Jones, B.F., 1998. A reappraisal of the use of infrared thermal image analysis in medicine. *IEEE Transactions on Medical Imaging* 17(6):1019–1027.

Jones, B.F., and P. Plassmann. 2002. Digital infrared thermal imaging of human skin. *IEEE Engineering in Medicine and Biology* 21:41–48.

Juneja M., R. Jain, S. Singhal, D. Mishra, and S. Singh. 2009. Locked-in syndrome: A rare manifestation of pediatric stroke. *Indian Journal of Pediatrics* 76(10):1053–1055.

Kennedy, P. R., and K.D. Adams. 2003. A decision tree for brain-computer interface devices. *Neural Systems and Rehabilitation Engineering* [See also *IEEE Trans.on Rehabilitation Engineering*] 11(2):148–150.

Kistler, A., C. Mariauzouls, and K. von Berlepsch. 1998. Fingertip temperature as an indicator for sympathetic responses. *International Journal of Psychophysiology* 29(1):35-41.

Koester Performance Research, 2007. *Compass Assessment Software* [online]. http://www.kpronline.com/products.html (accessed February 2009).

Krogstad, A., M. Elam, T. Karlsson et al. 1995. Arteriovenous anastomoses and the thermo-regulatory shift between cutaneous vasoconstrictor and vasodilator reflexes. *Journal of Autonomic Nervous System* 53(2–3):215–222.

Lacey, B.C., and J.I. Lacey. 1980. Cognitive modulation of time-dependent primary bradycardia. *Psychophysiology* 17(3):209–221.

Lancioni, G., and S. Lems. 2001. Using a microswitch for vocalization responses with persons with multiple disabilities. *Disability & Rehabilitation* 23(16):745–748.

Lancioni, G., M. O'Reilly, and G. Basili. 2001. Use of microswitches and speech output systems with people with severe/profound intellectual or multiple disabilities: A literature review. *Research in Developmental Disabilities* 22(1):21–40.

Lancioni, G., N. Singh, M. O'Reilly, D. Oliva, and J. Groeneweg. 2005. Enabling a girl with multiple disabilities to control her favourite stimuli through vocalization and a dual-microphone microswitch. *Journal of Visual Impairment and Blindness* 99(3):133–140.

Langley, M., and L. Lombardino. 1991. *Neurodevelopmental strategies for managing communication disorders in children with severe motor dysfunction*. Austin, TX: Pro-Ed Publishers.

Leung, B., and T. Chau. 2010. A multiple camera tongue switch for a child with severe spastic quadriplegic cerebral palsy. *Disability and Rehabilitation: Assistive Technology* 5(1):58–68.

Lund, S., and J. Light. 2007. Long-term outcomes for individuals who use augmentative and alternative communication: Part III — Contributing factors. *Augmentative and Alternative Communication* 23(4):323–335.

Madeleine, P., and L. Arendt-Nielsen. 2005. Experimental muscle pain increases mechano-myographic signal activity during sub-maximal isometric contractions. *Journal of Electromyography and Kinesiology: Official Journal of the International Society of Electrophysiological Kinesiology* 15(1):27–36.

Madeleine, P., P. Bajaj, K. Sogaard, and L. Arendt-Nielsen. 2001. Mechanomyography and electromyography force relationships during concentric, isometric and eccentric contractions. *Journal of Electromyography and Kinesiology: Official Journal of the International Society of Electrophysiological Kinesiology* 11(2):113–121.

Madeleine, P., L.V. Jorgensen, K. Sogaard, L. Arendt-Nielsen, and G. Sjogaard. 2002. Development of muscle fatigue as assessed by electromyography and mechanomyography during continuous and intermittent low-force contractions: Effects of the feedback mode. *European Journal of Applied Physiology* 87(1):28–37.

Memarian, N., A.N. Venetsanopoulos, and T. Chau. 2009. Infrared thermography as an access pathway for individuals with severe motor impairments. *Journal of NeuroEngineering and Rehabilitation* 6(11):1–8.

Miller, N.E. 1969. Learning of visceral and glandular responses. *Science* 163(3866):434–445.

Miller N.G., W.E. Reddick, M. Kocak, J.O. Glass, U. Lobel, B. Morris, A. Gajjar, and Z. Patay. 2010. Cerebellocerebral diaschisis is the likely mechanism of postsurgical posterior fossa syndrome in pediatric patients with midline cerebellar tumors. *American Journal of Neuroradiology* 31(2):288–294.

Morgan, A.T., and A.P. Vogel. 2008. Intervention for dysarthria associated with acquired brain injury in children and adolescents. *Cochrane Database Systematic Reviews* 16(3):CD006279.

Moriyamashi, T., H. Tagucihi, and Y. Mishima. 1996. Relation between the brain waves, face temperature and blood pressure using nonintrusive blood pressure monitor and the environments. *35th SICE Annual Conference (International Session Papers)*, 1205–1208, July 24–26, 1996, Tottori, Japan.

Ng, A.R., K. Arimura, K. Akataki, K. Mita, I. Higuchi, and M. Osame. 2006. Mechanomyographic determination of post-activation potentiation in myopathies. *Clinical Neurophysiology: Official Journal of the International Federation of Clinical Neurophysiology* 117(1):232–239.

Nhan, B.R., and T. Chau. 2009. Infrared thermal imaging as a physiological access pathway: A study of the baseline characteristics of facial skin temperatures. *Physiological Measurements* 30:N23–N35.

Noda Y., K. Sakai, M. Tojo, N. Sakuragawa, and M. Arima. 1990. Nemaline myopathy of severe infantile type: A case report of a 9-year-old girl. *No To Hattatsu* 22(1):82–85.

Noyes, J.M., and C.R. Frankish. 1992. Speech recognition technology for individuals with disabilities. *Augmentative and Alternative Communication* 8(4):297–303.

Orizio, C. 1993. Muscle sound: Bases for the introduction of a mechanomyographic signal in muscle studies. *Critical Reviews in Biomedical Engineering* 21(3):201–243.

Orizio, C., R.V. Baratta, B.H. Zhou, M. Solomonow, and A. Veicsteinas. 1999. Force and surface mechanomyogram relationship in cat gastrocnemius. *Journal of Electromyography and Kinesiology: Official Journal of the International Society of Electrophysiological Kinesiology* 9(2):131–140.

Palisano, R., P. Rosenbaum, S. Walter, D. Russell, E. Wood, and B. Galuppi. 1997. Development and reliability of a system to classify gross motor function in children with cerebral palsy. *Developmental Medicine and Child Neurology* 39(4):214–223.

Patel, R., 2002. Phonatory control in adults with cerebral palsy and severe dysarthria. *Augmentative and Alternative Communication* 18(1):2–10.

Patel, R., and J. Brayton. 2008. Identifying prosodic contrasts in utterances produced by 4, 7, and 11 year old children. *Journal of Speech, Language, and Hearing Research* 52:790–801.

Shinohara, M., and K. Sogaard. 2006. Mechanomyography for studying force fluctuations and muscle fatigue. *Exercise and Sport Sciences Reviews* 34(2):59–64.

Silva, J., and T. Chau. 2003. Coupled microphone-accelerometer sensor pair for dynamic noise reduction in MMG signal recording. *Electronics Letters* 39(21):1496–1498.

Silva, J., and T. Chau. 2005. A mathematical model for source separation of MMG signals recorded with a coupled microphone-accelerometer sensor pair. *Biomedical Engineering, IEEE Transactions on* 52(9):1493–1501.

Silva, J., W. Heim, and T. Chau. 2005. A self-contained, mechanomyography-driven externally powered prosthesis. *Archives of Physical Medicine and Rehabilitation* 86(10):2066–2070.

Smith, M. 1994. Speech by any other name: The role of communication aids in interaction. *European Journal of Disorders of Communication* 29:225–240.

SPi Infrared. 2008. RAZ-IR mini thermal camera [online]. SPi Infrared. http://raz-ir.com/ (accessed October 2008).

Statistics Canada. 2007. Social and aboriginal statistics division. Participation and activity limitation survey 2006. Analytical Report. http://www.statcan.gc.ca/bsolc/olc-cel/olc-cel?catno=89-628-X (accessed January 2009).

Tai, K., S. Blain, and T. Chau. 2008. A review of emerging access technologies individuals with severe motor impairments. *Assistive Technology* 20:204–219.

Titze, I. 1994. *Principles of voice production.* Englewood Cliffs, NJ: Prentice Hall.

Vetrugno R., R. Liguori, P. Cortelli, and P. Montagna. 2003. Sympathetic skin response: Basic mechanisms and clinical applications. *Clinical Autonomic Research* 13(4):256–270.

Wang, J., and E. Sung. 2007. Facial feature extraction in an infrared image by proxy with a visible face image. *IEEE Transactions on Instrumentation and Measurement.* 56(4):2057–2066.

Watakabe, M., Y. Itoh, K. Mita, and K. Akataki. 1998. Technical aspects of mechanomyography recording with piezoelectric contact sensor. *Medical & Biological Engineering & Computing* 36(5):557–561.

Watakabe, M., K. Mita, K. Akataki, and Y. Itoh. 2001. Mechanical behaviour of condenser microphone in mechanomyography. *Medical & Biological Engineering & Computing* 39(2):195–201.

Yorkston, K., D. Beukelman, E. Strand, and K. Bell. 1999. *Management of motor speech disorders in children and adults*. Austin, TX: Pro-Ed Publishers.

4 Advances in Technologies to Support Children with Communication Needs

Gail Teachman and Cynthia Tam

CONTENTS

At the front of the classroom, a group of first-grade children sit quietly on the carpet, excitedly waving their hands, hoping to get the teacher's attention so that they will be picked to be the next student who goes up to the whiteboard. It is circle time and the students know that this classroom activity always starts with a discussion about the calendar. Each student is hoping to earn a turn to 'magically' write the name of the month on the large, interactive screen at the front of the class, beside the teacher. As the teacher scans the quiet group, a voice interrupts, calling out 'I have something to say!' The children turn to regard Sami,* one of their classmates, who is sitting in a wheelchair beside the group of children on the carpet. Sami is beaming with excitement,

---

* Names and any identifying details in these case studies have been changed to protect the children's privacy.

anxious to show that he knows the answer. Although Sami has cerebral palsy and is unable to speak, he has just used his speech-generating device to capture the attention of his teacher and to request a turn to give the correct answer. 'OK, Sami, it's your turn. Tell us the name of this month,' says his teacher. Sami reaches with a shaky hand toward the laptop-sized device that is secured to his wheelchair tray. His extended finger wobbles in the air as he works to target a precise location on the screen in front of him. As he touches the screen, a digitised voice emerges from the device: 'October.' Simultaneously, the word 'October' appears on the whiteboard in front of the children, sent via a cable from Sami's device to the computer controlling the whiteboard. 'That's right, Sami,' says his teacher. 'This is the month of October.' Sami grins proudly as his classmates look on impressed — and in the next instant, their hands are up again, waving to gain the teacher's attention, eager to take their turn.

This chapter provides an overview of communication-related assistive technologies. We use case examples, such as this introductory case about Sami, throughout the chapter to highlight the enabling role of assistive technology (AT) in supporting children to communicate within a variety of everyday environments — home, school and community. Individual children interact with these technologies via an access pathway. For some children, this might involve using their hand to hit a mechanical switch or press a key on a keyboard. Other children might use their voice or blink an eye to activate and control technologies. We will not discuss these access pathways because Chapter 3 in this book is dedicated to that topic.

CHAPTER OBJECTIVES

1. The reader will learn about key issues and considerations related to communication needs throughout childhood and into young adulthood.
2. The reader will learn about the latest assistive technology trends in supporting communication.

The overall organization of this chapter is depicted in Figure 4.1. We begin by providing some background and context that will set the stage for discussion of technologies that may be of assistance to children who communicate differently. Following the introduction, we have organised the information about these technologies within four groupings: Engagement, Literacy, Participation, and Training and Support. This way of thinking about AT is our own construction and is intended to emphasise a functional, outcomes-based approach. We have selected examples to illustrate the ways that specific technologies can make a difference to a child's ability to engage fully, to master and demonstrate his or her literacy and to be provided with essential training and support. We acknowledge that many new devices and technology solutions incorporate designs and features that address needs in more than one of these areas. As noted, this chapter serves as an introductory overview and is not intended to provide a complete or exhaustive listing of the many current technology trends and innovations that address the communication needs of children.

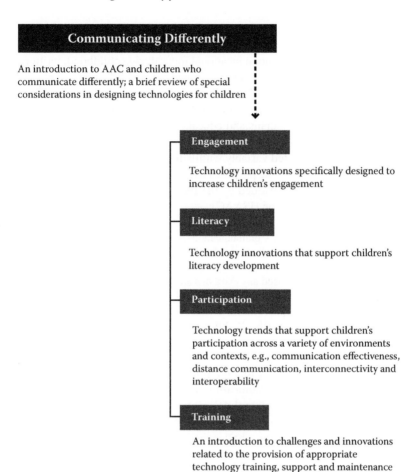

Communicating Differently

An introduction to AAC and children who communicate differently; a brief review of special considerations in designing technologies for children

Engagement

Technology innovations specifically designed to increase children's engagement

Literacy

Technology innovations that support children's literacy development

Participation

Technology trends that support children's participation across a variety of environments and contexts, e.g., communication effectiveness, distance communication, interconnectivity and interoperability

Training

An introduction to challenges and innovations related to the provision of appropriate technology training, support and maintenance

FIGURE 4.1   Conceptual roadmap of chapter content.

COMMUNICATING DIFFERENTLY

Learning to communicate is a critical developmental activity throughout childhood. Communication skills play a vital role as children form relationships and begin to make sense of their world. Parents intuitively and keenly observe their child's developing communication skills: delighting in that first social smile, eagerly anticipating those first words. Indeed, most would agree with Janice Light, a leader in the fields of education and augmentative and alternative communication, who noted, 'Communication is the essence of life' (Light 1997).

Many children with disabilities learn to communicate differently, however, and their communication attempts may be difficult for others to recognise and interpret. These children are unable to communicate in the same ways as their 'typically' developing peers. They may encounter limitations and difficulties either related to speaking, which is our most typical form of face-to-face communication, or related to the many skills involved in learning to communicate through writing. Certainly, the development of speech and language skills during childhood is critical to a child's ability to navigate his or her world successfully. It is also critical to consider that learning to write is one major educational focus during childhood; written communication is a key task that is required throughout a child's education and is an important factor supporting school success.

To meet the communication needs of children with limitations and difficulties in this area, their families, clinicians and educators often explore tools and strategies known as augmentative and alternative communication (AAC) systems. The scope of the term AAC is interpreted variably within different fields of study and in different international settings. For the purposes of this chapter, we will use the broad and inclusive definition that is forwarded by the International Society for Augmentative and Alternative Communication (ISAAC):

> Augmentative and Alternative Communication (AAC) are the words used to describe extra ways of helping people who find it hard to communicate by speech or writing. AAC helps them to communicate more easily. AAC includes many different methods. Signing and gesture do not need any extra bits and pieces and are called unaided systems. Others use picture charts, books and special computers. These are called aided systems. AAC can help people understand what is said to them as well as being able to say and write what they want. (ISAAC 1983)

People whose communication challenges involve significant neurological limitations and who have difficulty with both speaking and writing are often described as persons with 'complex communication needs,' a term that is frequently found in current literature. This functional description is difficult to define comprehensively, but it is useful because it offers an inclusive way of describing people with very significant communication challenges and it includes those with met and unmet needs.

Persons who are able to speak functionally but who encounter difficulty with writing often do not identify themselves as using AAC; instead, they may relate writing technologies more closely with the more general term 'assistive technology.' In this chapter, trends related to AT and AAC targeting both writing and speech are reviewed. Both of the terms AAC and AT will be used, depending on the focus of the technology being discussed.

WHICH CHILDREN BENEFIT FROM COMMUNICATION-RELATED ASSISTIVE TECHNOLOGIES?

In the case study above, we introduced 'Sami.' Sami was born prematurely and diagnosed with cerebral palsy (CP), which is a developmental condition characterised by movement and learning disorders. He has a type of CP called quadriplegia, which means that all four of his limbs are affected by significant movement limitations. A small bleed occurred around the time of Sami's birth, damaging areas of his brain. As a result, he is not able to control the muscles of his arms and legs, his core musculature is weak and he needs to use a wheelchair with supportive seating. He is also unable to control the very complex motor tasks that are required to produce speech.

Even the very discreet muscle control needed to control his eye movements can be challenging for Sami.

Although Sami cannot speak and is not able to raise his hand to ask for a turn, he is able to communicate actively within his classroom setting. In the case study scenario, he is described using a speech-generating device (SGD) to augment his other, non-verbal modes of communication. Children like Sami may sometimes use their eyes to communicate. For example, Sami will rest his gaze on one of a series of pictures, words or symbols that his educational assistant presents to him in order to indicate the one that he wishes to select. He can smile to say 'Yes' and he gazes downward to say 'No.' Sometimes he will repeatedly look at objects or people in his classroom to indicate that he is trying to communicate something related to those objects or people. Sami has a book full of picture symbols, photographs and words that are organised in categories (e.g., food, places and people). With some assistance to open the book to the page he wants, he is able to point to the symbols to get his message across. However, Sami finds that one of the best ways to engage his classmates is to use his new speech generating device. Even though it can sometimes be quite slow for him to use, when compared to his other methods of communicating, the device gives him a voice that can be heard across the room, that can capture the attention of his classmates and that allows him to show his peers that he is learning to read and write, just like them.

This case study of Sami provides a snapshot of a child with CP who experiences complex communication needs. It has been our experience that CP is the most common diagnosis among the population of children who need AAC. Epidemiological study in the area of communicative disorders, specifically of the population who use AAC, is greatly needed in order to better describe and define issues related to incidence and prevalence. Many diagnostic conditions can impose significant barriers to the development of communication in childhood.

Developmental or intellectual delays may also affect a child's ability to speak or write. In a recent review study, Wilkinson and Hennig (2007) commented on the very considerable body of work focusing on the use of AAC with this population of children. Some children with developmental delay may be able to speak, but their speech may be unclear and they may have language deficits, making it hard for the communication partner to understand their meaning. These children sometimes use a speech-generating device to 'repair' the conversation (Sigafoos et al. 2004). For example, they might use the device to clarify their topic or to repeat part of the message.

Children who are born prematurely, as well as extremely low-birth-weight babies, often develop functional sequelae that include communication disorders (Msall and Tremont 2000).

Children with congenital or traumatic amputations may have difficulty with the physical task of holding and manipulating a writing utensil, or hitting keys on a computer keyboard.

Childhood neurological conditions that impair the development of communication skills include brain injury, spinal cord injury and stroke. Degenerative conditions such as Rhett's syndrome, muscular dystrophy, amyotrophic lateral sclerosis (ALS) and juvenile arthritis can result in limitations in writing, speech or both. Autism is a neurodevelopmental disorder characterised by difficulties with social and communication skills. Landa (2007) provides a comprehensive review of communication development and communication issues related to autism.

Children who experience severe and traumatic illnesses, such as cancer, may encounter temporary or long-term communication limitations. In one study, it was reported that 62% of people who are mechanically ventilated experienced a high level of frustration in trying to communicate their needs (Patak et al. 2006). In another study, Reinders-Messelink et al. (2001) found that children treated with neurotoxins for acute lymphoblastic leukaemia experienced subsequent difficulty with handwriting, becoming slower, needing to take longer pauses and needing to exert greater pressure on the writing utensil.

Another emerging population of children who present with communication disorders is found among those exposed to human immunodeficiency virus (HIV). McNeilly (2000, 2005) provides an overview of conditions related to HIV that lead to communication deficits and suggests a range of strategies for intervention.

A wide variety of conditions and developmental issues may contribute to language disorders in children (Simms 2007). Language and learning deficits can significantly limit a child's success in developing functional speech and writing abilities.

How Large Is the Need for Communication Technologies That Are Designed for Children?

In a study of pre-school children, Binger and Light (2006) found that 12% of those receiving special education services required some type of AAC intervention. In another study, Kent-Walsh, Stark and Binger (2008) found that up to 50% of speech language pathologists working a school-aged caseload served children with AAC needs.

Other studies, not specific to AAC needs alone, can provide some insight into the potential need for technologies that can support written and face-to-face communication. In a large demographic study of over 14,000 students who were identified as having learning needs, a communication disorder was the second most prevalent need, comprising 13% of the group (McLeod and McKinnon 2007). In a large population study conducted in Utah in 1994, it was found that the prevalence of communication disorders among 8-year-olds was 63.4 per 1000 (95% confidence interval = 60.4–66.2) (Pinborough-Zimmerman et al. 2007).

Communication Issues and Design Considerations Specific to Childhood

During childhood, communication skills and expectations change, perhaps more than in any other stage of life. Interventions targeting communication must therefore take into account the need for a device to change and 'grow' with the child. Designers must also consider the typical occupations of childhood, which are focused on learning, play and the mastery of self-care. Technologies that support communication need to be designed with consideration of their fit within the real-world environments of childhood — at the dinner table and at the park, in the classroom and on the school bus, on the playground and in the shopping mall.

Children are also developing a sense of self-identity, finding ways to make sense of the world and exploring their place in the world. Communication is one of the vital ways that children can engage in these developmental tasks. As children grow up, become adolescents and begin to navigate the transition to young adulthood, they need, more than ever, to communicate effectively. They need communication solutions that support them in connecting with the world, engaging in higher level education, seeking out careers, planning for independent living, managing their own affairs including directing their care if necessary, managing finances, interacting in new spheres of community living, and expanding their social networks. For youth with communication challenges, these tasks can seem insurmountable and, therefore, progressively more customised and comprehensive solutions are needed (McNaughton and Bryen 2007).

Although this chapter is focused on innovations and trends related to specific technologies, there are important environmental and human factors to consider outside of the technology itself. After all, 'technology is a tool ... not the end goal itself' (Light 1997). The end goal is to support children to communicate successfully and participate meaningfully across a variety of environments. Changing paradigms and innovative practices in AT service delivery are paramount in any discussion of the effectiveness of communication AT solutions. Studies have demonstrated that many factors outside of the technology itself can lead to inadequacies and reduce the effectiveness of the technology solution. In summarizing an extensive review of literature related to inadequacies in computer access solutions for individuals with profound disabilities, Hoppestad (2007) noted that recent paradigm shifts to more person-centred approaches could result in solutions that better match individuals' abilities and aspirations. A smaller study that surveyed the families of six AAC users noted the importance of gaining families' perspectives about the barriers and supports, expectations and benefits related to AAC devices, especially since these factors may affect whether environments are conducive to use of the device (Bailey et al. 2006).

Communication technology needs to be selected using 'a process which is affected by a broader societal climate that determines, in part, unique personal climates which then foster unique provider and consumer perspectives predisposing each to the selection of a particular assistive technology device' (Scherer et al. 2007). Designers and clinicians must consider a range of human factors that affect successful access and use of AAC devices (Higginbotham et al. 2007). A guide can be found in the comprehensive model provided by Schlosser (1999), wherein he proposes considerations for AAC interventions that will have social validity. He suggests that interventions be evaluated from various stakeholder perspectives and using either social comparisons or subjective evaluation, with respect to three validation components: goals, methods and outcomes (Schlosser 1999).

ENGAGEMENT

In the competitive marketplace, toys, games, computer software and learning materials for typically developing children are designed to be desirable, attractive, 'cool' and engaging. Recently, researchers have highlighted the need for children's communication devices and tools to be designed with consideration of children's perspectives. Allen (2005) noted that communication device designers too often fail to take into account the sociological and psychological impact that the device has on the user. He stressed the importance of device desirability, recommending the use of a participatory framework in both the design and selection of devices. In a study that focused on eliciting children's perspectives, Light et al. (2007) invited six children without disabilities to collaborate in the design of prototypes for a speech-generating device. The children incorporated multiple functions into their devices, such as communication, social interaction, companionship, play, artistic expression and telecommunications. They also integrated features that would engage and support interactions with their peers. The researchers noted that the children characterised the systems as companions, assigning names to their devices. They reported that the children designed systems that could be personalised to reflect their own age, personality, attitudes, interests and preferences. The children incorporated bright colours, lights, transformable shapes, popular themes, humour and amazing accomplishments, all of which were noted by the researchers to capture interest, enhance appeal, build self-esteem and establish a positive social image. Light and Drager (2007) identified the need for future research to determine whether implementation of the design specifications valued by children would result in increased engagement, use and peer interaction. Craddock (2006) surveyed 45 students to identify factors that promote the journey from novice to 'power' user of AT. He found ample evidence that students who progressed to become 'power' users of their AT were highly engaged and identified positively with their AT, feeling that it provided them with added 'social credit.' Technology that is able to attract and engage a child's peers has the potential to increase that child's opportunities to model language and to practice his or her developing communication skills. In a study examining communication interventions for children with autism, Paul (2008) stressed the need for less adult-directed intervention and suggested that peer-mediated communication interactions are one of the most critical elements to ensure communication skills are integrated and generalised.

Mai is a 12-year-old girl who attends grade seven at her neighbourhood school. Class will begin in a few minutes, but a small group of girls is huddled, giggling and chatting in a group around Mai's desk. With her new communication device, the Tango®, Mai is showing off pictures from a concert that she attended on the weekend. The girls gasp as Mai proudly displays a picture of herself meeting one of the boy band members. Mai touches the screen and it changes — no longer displaying photos but instead displaying words and illustrations. Mai scrolls through until she finds the one she wants, touches it again and immediately a whispering girl's voice is heard from the device: 'I won a backstage pass in a fan club contest!' Mai especially loves to use the 'whisper' voice feature on her new device — she loves secrets just as much as all of the other girls. She used her Tango® to introduce herself to her teen idol and to take pictures while she was at the concert.

Mai has developmental delay and although she tries to use her speech, her words come out sounding slurred. Because her language skills are delayed, she often has trouble thinking of the words that can get her message across. She is learning that her new speech-generating device helps her to talk with her classmates about a wider variety of topics and it helps them to understand that she has lots to say. Mai's device is set up with language software that was designed with teenagers' communication needs and desires in mind. She can quickly access jargon and other 'cool' words and phrases that help her to fit in with her peers. Mai can plug her Tango® into the desktop computer in her classroom and use it like a keyboard to work on classroom writing projects. This feature is very helpful to Mai because her handwriting is very slow and illegible. Since she started using her Tango® as a keyboard, Mai writes more and includes more details in her writing assignments.

The Tango® (Blink Twice, Inc. © 2007) is one example of newer speech-generating devices that are innovative, in particular, because of the way they have been designed to integrate many of the features that children identify as engaging. The Tango® was developed by Blink Twice, Inc. in partnership with companies that already had proven experience and success in the children's toy and entertainment markets. As a result, the device does not look or feel like a laptop computer; instead, it looks like an elongated gamepad — all curves and smoothed-out edges with attractive silver control buttons and a touch screen that displays a single row of colourful message choices. The Tango® software supports multimedia options such as a camera function, story-telling and photo album modes. These features can facilitate improved access to interactional conversations, addressing the need identified in the literature for technologies to more readily allow children to engage their peers and participate in conversational narratives (Waller 2006). The software illustrations in the Tango® incorporate a choice of characters that can be matched to the sex and age range of the child user, a nod to some children's preferences to view the device as a companion. Vocabulary options built into the device software include socially age-appropriate language, such as lingo, slang and informal speech styles that sound like other children in the social setting and age range. This has been shown to positively change the perception of peers about children who use AAC devices (Becket al. 2006; Beck et al. 2000).

Another innovation that has been incorporated into newer speech-generating devices is the design of communication software that incorporates a whole-utterance-based approach to communication (Todman et al. 2008) where phrases or sentences are preprogrammed. The developers of the Tango® elected to default their device software design to a whole-utterance approach. In choosing this approach, they departed from more conventional software designs where the user composes a message by selecting individual words to build a sentence or phrase in a message window and then selects the message window to command the device to speak the message. This multistep approach has the advantage of allowing children to learn to use language by composing their own unique utterances. However, it can be very slow and there is a risk that the audience for the message will lose attention and will move on before the person using AAC has a chance to take his or her turn in the communication exchange. This is very real limitation for children and teens who are trying to engage their peers in a conversation. There is evidence that the use of whole-utterance approaches has the potential to deliver faster rates of communication without loss of coherence (Todman et al. 2008). Another example of software that is designed to incorporate whole-utterance approaches is InterAACT® from DynaVox Mayer-Johnson (InterAACT 2008). This software, described as a language framework, offers features called 'My Phrases' and 'Quickfires' to provide faster message delivery in specific communication contexts. However, the software also includes more traditional message construction options to support the development of children's language and literacy skills. This merging of approaches is an attempt to acknowledge the need for devices to grow along with the children who use the device.

InterAACT® also incorporates another innovative approach in its communication software that is based on emerging evidence that there is a need for AAC devices to engage children by supporting social interaction in specific child-oriented contexts (Light et al. 2007). These contexts might include a child's classroom, school playground, bedroom or the neighbourhood grocery store. InterAACT® software includes options to organise access to context-dependent language within the framework of 'visual scenes' (i.e., illustrations or photographs of those specific contexts).

As they develop communication skills, young children are more reliant on visual cues than are older children (Doherty-Sneddon and Kent 1996). Drager et al. (2005) studied 10 typically developing children who were randomly assigned to three different groups according to the organization and presentation style of three different dynamic screen speech-generating devices. Children did best when using a device where language was organised using a contextual scene format as opposed to a grid format. In a different study (Drager et al. 2003), 30 two-and-a-half-year-old children were randomly assigned to three different conditions: vocabulary in a grid format organised taxonomically, vocabulary in a grid format organised schematically, and vocabulary in an integrated scene organised schematically. The children did poorly in all conditions but were able to locate more items when vocabulary was organised using a schematic integrated scene.

Kevin sits in his wheelchair by the open classroom window with his Vmax® speech-generating device turned on and 'ready-to-go.' It is recess and he is waiting for his friend to appear outside the window in the playground. They are going to play 'donut-shop' and Kevin is pretending to be the clerk at the drive-up shop window. Kevin can't go outside today because it is a muddy, rainy spring day and his wheelchair just gets stuck out on the playground. Today, though, Kevin doesn't mind because he loves this new game. On his device display, there is a photograph of the local donut shop drive-up service area taken by Kevin's mother. Together, they decided on 'hot-spots' in the photographic scene where groups of phrases or sentences would be 'linked.' As Kevin's friend Sara approaches the window outside of the school, she is pretending to drive a car. She 'pulls up and stops her car' in front of Kevin who reaches out and touches the open window depicted in the scene on his device. Immediately, a boy's voice speaks, 'How can I help you today?' Sara giggles and responds: 'I'll have 5 coffees and 10 donuts, please.' Kevin then touches the donuts depicted in the visual scene and the device speaks out for him: 'What kind of donuts do you want today?' Sara hesitates a moment and then begins to name all of her favourite types of donuts. Soon, other schoolmates are lining up behind Sara to take a turn ordering donuts from Kevin. The children remain engaged and focused in their make-believe game until a bell sounds, signalling the end of recess.

Kevin is in grade four and although he has had a speech-generating device since he was in pre-school, he had never used it consistently. He had not become competent at composing novel messages by navigating throughout the many pages of words in his device and, as a result, his communication rate using the device was very slow. He became frustrated and lost interest. In an attempt to renew Kevin's interest and increase his opportunities to communicate, especially with his peers at school, Kevin's older device was replaced with the newer Vmax® device and InterAACT® software. The new device better accommodated Kevin's needs by providing quick access to whole-utterances, organised and represented within the framework of a selection of visual scenes. Kevin is now enjoying increased social interaction and his peers are beginning to learn that Kevin has a lot to say!

Just as we now carry phones that allow us to take pictures, check our calendars, and play music or a game, innovative technologies supporting children with communication needs are beginning to address the need to offer a variety of highly engaging functions and features.

LITERACY

Most children who use AAC do not develop literacy (defined here simply as reading and writing) in the same way as their non-AAC-using peers, nor do most achieve the same levels of mastery. There is a profound need to design and implement technologies that can provide support for the development of reading and writing in the early years. Some mainstream technologies that have demonstrated high appeal in the marketplace are now being applied innovatively to support children with communication needs.

Light and Drager (2007) reported that children with developmental disabilities, between the ages of 1 and 3 years, demonstrated substantial increases in vocabulary acquisition when dynamic display AAC technologies were introduced. Vocabulary acquisition is an important component of language development. Some parents express concern that early use of any type of SGD may have a detrimental effect on communication, fearing that use of the device will cause their children to stop making attempts to speak. However, studies have demonstrated that the use of SGDs assists children who use AAC to become more effective communicators, in some cases even contributing to speech improvements (Binger et al. 2008).

Early access to AAC technologies can build foundation skills to support the development of literacy, allowing very young children with complex communication needs to explore communication and learning applications in ways that are contextualised within play. This can be done long before they have the skills to use a keyboard and a mouse. Vocabulary on the device can be constantly expanded and modelled in meaningful, fun and timely ways, within the child's daily environments. This early access to technology provides an important head start, allowing exposure to a wider variety of vocabulary and involving learning concepts, such as cause and effect or turn-taking, that are basic to communication. Light and Drager (2007) stated that this early access to dynamic screen AAC technologies 'is critical to maximise opportunities for language development in the early years when children are neurologically primed for learning.' They also noted that expectations for very young children are often too low.

To better understand the foundational experiences important to literacy learning, Sturm et al. (2006) used survey methods to examine the reading activities of general education students and teachers during primary grade instruction. The results of the survey provided evidence to guide the development of software and hardware that is able to more closely reflect typical classroom demands and provide children with access to repeated opportunities to participate in reading, over time, for as long as instruction is needed. The authors pointed to the need to address universal design, cognitive models of literacy training and access to a wide variety of literacy activities at varying grade levels. The authors also stressed the need for literacy tools that support opportunities for children to express, orally and in writing, their thoughts about, and understanding of, reading materials.

In the case study of Sami provided at the beginning of this chapter, we highlighted the role that technology can play in providing opportunities for children who use AAC to demonstrate their developing literacy skills through the integration of communication devices and interactive whiteboards in the classroom setting. The range of potential applications of whiteboard technologies for children with disabilities is just beginning to be studied and very little material on this topic is published. In an article from mainstream educators who addressed the use of interactive whiteboards and interactive whole class teaching methods, Tanner et al. (2005) highlighted the need to consider the mediating effect that teachers have in facilitating the opportunities afforded by this type of technology for all students to engage in classroom discourse. They pointed out that while interactive whiteboards are attractive in relation to potential improvements associated with pace, motivation, engagement, involvement, participation and collaboration, it cannot be assumed that these will directly contribute to improvements in learning. Nonetheless, it is vital that children who use assistive technology for communication are provided with the same access to this type of classroom interaction as their peers. For children who encounter difficulty with communication, many newer technology designers have ensured that AAC technology is readily able to connect with interactive whiteboard systems and have explicitly highlighted this option in information materials about the devices.

The impact of dynamic visual cues and supports are well known in the broader field of cognitive neuroscience, but less well known and considered in the design of technologies for children with communication disabilities (Jagaroo and Wilkinson 2008). Jagaroo and Wilkinson (2008) suggested several potential uses of different types of motion that may be applicable, for example, for communication symbols sets where verbs become dynamic when the child selects them. Animated symbol sets are being integrated into software for writing and for dynamic screen SGDs.

Aiden is a 16-year-old boy who has muscular dystrophy, a degenerative disease that causes progressive and eventually profound muscle weakness. Over the years, Aiden has struggled to complete writing activities. Aiden is no longer able to walk and he uses a power wheelchair to get around. He tires very easily and is not able to use handwriting, except to complete a signature. When he began to type instead of handwriting his schoolwork, he was introduced to a word prediction program called WordQ™.

This type of software can reduce the effort that it takes for Aiden to write by predicting words as he types, thus saving keystrokes. Aiden can also use the text-to-speech features to listen to and edit his work. This auditory feedback is especially helpful to Aiden because he has a learning disability associated with his muscular dystrophy. Many aspects of reading and writing have been a struggle for Aiden during his school career, and at times, he has struggled to remain motivated and engaged. Aiden is no longer able to carry or manipulate print materials such as textbooks or novels. Instead, he now uses a software program called Kurzweil 3000™. This software offers integrated access to reading, writing and learning. Aiden especially loves the 'read-the-web' feature that allows him to explore the Internet, researching school projects, reading popular Web blogs and checking out the latest sports news. Using Kurzweil 3000™, Aiden is able to access electronic textbooks; he can choose to import text from thousands of online sources or, with some assistance, reading materials can be scanned directly into the program.

In the past year, Aiden has started to tire easily when using a keyboard and mouse. He has just started using an on-screen keyboard called WiViK®, which allows him to select letters or predicted words as he writes by pointing and clicking on-screen. WiViK® and WordQ™ were developed to work together so that Aiden's on-screen keyboard incorporates word prediction and auditory feedback. Aiden's wheelchair electronics have been integrated with mouse emulation software, using an electronic hardware solution called DrivePoint®, which allows him to change modes and use his wheelchair joystick to control the computer cursor on-screen. When Aiden points for more than 2 seconds on a key within WiViK®, that key is selected and appears in the word processing document. Aiden is beginning to lose his ability to speak because his breath control has been significantly reduced as his disease has progressed. He knows that he may one day lose his ability to speak, either because it is just too much effort or due to a need for mechanical ventilation. He sometimes feels overwhelmed by what his future may hold, but he knows that there are technologies that can assist him to communicate if he needs them. Aiden spends a lot of time surfing the Web in search of innovative, new technologies that may help him to continue to express himself and stay connected with family and friends.

Aiden represents many children and youth whose disability requires them to use a wide variety of technologies simultaneously in order to be successful in developing and demonstrating their literacy skills. Each of these technologies must be integrated to work together using innovative and thoughtful approaches, considering the users' preferences and aspirations.

Nearly all newer dynamic screen SGDs are integrated computer systems that are designed to facilitate access to specialised communication software for speaking. They also include comprehensive software options to support children's participation in writing, reading and learning activities, including Web browsing. 'With the realization of improved AAC technologies, young children with complex communication needs will have better tools to maximise their development of communication, language, and literacy skills, and attain their full potential' (Light et al. 2007 p. 204).

PARTICIPATION

The increasing use of computers in educational and public sectors and the enhanced power of assistive technologies have provided opportunities for young people with communication challenges to participate in a wide range of environments (e.g., school, online environments and community). To further support community participation, research and development in technology need to focus on improving the following four areas: communication effectiveness, distance communication, interconnectivity and interoperability (Higginbotham et al. 2007; McNaughton and Bryen 2007). We describe technologies that support increased participation, according to the four areas identified by these authors.

Communication Effectiveness

Communication is not a solo act. It is, by nature, a social event. Researchers have critiqued the development of AAC devices in the past, noting too great a focus on the functions of the devices instead of on the needs of the users (Higginbotham et al. 2007). The design of AAC devices often puts emphasis on supporting users to generate text rather than promoting social interactions. Current and emergent technologies continue to place significant physical, cognitive and linguistic demands on the user. Due to these limitations, individuals who use AAC devices often require considerable time to generate a message. The resulting slow communication rate limits their participation in the community (McNaughton and Bryen 2007).

Recognizing the need for individuals who use AAC devices to communicate in a 'fast, relevant, informative, truthful, and clear' manner (Higginbotham et al. 2005), researchers developed utterance-based AAC devices (Todman 2000). One international research team produced Contact™, a device that allows users to (1) generate and modify whole utterances that they can speak quickly in communication situations, and (2) type their own messages with the support of word prediction (Higginbotham et al. 2005).

McNaughton and Bryen (2007) proposed that, to fully support young people with communication difficulties to assume societal roles, AAC devices need to (1) provide quick access to a wide range of vocabulary items, (2) easily handle multiple functions (e.g., face-to-face communication, support for written communication, access to email and Internet functions), and (3) provide integrated cognitive tools (e.g., calendars). DeRuyter et al. (2007) provided one example of how this technology may work.

Consider an adolescent who uses AAC and is attending a high-school social studies class. The AAC device would automatically upload the relevant vocabulary for the day's lecture as the individual walked into the class, so that questions could be asked or answered easily during class. Notes being taken by a peer note-taker elsewhere in the classroom would be visible on the AAC device to the user in real time. The student might even privately exchange Instant Message gossip with a peer as the teacher writes the homework assignment on the board.

Gaining greater independence and being out in the community increases the need for privacy and confidentiality of communication. Support for security is particularly important for youths as they learn to manage their own financial activities such as using a credit card or a bank machine (McNaughton and Bryen 2007). AAC devices are often mounted on the users' wheelchair so that they are readily available. However, parents of the children who use these devices remind us that mounting the equipment on the chairs means that children do not have use of the devices when they are not seated in their wheelchairs (McNaughton et al. 2008). This is of particular concern because many places that children like to go, such as to the park or a relative's or friend's home, may not be wheelchair accessible. Innovative solutions that allow devices to be securely mounted but also easily removed from the chair are necessary.

In the area of written communication, the concern for effectiveness of communication often focuses on the choice of input software. With the enactment of the Americans with Disabilities Act (Americans with Disabilities Act 1990), the software industry began to add accessibility options to their products. Microsoft Windows provides one example. Microsoft added Accessibility Options to its Windows environment to support users with visual, hearing and physical impairments to use a Windows-based computer (Microsoft 2009a). On its Web site, Microsoft illustrates its products with some successful case studies. Hayabusa is a young person who has been described in a case study to highlight Microsoft's speech-recognition technology (Microsoft 2009b).

> In a wrestling match in Japan, Hayabusa suffered an injury to his cervical spine that caused paralysis of his upper extremities. He is able to use a mouse, but typing with a keyboard is too slow to meet his needs. Hayabusa prefers to use speech recognition to type. After trying a number of speech recognition packages, he was happy to find that speech recognition was built into the Microsoft operating system. He said then, 'For me it was significant that speech recognition was part of the purchase price. As well as saving me money, it meant that I didn't have to go through all the installation and initial setup procedures. And Windows Vista offers a wide range of options right out of the box.' Recognition errors sometimes occur, but Hayabusa finds the error correction methods on the Vista speech-recognition module to be better than those of other speech-recognition software that he has tried.

The case example of Hayabusa highlights some of the advantages, including lowered cost and ease of integration, that come about when adaptive technology is incorporated into mainstream technology. However, for other individuals, specific software developed for speech input, such as NaturallySpeaking (Nuance 2009), while more costly, is still preferable.

> Tim is a 17-year-old young man who lost the control of his four limbs due to transverse myelitis. His respiratory muscles are also affected, which means he has very short breaths and a lower volume of speech. Tim tried using both Vista speech recognition and NaturallySpeaking. He was able to control a mouse with the Headmouse (Origin 2007) and a sip-and-puff switch, but because of limited respiratory support, he prefers to use voice commands to control the applications. Given his need for almost 100% hands-free control, Tim finds NaturallySpeaking Professional edition to be a better fit for his needs as it supports the scripting of custom commands.

In the early 1990s, speech recognition was marketed mainly as an adaptive technology software because it offered a potentially easy and fast method of accessing the computer. Individuals who were unable to effectively operate a computer with a standard keyboard, mouse or other input device found that speech recognition systems offered an alternative method of access (Ferrier et al. 1995; Hux et al. 2000; Kambeyanda, Singer and Cronk 1997). Although it may be counterintuitive to recommend the use of speech recognition to individuals with speech differences (i.e., individuals with articulation difficulties and/or poor breath support), speech recognition has been considered to be a viable tool for these individuals since the time it became widely available (Noyes and Frankish 1992). Hawley (2002) described the experience with speech recognition by an individual with severe dysarthria. Recognition accuracy for this individual was, on average, 46%. Although typing 100 words with speech recognition and using switch input or joystick to correct misrecognition took 44 minutes, typing the same number of words with switch input or joystick alone would have taken 1 hour 40 minutes.

Early speech recognition studies showed that when speech recognition was used as an adaptive technology, adjustments were available in the software to allow it to be used by individuals with communication difficulties (Kotler and Thomas-Stonell 1997). However, as speech recognition technology moved into mainstream use, development focused more on the needs of the professional and business market than on the needs of people with disabilities. To achieve the speed required for professional use, currently available speech recognition software programs are being developed for continuous speech. The previously available discrete speech recognition systems are no longer an option. However, studies conducted with individuals with communication difficulties find that discrete speech systems adapt more easily to effortful speech production (Bruce, Edmundson and Coleman 2003). Rosen and Yampolsky (2000) found that speaking in a discrete manner facilitates articulation and intelligibility, and thereby can potentially positively affect recognition accuracy. In general, continuous speech recognition software, as offered on the mainstream market, requires users to speak in phrases without pausing between words and is therefore not suitable for individuals with significant speech difficulties or poor breath support. Recognizing the gap between mainstream speech recognition software and the needs of people with communication difficulties, researchers are exploring how speech recognition software can better accommodate speech differences (Kim et al. 2008; Morales and Cox 2007). Hopefully, the new understanding will help to broaden the voice models that are currently behind the mainstream speech recognition software and influence the development effort of mainstream technology developers to consider the needs of people with communication difficulties.

When adaptive technology is designed for application in the mainstream community, it is not only helpful to individuals who need the adaptive technology, but also it benefits the general population. Intellitools Classroom Suite™ (Intellitools 2006) is a good example of how the development of adaptive technology gained wide acceptance and application in mainstream education environments. The Classroom Suite was designed to improve the effectiveness of children's communication in mainstream classrooms. Simmons et al. (2008) surveyed pre-service teachers on their views of the use of the Classroom Suite in general classrooms. The pre-service teachers in Simmons et al.'s (2008) study agreed that the Classroom Suite was a flexible instructional tool that could meet the broad learning needs of all students, with or without disabilities. Importantly, the inclusion focus of the design allows content to be modified easily and used for all students in the general classrooms. The incorporation of educators' input in the development likely contributed to this product's success as a mainstream education technology (Simmons et al. 2008).

Written communication effectiveness is an important issue for students who must take notes. Research indicates that the ability to take proper notes in class, and to review the notes afterward, has a significant impact on students' learning (Piolat, Olive and Kellogg 2005). Note-taking is a complex task that involves comprehending new and often unfamiliar information, selecting the appropriate information to take note of, transcribing that information quickly enough to keep pace with the lecture and deciding how to organise the material to reflect the relationships stated by the speaker (DeZure, Kaplan and Deerman 2001; Piolat et al. 2005). Students with communication disorders are challenged in all aspects of note-taking. Many students with communication disorders also have motor impairments and are not able to produce written text fast enough to take notes. They may also have learning and cognitive difficulties that make selection of appropriate content and arrangement of the information into meaningful notes challenging, even when they can use computer-based equipment to help with the writing processes.

Technology development to aid in note-taking is scarce. Interestingly, while note-taking is a universal issue for many individuals with a wide range of disabilities, technological interventions have only been addressed for the deaf and hard-of-hearing population. The C-Print™ is a transcription system that provides both real-time text display in class for students who are deaf or hard-of-hearing and copies of notes for them to review and study at home (Stinson and McKee 2000). The system consists of a computer that the transcriptionist uses to type the notes and a second computer or video display to show the text in real time. Specialised software employing phonetics-based abbreviation strategy allows transcriptionists to type at a faster rate. Transcriptionists are trained to use listening strategies to identify important points, and organization strategies to eliminate redundancies and present the information. In a study that examined the effectiveness of the C-Print system from students' perspectives, the students reported that the system enhanced their learning experience and made them more confident with their studies (Elliot et al. 2001).

The Liberated Learning Consortium is a group of universities and industrial partners from around the world, whose goal is to improve information accessibility in the school system through the use of speech-recognition technology (Bain et al. 2005). Bain et al. (2005) described and reported on one of the group's on-going projects, which has involved the use of custom speech-recognition software to provide real-time transcription for students who are deaf or hard-of-hearing. In the project, teachers speak directly into the speech-recognition software. While students have found reading the captions and receiving the notes to be helpful, the reported mean dictation accuracy of 77% is less than desirable. Errors in the transcripts are particularly problematic as they can distort the content, either making it difficult to understand or, worse, imparting incorrect information. It is encouraging to see that researchers are beginning to address the difficult issue of note-taking. There is also an increasing awareness that the technology not only benefits students who are deaf and hard-of-hearing; it can also be helpful to students with a wide range of disabilities (Wald and Bain 2008). Until recently, studies on the use of speech recognition technology for note-taking have focused on providing assistance to college/university students. In fact, the only study reporting the trial of this technology in the high school environment was provided by Leitch (2008). Although speech recognition is a promising mainstream technology, before it can be used widely as a note-taking tool to help students with communication difficulties, technological breakthrough is required to improve recognition accuracy.

Distance Communication

Children with communication difficulties can be absent from school for extended periods of time due to illnesses and may need home-schooling. These children often lack opportunities to interact with other children socially and academically. Cooperative and collaborative learning interactions have been shown to be important for the development of social and communication skills, as well as for self-confidence and independence (Kumpulainen and Wray 2002). Recognizing the importance of collaborative learning, educators have explored the use of computer networking technology to enhance students' learning experience (Lehtinen 2003).

> Allen and Ricky are two brothers who were born with a condition that affects all the joints in their bodies. Allen is 15 and Ricky is 11. They cannot write without dislocating finger joints or walk without the risk of dislocating their hip joints. Allen and Ricky both require the use of an adaptive keyboard and mouse because the physical requirements of typing and mousing can lead to painful dislocations of the joints in their upper limbs. The brothers also suffer from a very significant latex allergy. Therefore, both boys were home-schooled after a brief trial of attendance at a local public school in grade one which ended with life-threatening allergic reactions. With the assistance of a PEBBLES system (Weiss et al. 2001), the brothers 'attended' their school virtually. Widely available Web-based communication has also allowed them to communicate with other people outside their home and participate in community activities, such as tutoring other children, sitting on the advisory board of the local library, assisting with events at their church and hosting a clean-up party at a local park. In a recent science fair, Allen answered questions posted to him by the judges through Skype, related to an environmental care project he conducted. His responses earned him an award in the regional science and engineering fair.

Videoconferencing technology is becoming a more commonly used form of communication. The technology provides opportunities for individuals to interact even when they are separated by long distances (Fels and Weiss 2000). Global SchoolNet, an initiative that links students and teachers worldwide to work collaboratively on projects, was launched in 1984 (Global SchoolNet 2009). A development team at Ryerson University in Toronto, Canada, is using videoconferencing technology, together with robotics, to enable students with disabilities to have a virtual presence in their classrooms and to interact with their peers and teachers (Weiss et al. 2001). The system they developed, called PEBBLES, was initially designed for use by elementary school students. However, with the need for a higher level of collaboration in the high school environment, a modified version, incorporating a set of specific collaboration tools similar to that of the electronic whiteboard, was developed for use in a high school classroom (Yeung, Konstantinidis and Fels 2005). Yeung et al. (2005) reported on the effectiveness of PEBBLES, noting that it was a promising development for linking students who were absent from the classroom and for enabling them to participate in classroom activities. However, they recommended further usability studies and development work to enhance the audio functions and portability of the system.

The tremendous growth of distance education programming has opened up many opportunities to students with communication and physical difficulties, allowing them to study in the leisure of their own homes and at a pace that is more manageable. However, distance education poses a different set of challenges for students with communication difficulties. Most distance education is Web-based. Students may encounter difficulties accessing and navigating through enrolment, course selection and grade reporting. Additionally, they must navigate Web-based courseware packages, such as Blackboard®, that furnish the general framework for instruction, electronic discussion forums for online class meetings, and online library services. These navigational challenges may be too rigorous for some students (Schmetzke 2001). For example, if the course requires extensive use of chat rooms, students using AAC devices may have difficulties with the speed of communication required for synchronous online communication (Burgstahler, Corrigan and McCarter 2004). Instead, instructors could consider providing accessible alternatives such as the use of email instead of chat rooms for discussion (Keeler and Horney 2007). For students with communication difficulties, tasks are made easier when institutional Web pages and all coursework-related materials are designed in strict adherence to Web accessibility guidelines and with consideration of the specific assistive technology needs of students (Keeler and Horney 2007; Edmonds 2004).

Making sure that the library is totally accessible online by students with communication difficulties is vital in supporting them to pursue distance education. This includes support for online searches of catalogues, indexes to journal articles and other electronic references, as well as reservation of books (Burgstahler et al. 2004). Schmetzke (2003) alleged that while much of the discussion about library access occurs around the provision of adaptive technology, what is often neglected is the accessibility of the library Web site. He reviewed five studies that investigated the accessibility of libraries of major universities and found that only 31% to 43% of the libraries' Web pages were considered to be accessible.

Accessibility to library resources can be an issue even when a student is able to physically go to the library (Oravec 2002). Organizational policies, such as those related to network security, can create obstacles for accessibility. Students requiring the use of adaptive technology need a computer workstation that is equipped to meet their needs (Moisey and Van de Keere 2007).

'Libraries for all' was a project initiated in Australia and replicated in Canada (Shepherd and McDougall 2008). The program provided printed communication displays to local libraries to facilitate communication between people who use AAC and librarians. A train-the-trainer model was used to ensure that library staff were familiar with the use of this AAC tool. Shepherd and McDougall (2008) found that use of the displays facilitated access to a range of resources including books, Internet and audiotapes. Furthermore, the libraries involved in the project continued to use the displays after completion of the project, indicating that the project was well received.

Interconnectivity and Interoperability

Telephone use is taken for granted by most people in our society. However, communicating on the phone can be very challenging for individuals with communication difficulties. Unable to see one another and use gestures and facial expressions to convey meaning, individuals with speech differences may find it harder to get their messages across to their listeners over the phone. The reduced bandwidth of the telephone line and the background noise can further degrade the quality of the voice signals over the telephone (Drager, Hustad and Gable 2004). While use of AAC devices for telephone communication may be a viable option, it is very common that the conversation partner, or telephone operator, has limited experience with AAC users and is not patient enough to wait and listen to the voices generated by an AAC device. This is especially true when keying in messages is a slow and laborious task for the AAC users (Drager et al. 2004). Pre-stored introductory messages alerting people to their speech differences and needs would be helpful in these scenarios. Currently, a wireless phone connection is available on some AAC devices to facilitate telephone use. For example, the ECO of Prentke Romich Corporation utilises ECO2 integrated Bluetooth® connectivity to provide a phone connection.

'Going online' has become part of daily life. In 2003, 64% of Canadians (Statistics Canada 2004) and 63% of the U.S. population (Fallows 2004; Madden 2003) reported regular use of the Internet. Adults reported that they accessed the Internet for four main reasons: information seeking, communications, transactions and entertainment (Fallows 2004). However, people with disabilities are disenfranchised by the limited accessibility of many Web pages and are thus not able to access important information on the Web such as health information (Davis 2002). In a study that compared Internet use across Canada and in countries around the world, Veenhof, Clermont and Sciadas (2005) confirmed this 'digital divide.' Technology has the potential to narrow the gap of the digital divide by providing a match between the technology and the individual needs of the user. For example, one software solution called ICanEmail® guides the user through the email process by 'speaking' questions such as, 'Who would you like to send this to?' To create a message, the user can record a voice message. This software will accept voices sent from an AAC device. For incoming mail, the user can choose to have the email read by text-to-speech software. Moisey and Van de Keere (2007) studied the effectiveness of ICanEmail software when used in this way and found that the technology compensated for low literacy skills and allowed individuals with developmental disabilities to access the Internet.

Acknowledging that poorly designed Web pages are often what limit the accessibility of Internet-based information for people with disabilities, researchers have invested effort into improving Web-page design. A unified Web site accessibility guideline that combines input from many researchers involved in projects on Web accessibility is now available to Web-page designers (Web Accessibility Initiative 2006). In general, Web access relies heavily on mouse-navigation and selection. Some children with physical disabilities cannot use a mouse and may need to use mouse emulation via single-switch scanning (Blackstein-Adler et al. 2004). Several scanning methods (i.e., rotational or Cartesian) are available, but all require the user to scan the desktop to direct the mouse towards the target before scanning some buttons to send a mouse click. Some Web pages are designed with full keyboard access, but accessing a Web page with keyboard commands can also be impractical. Kasday, Bryen and Bohman (2005) examined the Yahoo Internet portal and found that there were 270 links on its homepage. Therefore, accessing a particular link could take up to 270 activations of the tab key. Assuming that it may take a person with significant motor difficulties up to 2 seconds to activate a key, they noted that it could take more than 6 minutes for that person to reach a link at the bottom of the Yahoo homepage. Kasday and associates (2005) at Temple University concluded that improved Web accessibility for people with physical and communication difficulties could be achieved by changing the Web-page design. The Accent online tool was the result of collaboration between the Institute on Disabilities at Temple University and WebAIM at Utah State University. Users can submit a Uniform Resource Indicator (URI) to this online tool, which processes the content of the pages in the URI and displays the information in an easier format for the users to navigate.

Emiliani and Stephanidis (2005) describe universal access and highlight the need for this access across environments:

> Universal access implies the accessibility and usability of information technologies by anyone at any place and at any time. Universal access aims to enable equitable access and active participation of potentially all people in existing and emerging computer-mediated human activities by developing universally accessible and usable products and services. These products and services must be capable of accommodating individual users' requirements in different contexts of use, independent of location, target machine, or runtime environment. (p. 606–607)

We have already noted that students with communication difficulties who are dependent on adaptive computer software may not be able to use public computers (e.g., in the library or at school). In these cases, carrying a complete portable system is necessary, but AT software developers are beginning to address this issue. The growing need by the business sectors to gain instant access to files and to collaborate with global team members has led to the development of Web-based storage and collaboration tools (Chen et al. 2009). The same concept is beginning to influence the availability of adaptive technology for people with communication difficulties. One example is the WriteOnline® software developed by Crick Software in the United Kingdom. This online word processing software includes word prediction, auditory feedback, assistance with visual access and an on-screen keyboard. Students who need these features are now able to use this software anywhere they are, anytime they need to write, simply by logging in. They are also able to store and retrieve their document files from the online storage space provided by the software developer.

Instead of utilizing Web-based storage options, other developers are using USB flash drives to make adaptive technology more available to users. Kurzweil Educational Systems have developed the Kurzweil 3000 V11 USB®, ensuring that the Kurzweil 3000 software is available to students and teachers without the need to install the software on any computer. Users can also store their settings and document files on the same flash drive.

As illustrated in the previous examples, current efforts to make adaptive technology more portable are limited to software-based solutions and mostly address learning issues. The challenge for the AAC field is to provide innovative solutions that will allow young people with significant physical disabilities to use any computer for communication from anywhere they are. As an example, current switch-based access methods rely on the compatibility between hardware (i.e., the switch interface) and software (e.g., single or multiple switch scanning software), which limits the universality of access. A universal switch access box and standard keyboard emulation for switch access needs to be developed so that students with disabilities can plug in their switches to any computer and then use available Web-based access software to carry out their computing needs.

In the past 20 years, mainstream technology has undergone a digital revolution. Digital communication technologies and wireless connectivity have become the essential features of the information society (Emiliani 2006). Today's telephone is not simply a telephone; wireless telephones, such as the BlackBerry®, can incorporate Web browsing, global positioning, instant messaging, email, and camera, organiser and media player functions. At present, however, the majority of stand-alone AAC devices support only face-to-face communication (DeRuyter et al. 2007). Individuals with communication difficulties continue to require multiple devices to perform the various other functions that they may require.

> Tina is sitting with her friends in the cafeteria of the high school. She wants to call her mother and let her know that things are going well at school. Tina sends an email to her mother's Blackberry. Then, she turns on the webcam that is clamped onto the AAC device that she is using and logs on to Skype to wait for her mother to call. Tina has cerebral palsy and epilepsy that is not well controlled. Her mother likes to be able to see Tina, face-to-face, while talking with her. However, Tina's AAC device does not include telephone and camera features. As a result, a separate webcam has been attached to the top of her AAC device and a wireless telephone has been mounted on the side. In addition, because the device has very limited memory capacity, and because Tina needs to access graphic software and music requiring sizable storage space, an external hard drive has also been added. With the requirement that these various devices be mounted together, Tina's mounting system is complex and wires dangle at the back of the device. An additional issue involves the constant crashing of the system as it struggles to meet the power and memory demands of the devices and software that have been added to it.
>
> Tina's family eventually purchased a computer with multimedia capability, a built-in camera and sufficient power and memory to support her computing needs. Voice output software is used to support Tina's communication needs. The mounting of this new computer is much less cluttered and use of the new computer makes Tina feel more like her peers who carry their portable computers to school. Tina is also more relaxed knowing that her computer will be able to deliver the necessary functions when she needs them.

Individuals who use AAC devices for communication have identified the importance of interoperability between AAC devices and mainstream technologies (Bryen,

Carey and Potts 2006). Traditionally, the approach to enable users with disabilities to access mainstream technologies was a reactive one involving the reconfiguration of the physical interaction of devices or adaptation of the visual interface (Emiliani 2006). The major pitfall of the reactive approach in the face of a rapidly changing technological environment is the constant issue of compatibility with new technologies. Emiliani therefore proposed that a proactive strategy be adopted, whereby access features are built into a product right at the conception or early phases of design (Emiliani and Stephanidis 2005).

TRAINING AND SUPPORT

Successful communication requires skilled participation by both the person with communication challenges and the communication partner (Blackstone et al. 2007). Training and support are important to give AAC device users the confidence to accept and use their devices (McNaughton and Bryen 2007). In a focus group, parents expressed that in addition to training the children how to use their devices, there is a need to provide training to parents and professionals (e.g., speech-language pathologist and teachers) who work with the children (McNaughton et al. 2008). Training of teachers and other educational staff in AAC technology operation and programming is vital in supporting children's learning at school. If the teaching staff has no knowledge of the basic operation of AAC devices and does not know how to assist the children when technical problems occur, children could be left with no way to communicate and participate in classroom interactions (McNaughton et al. 2008).

McDonald et al. (2007) evaluated whether provision of communication devices facilitated the success of young children with communication difficulties in education. The results were disappointing. Only 36% of the children in the study achieved the educational targets. Inappropriate provision of equipment and lack of appropriate support were among the reasons that are believed to have contributed to the poor outcomes. In a review study of training strategies for teaching young children to use assistive technology devices, Campbell et al. (2006) found that providing the children with opportunities to access and use the devices in everyday real-world situations was the most significant factor encouraging use. A lack of consistent support was the key factor determined to limit successful implementation of AAC devices (Hodge 2007). Similarly, in a study called the Communication Aids Project (CAP), a 4-year initiative by the U.K. Department for Education and Skills, outcomes for 60 children aged 3 to 18 years, who used a communication aid, indicated that only 38% of communication goals were met at 6 months following receipt of the aid. Reasons identified for this poor goal attainment included 'inappropriate provision of equipment, demands of the equipment, [and] lack of appropriate support and targets' (McDonald et al. 2008).

Lebel, Olshtain and Weiss (2005) alleged that online training courses are particularly useful for learning in the field of AAC. Appropriate delivery of communication services requires a multidisciplinary team (e.g., occupational therapists, speech-language pathologists, engineers, etc.). An online training format makes it easier to bring together experts from different fields and various locations. Furthermore, because AAC is a fast-changing field, keeping up-to-date is extremely important.

Delivery of training online not only allows content to be kept current, but also allows professionals to participate in training at a time that is most suitable to them.

Recognizing the benefits of online learning, the Central Equipment Pool, an organization responsible for the management of AAC equipment leasing in Ontario, Canada, is now offering online training and electronic discussion forums to speech-language pathologists and occupational therapists.

> Allison and her family live in a little town that is a 3-hour drive from the communication technology clinic where she receives her equipment and support. With significant visual and physical limitations because of cerebral palsy, Allison needs to use an IntelliKeys keyboard (Synapse Adaptive 2009), with a custom-designed layout, to access her computer. Since purchasing a new computer, Allison's family has experienced many technical problems with the software and peripherals that they previously owned. Through the use of Webex Support Center (Cisco 2009), the technical team in the clinic has been able to remotely control Allison's computer and help the family resolve technical conflicts. However, Allison also experienced difficulties at school. Unfortunately, the technical support person at school was not able to load the custom keyboard layout onto the IntelliKeys keyboard at school and with the school network security, the technical team at the clinic was not able to connect to Allison's computer at school to provide assistance. When the issues could not be resolved through telephone conversations, the technical team had to visit the school to rectify the problem. Although the issue was eventually resolved, the lack of connectivity with the school system delayed implementation of the technology at school for almost 2 months.

The recent advancements in computer and Web technologies make the implementation of Web-based support feasible (Yao 2008). With the infrastructure provided by the World Wide Web, researchers have explored the possibility of gathering information from a remote computer to provide support through remote control. The need to provide remote support has been well recognised in the field of AAC for many years (Hine et al. 2002). A lack of immediately available and on-going support can lead to technology abandonment, while travelling to users' homes to provide support is costly and time-consuming. Hine et al. (2002) developed an online support system through a videophone link and software that synchronised the two computers in the remote link. The project successfully delivered remote support to users. Further exploration of a secure way for connections to be made is necessary so that organizations will be more likely to allow support activities to be carried out at schools and in workplaces. It is hoped that the timely provision of technical support will allow children to participate more successfully in their chosen activities in the community.

There is an increasing call for more durable and reliable AAC technology to ensure that breakdown and maintenance concerns do not limit the participation of AAC users (McNaughton and Bryen 2007). To this end, devices that utilise mainstream technology tend to lend themselves to a wider availability of maintenance and support. The Toughbook series of notebook computers produced by Panasonic is one example of mainstream technology adapted for use as an AAC device. These rugged notebooks were originally designed for use by individuals, such as fire officers, who work in demanding situations. However, the rugged, shockproof design also makes these computers particularly suitable for mounting on powered wheelchairs.

CONCLUSION

The World Health Organization (2001) has proposed a new framework and classi-fication system to inform our thinking about constructs such as disability, function and health. One major shift in perspective that the model suggests is to look at indi-viduals within the context of their ability to participate meaningfully in all aspects of everyday living. Since it was first introduced, researchers have proposed ways that the framework may guide research, education and interventions targeting assess-ment of communication (Simeonsson 2003; Raghavendra et al. 2007). Hammel et al. (2008) concluded, following a survey of 63 people with diverse disabilities, that par-ticipation is conceptualised differently by different people. As a result, they stressed the need to support individuals to pursue this end goal of participation on their own terms. When people who use AAC were asked to talk about their wishes and desires related to future AAC research priorities, it was identified that:

> People who use AAC and their facilitators appear to perceive research priorities in more pragmatic terms than some researchers. They want to see research that, for example, results in the development of intervention programs that lead to the acquisi-tion of new life skills. They seek abilities that allow them to do the everyday things in life, such as to (a) travel more easily, (b) communicate with a doctor better, (c) direct their attendants more successfully, (d) make more of their leisure time, and (e) make and keep new friends. It is not more research into new symbol systems or voice output communication aids per se that is of prime interest to them, but rather it is research designed specifically to provide key skills that result in greater functional success in those situations that are of importance to the individual and for those who interact with that individual. Researchers should, therefore, consider client-centred goals dur-ing service delivery that reflect individual functional and social outcomes that impact on quality of life. (O'Keefe et al. 2007, p. 95)

Many of the innovative technologies described in this chapter represent a shift toward design and service delivery that takes these considerations into account.

Key researchers in the fields of AT and AAC have proposed frameworks that can serve as useful guides for continued innovative work in this area. In an article reviewing needs related to enhancing connections with the world for people with communication differences, DeRuyter et al. (2007) proposed specific roles and activ-ities to guide future research for each of six different stakeholder groups, including individuals who use AAC; individuals who assist in selecting and supporting the use of AAC devices; AAC researchers; AAC device manufacturers, mainstream applica-tion developers and technology manufacturers; and public policy makers.

It is vital that we attend to these recommendations and perspectives as well as to the building evidence supporting the shift to newer ways of viewing AT and disabil-ity in general. Hartley and Wirz (2002) proposed that a paradigm shift to a 'commu-nication disability model' will be especially important toward supporting innovation that takes into account the need for feasible communication-related solutions for developing, poor countries.

In a compelling article titled 'Reach for the Star,' Williams et al. (2008) reviewed published writings of individuals who use AAC and proposed the following five principles to guide future AAC assessment, intervention, research and development: the time for AAC is now; one is never enough; my AAC must fit my life; AAC must support full participation in all aspects of 21st century life; and, nothing about me without me. These five simple but elegant principles serve as powerful reminders that in continuing the pursuit of innovative technologies for children and youth with communication needs, we need to seek out, listen to and be led by their voices.

REFERENCES

Allen, J. 2005. Designing desirability in an augmentative and alternative communication device. *Universal Access in the Information Society* 4:135–145.

Americans with Disabilities Act. 1990. 42 U.S.C.A. § 12101 et seq. http://www.usdoj.gov/crt/ada/statute.html (accessed May 20, 2009).

Bailey, R.L., H.P Parette, J.B. Stoner Jr., M.E. Angell, and K. Carroll. 2006. Family members' perceptions of augmentative and alternative communication device use. *Language, Speech, and Hearing Services in Schools* 37:50–60.

Bain, K., S. Basson, A. Faisman, and D. Kanevsky. 2005. Accessibility, transcription and access everywhere. *IBM Systems Journal* 44:589–603.

Beck, A.R., H. Fritz, A. Keller, and M. Dennis. 2000. Attitudes of school-aged children toward their peers who use augmentative and alternative communication. *Augmentative and Alternative Communication* 16:13–26.

Beck, A.R., S. Bock, J.R. Thompson, L. Bowman, and S. Robbins. 2006. Is awesome really awesome? How the inclusion of informal terms on an AAC device influences children's attitudes toward peers who use AAC. *Research in Developmental Disabilities: A Multidisciplinary Journal* 27:56–69.

Binger, C., J. Berens, J. Kent-Walsh, and S. Taylor. 2008. The effects of aided AAC interventions on AAC use, speech, and symbolic gestures. *Seminars in Speech & Language* 29:101–111.

Binger, C., and J. Light. 2006. Demographics of preschoolers who require AAC. *Language, Speech & Hearing Services in the Schools* 37:200–208.

Blackberry [smartphone] Research in Motion. http://www.blackberry.com/

Blackboard [Computer Software]. Blackboard Inc. http://www.blackboard.com/

Blackstein-Adler, S., F. Shein, J. Quintal, S. Birch, and P.L. Weiss. 2004. Mouse manipulation through single-switch scanning. *Assistive Technology* 16:28–42.

Blackstone, S.W., M.B. Williams, and D.P. Wilkins. 2007. Key principles underlying research and practice in AAC. *Augmentative and Alternative Communication* 23(3):191–203.

Bruce, C., A. Edmundson, and M. Coleman. 2003. Writing with voice: An investigation of the use of a voice recognition system as a writing aid for a man with aphasia. *International Journal of Language & Communication Disorders* 38(2):131–148.

Bryen, D.N., A. Carey, and B. Potts. 2006. Technology and job-related social networks. *Augmentative and Alternative Communication* 22:1–9.

Burgstahler, S., B. Corrigan, and J. McCarter, 2004. Making distance learning courses accessible to students and instructors with disabilities: A case study. *Internet and Higher Education* 7:233–246.

Cambium Learning. 2007. The research basis for Intellitools products. http://www.intellitools.com/about/research/pdfs/research_feb07.pdf

Campbell, P.H., S. Milbourne, L.M Dugan, and M.J. Wilcox. 2006. A review of evidence on practices for teaching young children to use assistive technology devices. *Topics in Early Childhood Special Education* 26:3–13.

Central Equipment Pool. http://courses.cepp.org/Welcome_to_the_CEP_Courses_Server.html

Chen, S., S. Nepal, J. Chan, D. Moreland, and J. Zic. 2009. A service-oriented architecture to enable virtual storage services: A dynamic collaboration context. *International Journal of Ad Hoc and Ubiquitous Computing* 4(2):95–107.

Craddock, G. 2006. The AT continuum in education: Novice to power user. *Disability and Rehabilitation: Assistive Technology* 1:17–27.

Davis, J.J. 2002. Disenfranchising the disabled: The inaccessibility of Internet-based health information. *Journal of Health Communication* 7:355–367.

DeRuyter, F., D. McNaughton, K. Caves, D.N. Bryen, and M.B. Williams. 2007. Enhancing AAC connections with the world. *Augmentative and Alternative Communication* 23:258–270.

DeZure, D., M. Kaplan, and M. Deerman. 2001. Research on student note-taking: Implications for faculty and graduate student instructors. http://www.math.lsa.umich.edu/~krasny/math156_crlt.pdf (accessed May 7, 2009).

Doherty-Sneddon, G., and G. Kent. 1996. Visual signals and the communication abilities of children. *Journal of Child Psychology & Psychiatry & Allied Disciplines* 37:949–959.

Drager, K.D.R., K.C. Hustad, and K.L. Gable. 2004. Telephone communication: Synthetic and dysarthric speech intelligibility and listener preferences. *Augmentative and Alternative Communication* 20(2):103–112.

Drager, K.D.R., J. Light, R. Carlson, K. D'Silva, B. Larsson, L. Pitkin et al. 2005. Learning of dynamic display AAC technologies by typically developing 3-year-olds: Effect of different layouts and menu approaches. *Journal of Speech, Language, and Hearing Research* 47:1133–1148.

Drager, K.D.R., J. Light, J.C. Curran-Speltz, K.A. Fallon, and L.Z. Jeffries. 2003. The performance of typically developing 2 1/2-year-olds on dynamic display AAC technologies with different system layouts and language organizations. *Journal of Speech, Language, and Hearing Research* 46:298–312.

Dragon NaturallySpeaking. 2009. [Computer program]. Nuance Communication Inc. http://www.nuance.com/naturallyspeaking/

DrivePoint [electronic hardware access solution] Ontario Rehab Technology Consortium. http://www. oise.utoronto.ca/ortc

ECO2 Phone Connection. [telephony access solution] Prentke Romich Corporation. http://prentrom.com/eco/specifications.

Edmonds, C.D. 2004. Providing access to students with disabilities in online distance education: Legal and technical concerns for higher education. *The American Journal of Distance Education* 18(1):51–62.

Emiliani, P.L., and C. Stephanidis. 2005. Universal access to ambient intelligence environments: Opportunities and challenges for people with disabilities. *IBM Systems Journal* 44:605–619.

Fallows, D. 2004. The Internet and daily life: Many Americans use the Internet in everyday activities, but traditional offline habits still dominate. http://www.pewinternet.org/reports/2004//The_Internet_and_Daily_Life.aspx. (Accessed August 25, 2010).

Ferrier, L., H. Shane, H. Ballard, T. Carpenter, and A. Benoit. 1995. Dysarthric speakers' intelligibility and speech characteristics in relation to computer speech recognition. *Augmentative and Alternative Communication* 11:165–174.

Friedman, M.G., and D.N. Bryen. 2007. Web accessibility design recommendations for people with cognitive disabilities. *Technology and Disability* 19:205–212.

Global Schoolnet. 2009. http://www.globalschoolnet.org/index.cfm?section=AboutUs (accessed May 20, 2009).

Hawley, M. 2002. Speech recognition as an input to electronic assistive technology. *British Journal of Occupational Therapy* 65(1):15–20.

Hammel, J., S. Magasi, A. Heinemann, G. Whiteneck, J. Bogner, and E. Rodriguez. 2008. What does participation mean? An insider perspective from people with disabilities. *Disability & Rehabilitation* 30:1445–1460.

Hartley, S.D., and S.L. Wirz. 2002. Development of a 'communication disability model' and its implication on service delivery in low-income countries. *Social Science & Medicine* 54:1543–1557.

Headmouse. 2007. [Computer hardware]. Grand Prairie, Texas: Origin Instruments.

Higginbotham, D.J., D. Beukelman, S. Blackstone, D. Bryen, K. Caves, F. DeRuyter et al. 2009. AAC technology transfer: An AAC-RERC report. *Augmentative and Alternative Communication* 25:68–76.

Higginbotham, D.J., G.W. Lesher, B.J. Moulton, K. Adams, and D. Wilkins. 2005. The Frametalker project: Building an utterance-based communication device. *Proceedings of Center on Disabilities Technology and Persons with Disabilities Conference*. http://www.csun.edu/cod/conf/2005/proceedings/2413.htm (accessed May 19, 2009).

Higginbotham, D.J., H. Shane, S. Russell, and K. Caves. 2007. Access to AAC: Present, past, and future. *Augmentative and Alternative Communication* 23:243–257.

Hine, N., P. Sergeant, P. Panek, W. Zagler, C. Beck, and G. Seisenbacher. 2002. RESORT — Providing remote support for PC based AAC systems. *Proceedings of 10th Biennial Conference of the International Society for Augmentative and Alternative Communication (ISAAC)*, Odense, Denmark.

Hodge, S. 2007. Why is the potential of augmentative and alternative communication not being realized? Exploring the experiences of people who use communication aids. *Disability & Society* 22:457–471.

Hoppestad, B.S. 2007. Inadequacies in computer access using assistive technology devices in profoundly disabled individuals: An overview of the current literature. *Disability and Rehabilitation: Assistive Technology* 2:189–199.

Hux, K., J. Rankin-Erikson, N. Manasse, and E. Lauritzen. 2000. Accuracy of three speech recognition systems: Case study of dysarthric speech. *Augmentative and Alternative Communication* 16:186–196.

ICanEmail [computer software] R J Cooper Inc. http://www.rjcooper.com/icanemail/index.html

Intellikeys [Computer hardware]. Intellitools. http://www.synapseadaptive.com/intellitools/IntelliKeys.html

InterAACT [computer software] DynaVox Mayer-Johnson. http://www.dynavoxtech.com/products/interaact/

International Society for Augmentative and Alternative Communication (ISAAC). 1983. http://www.isaac-online.org/en/aac/what_is.html (accessed May 12, 2009).

Jagaroo, V., and K. Wilkinson. 2008. Further considerations of visual cognitive neuroscience in aided AAC: The potential role of motion perception systems in maximizing design display. *Augmentative and Alternative Communication* 24:29–42.

Kambeyanda, D., L. Singer, and S. Cronk. 1997. Potential problems associated with use of speech recognition products. *Assistive Technology* 9(2):95–101.

Kasday, L.R., D.N. Bryen, and P.R. Bohman. 2005. Web browsing challenges, strategies, and tools for people with motor disabilities and users of AAC technologies. http://www.webaim.org/projects/whitepaper.htm (accessed May 18, 2009).

Keeler, C.G., and M. Horney. 2007. Online course designs: Are special needs being met? *American Journal of Distance Education* 21(2):61–75.

Kent-Walsh, J., C. Stark, and C. Binger. 2008. Tales from school trenches: AAC service-delivery and professional expertise. *Seminars in Speech & Language* 29:146–154.

Kim, H., M. Hasegawa-Johnson, A. Perlman, J. Gunderson, T. Huang, K. Watkin, and S. Frame. 2008. Dysarthric speech database for universal access research. Paper presented at the *Interspeech Conference*, Brisbane, Australia.

Kotler, A., and N. Thomas-Stonell. 1997. Effects of speech training on the accuracy of speech recognition for an individual with a speech impairment. *Augmentative and Alternative Communication* 13:71–80.

Kumpulainen, K., and D. Wray. 2002. *Classroom interaction and social learning: From theory to practice.* London: Routledge Falmer.

Kurzweil 3000 V11 USB [computer software] Kurzweil Educational Systems, Cambium Learning. http://www.kurzweiledu.com/kurz3000USB.aspx

Landa, R. 2007. Early communication development and intervention for children with autism. *Mental Retardation & Developmental Disabilities Research Reviews* 13:16–25.

Lebel T., E. Olshtain, and P.L. Weiss. 2005. Teaching teachers about augmentative and alternative communication: Opportunities and challenges of a web-based course. *Augmentative and Alternative Communication* 21:264–277.

Lee, H.Y., and C.M. Wu. 2003. Rapid prototyping of wireless augmentative and alternative communication system for speech impaired subjects. *Biomedical Engineering — Applications, Basis & Communications* 15(3):100–108.

Lehtinen, E. 2003. Computer supported collaborative learning: An approach to powerful learning environments. In *Unraveling basic components and dimensions of powerful learning environments,* E. De Corte, L. Verschaffel, N. Entwistle, and J.V. Merriëënboer, Eds. New York: Pergamon. pp. 35–53.

Light, J.C. 1997. Communication is the essence of human life: Reflections on communicative competence. *Augmentative & Alternative Communication* 13:61–70.

Light, J., and K. Drager. 2007. AAC technologies for young children with complex communication needs: State of the science and future research directions. *Augmentative and Alternative Communication* 23:204–216.

Light, J., R. Page, J. Curran, and L. Pitkin. 2007. Children's ideas for the design of AAC assistive technologies for young children with complex communication needs. *Augmentative and Alternative Communication* 23:274–287.

Madden, M. 2003. America's online pursuits: The changing picture of who's online and what they do. http://www.pewinternet.org/Reports/2003/Americas-Online-Pursuits.aspx (accessed June 24, 2010).

McDonald, R., E. Harris, K. Price, and N. Jolleff. 2008. Elation or frustration? Outcomes following the provision of equipment during the Communication Aids Project: Data from one CAP partner centre. *Child: Care, Health & Development* 34:223–229.

McLeod, S., and D.H. McKinnon. 2007. Prevalence of communication disorders compared with other learning needs in 14,500 primary and secondary school students. *International Journal of Language & Communication Disorders* 42:37–59.

McNaughton, D., and D.N. Bryen. 2007. AAC technologies to enhance participation and access to meaningful societal roles for adolescents and adults with developmental disabilities who require AAC. *Augmentative and Alternative Communication* 23:217–229.

McNaughton, D., T. Rackensperger, E. Benedek-Wood, C. Krezman, M.B. Williams, and J. Light. 2008. "A child needs to be given a chance to succeed": Parents of individuals who use AAC describe the benefits and challenges of learning AAC technologies. *Augmentative and Alternative Communication* 24:43–55.

McNeilly, L.G. 2000. Communication intervention and therapeutic issues in pediatric human immunodeficiency virus. *Seminars in Speech & Language* 21:63–77.

McNeilly, L.G. 2005. HIV and communication. *Journal of Communication Disorders* 38:303–310.

Microsoft Corporation. 2009a. Accessibility at Microsoft. http://www.microsoft.com/ENABLE/ (accessed May 20, 2009).

Microsoft Corporation. 2009b. Hayabusa: Composing with voice recognition technology. http://www.microsoft.com/enable/casestudy/hayabusa.aspx (accessed May 20, 2009).

Moisey, S., and R. Van de Keere. 2007. Inclusion and the Internet: Teaching adults with developmental disabilities to use information and communication technology. *Developmental Disabilities Bulletin* 35(1&2):72–102.

Morales, O.C., and S. Cox. 2007. Modelling confusion matrices to improve speech recognition accuracy, with an application to dysarthric speech. Paper presented at the *Interspeech Conference*, Antwerp, Belgium.

Msall, M.E., and M.R. Tremont. 2000. Functional outcomes in self-care, mobility, communication, and learning in extremely low-birth weight infants. *Clinics in Perinatology* 27:381–401.

Noyes, J.M., and C.R. Frankish. 1992. Speech recognition technology for individuals with disabilities. *Augmentative and Alternative Communication* 8:297–303.

Oravec, A. 2002. Virtually accessible: Empowering students to advocate for accessibility and support universal design. *Library High Tech* 20(4):452–461.

O'Keefe, B.M., N.B. Kozak, and R. Schuller. 2007. Research priorities in augmentative and alternative communication as identified by people who use AAC and their facilitators. *Augmentative and Alternative Communication* 23:89–96.

Patak, L., A. Gawlinski, N.I. Fung, L. Doering, J. Berg, E.A. Henneman et al. 2006. Communication boards in critical care: Patients' views. *Applied Nursing Research* 19:182–190.

Paul, R. 2008. Interventions to improve communication in autism. *Child & Adolescent Psychiatric Clinics of North America* 17:835–856.

Pinborough-Zimmerman, J., R. Satterfield, J. Miller, D. Bilder, S. Hossain, and W. McMahon. 2007. Communication disorders: Prevalence and comorbid intellectual disability, autism, and emotional/behavioral disorders. *American Journal of Speech-Language Pathology* 16:359–367.

Piolat, A., T. Olive, and R.T. Kellogg. 2005. Cognitive effort during note taking. *Applied Cognitive Psychology* 19:291–312.

Polur, P.D., and J.E. Miller. 2005. Effect of high-frequency spectral components in computer recognition of dysarthric speech based on a Mel-cepstral stochastic model. *Journal of Rehabilitation Research & Development* 42(3):363–372.

Raghavendra, P., J. Bornman, M. Granlund, and E. Björck-Åkesson. 2007. The World Health Organization's international classification of functioning, disability and health: Implications for clinical and research practice in the field of augmentative and alternative communication. *Augmentative and Alternative Communication* 23:349–361.

Ray, L. and S. Feit. 2001. Reading for results: A balanced approach to literacy. *Proceedings of Center on Disabilities Technology and Persons with Disabilities Conference*. Minneapolis, MN.

Reinders-Messelink, H.A., M.M. Schoemaker, T.A.B. Snijders, L.H.N. Göeken, J.P.M Bökkerink, and W.A. Kamps. 2001. Analysis of handwriting of children during treatment for acute lymphoblastic leukemia. *Medical and Pediatric Oncology [Electronic version]* 37:393–399.

Research in Motion. 2009. Features of BlackBerry. http://na.blackberry.com/eng/devices/features/ (accessed May 18, 2009).

Rollins, D.L. 2008. U.S. patent No. 7337404, 2008. Washington, D.C.: U.S. Patent and Trademark Office.

Rosen, K., and S. Yampolsky. 2000. Automatic speech recognition and a review of its functioning with dysarthric speech. *Augmentative and Alternative Communication* 16:48–60.

Scherer, M., J. Jutai, M. Fuhrer, L. Demers, and F. DeRuyter. 2007. A framework for modeling the selection of assistive technology devices (ATDs). *Disability and Rehabilitation: Assistive Technology* 2:1–8.

Schlosser, R.W. 1999. Social validation of interventions in augmentative and alternative communication. *Augmentative & Alternative Communication* 15:234–247.

Schmetzke, A. 2001. Online distance education — "anytime, anywhere" but not for everyone. Information Technology and Disabilities 7. http://people.rit.edu/easi/itd/itdv07n2/axel. htm (accessed June 24, 2010).

Shepherd, T.A., and S. McDougall. 2008. Communication access in the library for individuals who use augmentative and alternative communication. *Augmentative and Alternative Communication* 24(4):313–322.

Sigafoos, J., E. Drasgow, J.W. Halle, M. O'Reilly, S. Seely-York, C. Edrisinha et al. 2004. Teaching VOCA use as a communicative repair strategy. *Journal of Autism and Developmental Disorders* 34:411–422.

Simeonsson, R.J. 2003. Classification of communication disabilities in children: Contribution of the International Classification on Functioning, Disability and Health. *International Journal of Audiology* 42:S2–S8.

Simmons, T., D. Bauder, M. Abell, and W. Penrod. 2008. Delivering the general curriculum: Pre-service teacher perspectives regarding a technological approach for students with moderate and severe disabilities. *Information Technology and Disabilities Journal* 12. http://people.rit.edu/easi/itd/itdv12n1/simmons.htm (accessed May 12, 2009).

Simms, M.D. 2007. Language disorders in children: Classification and clinical syndromes. *Pediatric Clinics of North America* 54:437–467.

Statistics Canada. 2004. *Household Internet Use Survey.* http://www.statcan.ca/Daily/ English/040708/d040708a.htm (accessed May 19, 2009).

Sturm, J.M., S.A. Spadorcia, J.W. Cunningham, K.S. Cali, A. Staples, K. Erickson et al. 2006. What happens to reading between first and third grade? Implications for students who use AAC. *Augmentative and Alternative Communication* 22:21–36.

Tango [speech generating device] Blink Twice Inc. 2007. http://www.dynavoxtech.com/ products/tango/

Tanner, H., S. Jones, and S. Kennewell. 2008. Interactive whole class teaching and interactive white boards. *Journal of Computer Assisted Learning* 24:61–73.

Todman, J. 2000. Rate and quality of conversations using a text-storage AAC system: Single-case training study. *Augmentative & Alternative Communication* 16(3):164–179.

Todman, J., N. Alm, J. Higginbotham, and P. File. 2008. Whole utterance approaches in AAC. *Augmentative and Alternative Communication* 24:235–254.

Toughbook [Computer hardware]. http://www.panasonic.ca/english/Office/notebook/

Veenhof, B., Y. Clermont, and G. Sciadas. 2005. *Literacy and digital technologies: Linkages and outcomes.* Connectedness Series. Ottawa: Statistics Canada, Science, Innovation and Electronic Information Division. http://www.statcan.ca/english/research/56F0004 MIE/56F0004MIE2005012.pdf (accessed May 18, 2009).

Vmax [integrated speech generating device and computer] DynaVox Mayer-Johnson http:// www.dynavoxtech.com/products/v/

Waller, A. 2006. Communication access to conversational narrative. *Topics in Language Disorders* 26:221.

WebEx [computer software]. http://www.webex.com/product-overview/support-center/ remote-support.html

Wilkinson, K.M., and S. Hennig. 2007. The state of research and practice in augmentative and alternative communication for children with developmental/intellectual disabilities. *Mental Retardation & Developmental Disabilities Research Reviews* 13:58–69.

Williams, M.B., C. Krezman, and D. McNaughton. 2008. Reach for the stars: Five principles for the next 25 years of AAC. *Augmentative and Alternative Communication* 24:194–206.

WiViK [computer software] http://www.wivik.com/

WordQ [computer software] http://www.wordq.com/

World Health Organization (WHO). 2001. International classification of functioning, disability and health (ICF). Geneva: World Health Organization.

World Wide Web Consortium. 2009. Web Accessibility Initiative. http://www.w3.org/WAI/
    about-links.html (accessed May 19, 2009).
WriteOnline [computer software] Crick Inc. http://www.cricksoft.com/uk/writeonline/
Yao, J.T. 2008. An introduction to web-based support systems. *Journal of Intelligent Systems*
    17(1–3):267–281.
Yeung, J., B. Konstantinidis, and D. Fels. 2005. Videoconferencing system for high school class-
    room environments. *Proceedings of the Fourth International Cyberspace Conference on
    Ergonomics*. Johannesburg: International Ergonomics Association Press.

5 Optimal Web-Based Survey Design in the Youth Population

Enabling Access for All

T. Claire Davies and N. Susan Stott

CONTENTS

INTRODUCTION

Online Web-based surveys are becoming increasingly popular compared to paper-and-pen-based surveys when evaluating services or products. This is largely due to reduction in costs, the ease of reaching a geographically diverse population and the ability to analyze and report up-to-the-minute results (Schmidt 1997). Web-based surveys have been used to evaluate education (Layne, DeCristoforo, and McGinty 1999), healthcare (Grant et al. 2010) and public opinion (Angus Reid Global Monitor) and have proven very effective at identifying the needs of youth to allow for improvements to transitional services, educational access (Avery et al. 2006), healthcare access and employability (Grant et al. 2010). Children as young as 8 years appear capable of using the Internet to self-report on aspects of their life with their answers paralleling those given to the same questionnaire delivered in a paper-based format (Young et al. 2009). Thus, Web-based surveys have considerable promise in the youth population particularly for studies that require multi-site data collection or that target rural or distant populations. However, many researchers lack expertise in the technical aspects of Web-based survey development and thus either use readily available survey tools that do not adhere to standards of accessibility, or employ a graphic artist to design a survey that will appeal visually to the target group. In both scenarios, the importance of survey accessibility and ease of use may not be at the forefront of the design process. Poorly designed interfaces can act as barriers to participation and systematically exclude young people with impairments such as poor visual acuity or reduced manual dexterity from involvement in an online survey. Thus, when designing Web-based surveys to capture data that are truly population-based, one must consider not only whether all potential respondents have physical access to a computer and the Internet, but also the accessibility and ease of use of the graphical user interface (Sutter and Klein 2007).

Most information on Internet access in the youth population focuses on non-disabled youth. The percentage of youth accessing the Internet has risen sharply over the last 20 years and, in some areas of the world may be as high as 87% to 98% of all youth (Media Awareness Network 2009; Sutter and Klein 2007; de Haan, Duimel and Valkenburg 2007). Conversely, there is less information about access to and use of the Internet by youth with disabilities. In 2003, a study by the U.S. National Center for Education Statistics reported that disabled children between the ages of 5 and 17 were less likely to access the Internet than their counterparts without a disability (DeBell and Chapman 2006). However, a more recent study of 97 physically disabled adolescents in the Netherlands showed no difference in Internet access or frequency of use compared to adolescents without a disability (Lathouwers, de Moor and Didden 2009). Although studies of access by individuals with disabilities have small numbers, the results suggest that lack of a computer or Internet connection would be an unlikely reason to exclude most disabled youth from participation in a Web-based survey, at least in the developed world.

Benyon, Crerar and Wilkinson (2000) suggest three components to any computer system: interaction methods, interaction devices and interface design. Many interaction devices and methods exist to enhance physical access to a computer, ranging from accessibility options within the operating system through to modified input devices such as joysticks, touch screens and speech recognition software (for review, see Davies et al. 2009). However, the uptake of assistive technology to enhance computer use appears to be variable with many barriers to use. At school, insufficient funding, lack of staff training and negative staff attitudes all act as barriers (Copley and Ziviani 2004), while in the home environment, cost is often a contributing factor (Ellis 2007). As an example, our survey of youth with upper limb motor impairments (due to cerebral palsy) has shown that most prefer to use a typical mouse, either by hand for movement of the cursor on the screen with finger-clicking for selection of a target, or by using a modified access mechanism such as the foot in combination with toe-clicking (Davies, Stott and Ameratunga 2010). Only a small number use assistive technology, though most are aware of options such as trackballs or eye trackers, and some have even used them in the past. Although we did not ask participants why they decided to return to the use of a typical or modified mouse, the lack of available assistive technology in educational settings may contribute to the decision (Michaels et al. 2002). In addition, individuals use computers in a variety of locations including friends' homes and the public library where access to assistive technology is not always available. The most pragmatic decision may be to use a typical mouse at all sites.

While this data suggest that most youth with disabilities can access a computer and the Internet, the researcher needs to give consideration to the *physical ease of access*, including speed and accuracy, which will strongly influence the successful completion of an online survey. This chapter focuses on the part of the survey design process targeted toward ease of use and reducing the *physical* load in completion of an online survey. This review assumes that the reader is cognizant of other issues for survey design, such as question development and choice, order of questions and the cognitive load for participants, that is, the number and complexity of questions (Converse and Presser 1986; Jobe 2003). These issues apply equally to a paper survey that is posted, faxed or emailed and an online survey and need to be addressed as part of survey development.

In the next section, we discuss the affordances and limitations of Web-based surveys, contrasting them against traditional pen-and-paper delivery. Subsequently, we introduce the key design requirements for accessible Web pages and graphical user interfaces, covering both international guidelines and models of human movement and reaction times. Building on these ideas, we propose a collection of key considerations in the design of Web-based surveys. Finally, we close with four case studies ranging from simple to complex surveys, to illustrate the concepts and evaluations introduced in this chapter. Figure 5.1 provides a graphical roadmap to help orient the reader.

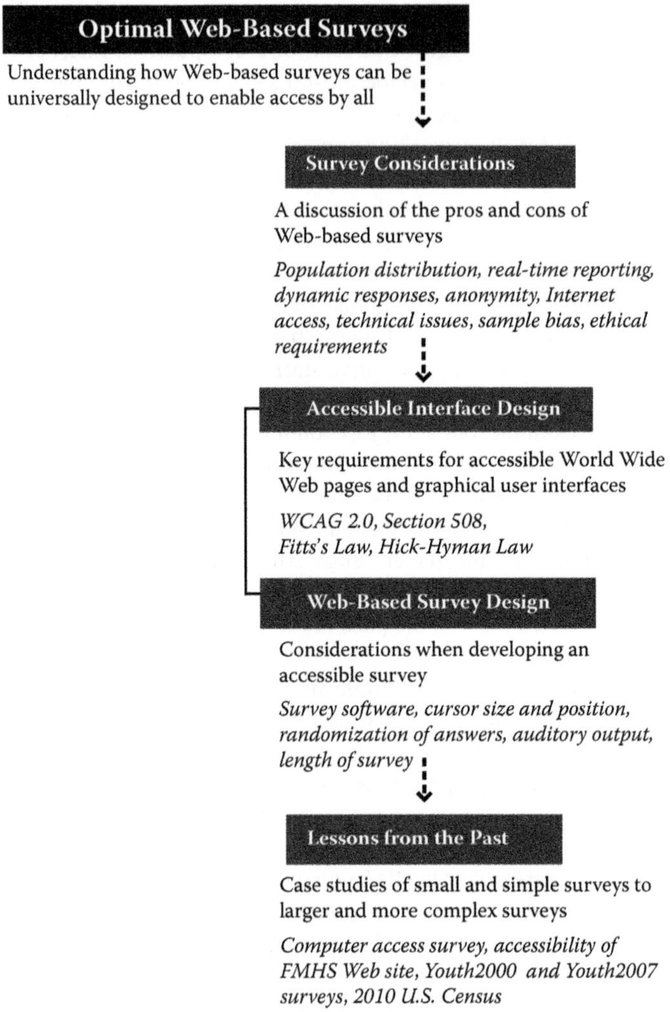

Optimal Web-Based Surveys

Understanding how Web-based surveys can be
universally designed to enable access by all

Survey Considerations

A discussion of the pros and cons of
Web-based surveys

*Population distribution, real-time reporting,
dynamic responses, anonymity, Internet
access, technical issues, sample bias, ethical
requirements*

Accessible Interface Design

Key requirements for accessible World Wide
Web pages and graphical user interfaces

*WCAG 2.0, Section 508,
Fitts's Law, Hick-Hyman Law*

Web-Based Survey Design

Considerations when developing an
accessible survey

*Survey software, cursor size and position,
randomization of answers, auditory output,
length of survey*

Lessons from the Past

Case studies of small and simple surveys to
larger and more complex surveys

*Computer access survey, accessibility of
FMHS Web site, Youth2000 and Youth2007
surveys, 2010 U.S. Census*

FIGURE 5.1   A graphical map representing the layout of the chapter.

SURVEY DESIGN CONSIDERATIONS: WEB-BASED SURVEYS VERSUS PEN AND PAPER

Before the 1990s, most surveys were conducted using paper-based methods. Researchers (or enumerators) provided the survey in paper format and either asked the participant to complete the questionnaire in their presence, or requested that it be returned physically or by mail to the researchers. The researchers would then be responsible for collecting and collating the results. This process could be very time consuming and costly for all involved. For example, the 1790 census in the United States started on August 2, 1790, but was not finally completed until March 1792, after South Carolina had obtained an extension from Congress (Clemence 1985). As the time for collection of data spanned almost 2 years, there were likely additional births that were counted and some deaths that were not counted. Since then, decennial censuses have been conducted in the United States. By 1990, the cost of the census was so great (a 400% increase over 1960 after adjusting for inflation) that a significant review was undertaken to evaluate ways in which these costs could be contained or reduced (Edmonston and Schultze 1995). Following this review, the U.S. Bureau of the Census has attempted to collect census information online. The 2000 census allowed some respondents to be surveyed online and over 65,000 were successful (Whitworth 2001). However, in 2010, an online census still remains experimental (U.S. Census Bureau 2010). The research and hurdles associated with the U.S. census will be discussed further in the case studies in the latter half of this chapter.

The easy availability of computer access over the last 2 decades has prompted researchers to look for electronic means of obtaining population-based data. Although delivering a survey by email rather than by post is cost-efficient for the researcher, there is little difference from the participant's viewpoint. The participant is still required to either print out the survey and post back the completed version to the researcher, or save the document to the hard drive and complete (and return it) electronically. Email return of completed survey documents can be particularly problematic as the email address will be attached to the returned document, negating anonymity. In contrast, there are many benefits to using an online survey to collect survey data, including (1) potential widening of the geographic distribution of participants, (2) the ability to collect data in real time, (3) the option of targeting the next question, depending on the answer to the previous question, and (4) greater participant and researcher anonymity. However, Internet access, technical design issues, sample bias and ethical consent must all be considered when developing an online survey. Some advantages and disadvantages of Internet survey data collection are discussed in more detail in the following sections while others can be found in reviews by Rhodes, Bowie and Hergenrather (2003) and Rew et al. (2004) .

POPULATION DISTRIBUTION

Web-based methods allow the researcher to be at a different location from the participant, thus reducing the costs of mailing. This allows worldwide surveying from a single location. The distribution of the survey is limited only by the number of individuals to whom you can supply the link. In addition to being able to access participants around the world, an online survey also allows respondents to be at a location and time convenient for them. While some individuals may feel comfortable filling out a questionnaire at the doctor's office or in the middle of a mall, others need more privacy. Privacy and comfort when completing the questionnaire can potentially increase the percentage of truthful responses (Watson et al. 2001).

REAL-TIME REPORTING

Online surveys allow answers to be coded for real-time reporting of results. Data collection and entry into a database is automated, meaning that data can be analyzed at any time as the survey proceeds. Often, once a survey is launched, an error will be found that was not picked up during usability testing. Real-time reporting helps the researcher identify an erroneous question in the survey, either through anomalous survey responses or through a survey feedback section. In contrast, transcription of answers from either a paper-based or an electronic word document into a separate database is cumbersome and often not undertaken until after the survey is completed.

If one learns that the right question is not being asked or that sufficient information is not being provided, then the question can be modified to ensure that future responses will collect the data that one desires.

On one of our surveys, FMHS was used as an acronym for Faculty of Medical and Health Sciences. As all of our usability participants who piloted the survey were aware of the acronym, we did not realise that we had not expanded the acronym. Two individuals who received an email requesting their participation in the survey contacted the researcher to request clarification of the acronym, even though all potential survey respondents were enrolled within the Faculty as students! Real-time analysis of data allows immediate changes to provide this information to future respondents.

Another benefit of real-time reporting is that the researcher can easily track the number of respondents, determine when to follow up and decide when the survey should be closed. The percentage of those respondents who started but did not complete the survey can also be identified by many software packages, including SurveyGizmo (Survey Gizmo 2005–2010) and SurveyMonkey (Survey Monkey 1999–2010). In a recent online survey that we conducted, 78% of participants responded within the first 72 hours. Tracking the number of responses over a given time period in real time can allow the researcher to program an automatic delivery of reminder emails/contact letters with the survey link to all participants to prompt those who have not yet completed the survey. It can also allow the researcher to determine whether and when to expand the search for additional participants.

DYNAMIC RESPONSES

Unlike respondent-completed paper-based surveys, Web-based surveys can be branched to allow skipping of irrelevant questions or targeting of follow-up questions to explore the meaning behind a specific answer (Figure 5.2). Using the example of a survey about access to computers and assistive technology, if a respondent answers 'Yes' to question 1, 'Have you ever used a computer,' the next screen can ask, 'Where have you used a computer,' whereas if the answer is 'No,' the following screen can instead ask, 'Would you like to use a computer?' Branching of a Web-based survey reduces the question load for the participant and ensures that he or she is only exposed to relevant questions (Sutter and Klein 2007). In a traditional survey format, all questions must be available to the respondent. This feature may lead the respondent to change his or her answer to an earlier question if the respondent decides that a different response would either better suit the end goal of the questionnaire or would help to avoid other questions.

In addition to being able to configure the questionnaire based on the response, a dynamic survey can be programmed to rotate the response categories and the order of questions to minimise skewing of the results. Prompts, either visual or audio, can

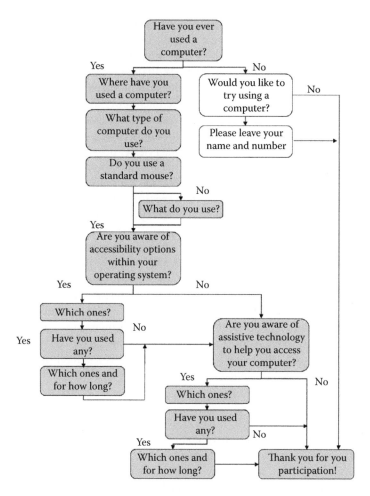

FIGURE 5.2   An example of question branching for Web-based surveys. A path through the darkened blocks represents the maximum number of possible questions.

also be inserted to draw attention to questions that have not been answered, thus minimizing gaps in data collection.

ANONYMITY

Traditional paper-based surveys are often conducted by an interviewer, either face to face or over the phone, with the interviewer guiding the interviewee through the complexities of the survey questions. This allows the interviewer to adapt the delivery of the survey questions, depending on the response, in the same way that a Web-based survey can be branched. However, the presence of an interviewer has been shown to affect how a participant chooses to answer a question, with interviewers of different ethnicity, gender or socio-economic background potentially eliciting differ-ent answers from the same sample population (Davis et al. 2009). More experienced

interviewers can also achieve different answers compared to less experienced interviewers due to more active engagement with the interviewee. These types of effects
have been termed the 'interviewer effect' and are particularly evident when surveys
involve sensitive material (Davis et al. 2009). Williams (1968) has argued that respondents to an interview survey are active participants in the process, seeking subcon-
scious feedback and non-verbal cues from the interviewer as to the 'right' response
and avoiding responses that may expose the respondent to humiliation or stigma.

By contrast, Web-based surveys are perceived as having greater anonymity and
can be answered anywhere at any time. An interviewer does not meet with the individual and can therefore not physically identify the individual. In many paper-based
surveys, the researchers code the response sheets to determine who has and who has
not answered, thus linking the response to a specific individual. The perceived (and
real) anonymity associated with electronic surveys is a major advantage of Web-
based surveys over traditional paper-based surveys, particularly in the younger adolescent population, as it is likely to enhance honesty of answers (Rew et al. 2004;
Webb et al. 1999). However, the respondent does not have the opportunity to give
feedback about a question while completing the survey, unless the survey designer
so chooses. This may introduce other problems if the intent of a question is unclear
to the reader or the survey design impairs access (e.g., a large number of possible
answers to one question). For this reason, all online surveys must be carefully piloted
for readability (considering reading age of the respondents as well as visibility of the
text) and usability, using the target population where possible. Real-time analysis of
response data is also recommended as discussed previously.

INTERNET ACCESS

Unlike paper-based surveys that can be completed almost anywhere, Web-based surveys require access to the Internet. While Internet access is becoming more prevalent
in all environments, there may be the occasional situation in which the researcher
may not have access to the Internet and is unable to conduct an online survey. Mobile
computing is becoming more popular (Blackberry, iPhone), but is still quite expensive for the average researcher and sometimes a paper-and-pen-based method of collecting data may still be most cost-effective.

In 2008, a report from the International Telecommunications Union reported that
in 24 countries worldwide, greater than 70% of the population had use of the Internet
(International Telecommunications Union 2008). In a fast response survey of U.S.
schools, it was found that, by 2005, almost 100% of the schools in the United States
had Internet access at the school, regardless of school size or parental income level
(based on number of students eligible for free or subsidised lunches) (Wells, Lewis
and Greene 2006). It was also found that 94% of instructional classrooms themselves had Internet access. In Canada in 2003, 79.5% of the population under 35
years used the Internet at home, school, work, library or another location (Statistics
Canada 2006). By 2005, a nationwide survey found that 94% of Canadian youth
were able to access the Internet at home (Media Awareness Network 2009; Norris
2007). In the Netherlands in 2007, 98% of a sample of 1566 adolescents, aged 13 to
18 years, accessed the Internet at home (de Haan, Duimel and Valkenburg 2007).

These statistics suggest that the presence and use of the Internet has become commonplace, especially by the youth of developed countries.

However, for some individuals with disabilities, access lags behind that of the general population. Individuals with disabilities may have limitations in the location of access due to the need to use assistive technology. One group that may have particular difficulty with access is the population with visual impairment or blindness. A study by Kaczmirek and Wolff (2007) noted that, in their survey of 235 older people who were either blind or visually impaired, only a small percentage (18.5%) accessed the Internet (Kaczmirek and Wolff 2007). Survey design for youth with visual impairments may require different and tailored strategies involving a mixed-mode approach (Kaczmirek and Wolff 2007) (discussed in more detail in section).

TECHNICAL ISSUES

One of the biggest challenges with Web-based surveys is the potential occurrence of programming errors that leave the participant stranded, without knowledge of how to respond or unable to complete the survey. Especially with individuals using a variety of different assistive technologies, the computer may be older than those with which the researcher is familiar. It may also use dated versions of certain programs. The individual continues to use these versions because they work effectively and do not necessitate additional training. A questionnaire may be developed to be accessible using a new computer or Web browser, but may not work effectively with an earlier version of the operating system or an older computer. It is therefore important to test the survey on a variety of different operating systems to evaluate backward compatibility.

Another technical difficulty may occur if a respondent presses the answer button multiple times, causing duplication of responses. When designing interfaces for individuals with inadvertent movements, for example, intention tremor or athetosis, this is a particularly important problem. Filter keys through Windows have been developed to combat this problem of repeated entry in a text environment. A similar approach can be taken in the design of questionnaires. Depending on the speed of the Internet connection, some individuals may become impatient waiting for the next screen and may hit the answer button several more times. By designing the survey to accept only one response, this problem can be reduced, but the designer of the survey must be informed that this is a potential issue that may be more prevalent in certain populations.

Unfortunately, there is always the possibility of the computer freezing or the Internet provider dropping the link temporarily. A short, concise survey may reduce the risk of these issues. Many technical glitches can be addressed most easily by testing and retesting the Web-based survey with a subset of the potential target population.

SAMPLE BIAS

Low response rates to a survey are said to introduce potential sample bias and may compromise the validity of the findings due to differences in demographics, attitudes and behaviours of the respondents compared to the non-respondents. Recent reports from the developers of telephone surveys have challenged this statement, reporting that a higher response rate does not necessarily improve survey accuracy or lead to samples that are more representative of the demographic characteristics of the target population (Keeter et al. 2006; Holbrook, Krosnick and Pfent 2007). Other studies have suggested that, in some groups at least, there is not as much difference between those who respond to surveys and those who do not respond as previously thought (Kellerman and Herold 2001). Despite this, most researchers (and journals publishing their research!) wish to know and report the response rate to their survey, together with an analysis of survey responders and non-responders.

This can raise some problems in online surveying. A survey response rate can be easily calculated if a researcher uses an address database (either paper or electronic) to distribute a paper-based survey with response sheets that contain numerically coded identifiers to determine who of the potential participants has responded. The response rate then equals the number of respondents divided by the number invited to respond. In an online survey, the true response rate may be difficult to calculate if the survey is available on a public-access Web site. In this scenario, the number of visitors to that site who were eligible to fill in the survey, but chose not to, is unknown.

The response rate to an Internet survey is more easily calculated if the population is defined, for example, all youth aged between 14 and 18 years enrolled in a local school, and only that group is invited by email to participate and supplied with the electronic link. However, the greater anonymity of the respondent means that problems arise if the link to the survey is distributed more widely than the researcher intends. Using the above example, youth can quickly distribute the survey link to their friends, particularly if the survey appeals to that age group. While a paper survey can also be emailed around, the coded identifier would give away the duplication of the answers. Youth may also be tempted to fill in a survey more than once if there is a potential reward (such as being entered into a drawing for an iPod at the end of the survey). While restricting responses to one per IP (Internet protocol) location may seem a sensible solution, in practice an IP address can belong to one Web host (e.g., an academic institution or commercial company) rather than a single individual (Sutter and Klein 2007). In addition, participants would still be able to reply from more than one IP location using the same link. To reduce the problems of multiple responses by one participant, potential participants can be anonymously assigned unique logins and passwords that can only be used once.

Regardless of the debate over the relationship between response rate and representative sampling, most researchers wish to increase the response to their survey as much as possible to provide greater power for statistical analyses. Increasing the response rate to surveys has been a subject of much research. A recent Cochrane systematic review (Edwards et al. 2009) has identified personalized messages, a picture with the email message and avoidance of the word *survey* in the email header as strategies for enhancing uptake of an electronic survey. Conversely, a male signature on the email seems to reduce the chances of uptake. Some work has also been done to assess whether online surveying per se changes response rate (Holbrook, Krosnick and Pfent 2007; Sutter and Klein 2007; Avery et al. 2006). In 1999, Pealer and co-authors used both a self-administered mailed survey and a Web-based survey version to test the response rate to the National College Health Risk Behavior Survey

(Pealer et al. 2001). They showed that, at least in their population of university students, the response rates to both types of survey were similar.

The greatest response rates may be obtainable by mixed-mode approaches (Greenlaw and Brown-Welty 2009). Mixed-mode approaches are those that provide a variety of means to collect the data (including online surveys, paper-based mailings, telephone interviews, etc.). Mixed modes can be provided sequentially or concurrently. For instance, electronic surveys can be followed by personal interviews with those who did not respond online (de Leeuw 2005). Another alternative would be to provide both the option to complete the survey online or with pen and paper. Research on the use of mixed-mode approaches is contradictory as to whether the demographics, health characteristics and behaviours of online respondents differ from those who respond to paper-based surveys or participate in telephone interviews (Link and Mokdad 2005a,b; Pealer et al. 2001). Further work is needed in this area to determine the validity and reliability of responses between online, paper-based and telephone interview methods.

Notwithstanding these concerns, in some populations a mixed-mode approach may be the only solution to enable access to the survey. An example of the need to use mixed-mode methodology for a disabled population is provided by Kaczmirek and Wolff (2007). They discuss the challenges of designing a self-administered survey for individuals who use enlargers to magnify text, have an impaired visual field (e.g., tunnel vision) or may read by means of a Braille display or electronic screen reader. The traditional layout of surveys makes it difficult for readers with visual impairments to gain an overview of the page, either paper-based or electronic. Reading aids act by magnifying single words or specific text. This means that questions or answer categories can be skipped inadvertently or the meaning can be lost. Similarly, restricted visual fields may make it hard to see answer boxes located to the periphery of the screen. Survey length can also be a barrier for those who answer with a Braille typewriter, with Kaczmirek and Wolff (2007) pointing out that it may take more than 1 hour to answer 20 questions. They recommended offering different modes of participation, including Web- and paper-based surveys as well as a Braille version and provide 12 design guidelines to enhance survey readability.

ETHICAL REQUIREMENTS

Ethical approvals for health-based research in the paediatric and adolescent population usually require both parental consent and child/youth assent if the child is over the age of 7 or 8 years. While an online survey approach provides greater anonymity of both researcher and participant, the research design must be subject to the same ethical review before survey release. Issues specific to online surveys that may need to be addressed by the researcher include (1) how to manage a respondent's discomfort or need for emotional support if the survey addresses sensitive issues, given that the researcher and participant are unlikely to be co-located, (2) protection of personal data transmitted online from viewing by a third party, and (3) secure storage of personal data online in a way that ensures on-going confidentiality and integrity of the data (Sutter and Klein 2007).

SUMMARY

While there are pros and cons to each method of surveying, many of the issues can be addressed with effective pre-testing of the survey. This involves both usability and accessibility testing at all stages of design to ensure that the survey can be used by all. While the listed benefits of Web-based surveying primarily appeal to the researcher, one of the most convincing arguments for use of a Web-based survey is the potential to provide superior access compared to pen-and-paper-based surveys due to the increased flexibility of design, while avoiding the perceived lack of anonymity that accompanies an interviewer-led survey.

ACCESSIBLE INTERFACE DESIGN

Have you ever wondered why a drive-through ATM has Braille on it?
To enable accessibility for all, without the need for adaptation.

Good interface design can seem intuitive in many ways; a larger target is more easily reached than a smaller one, black on white or white on black is more easily read than red on green, etc. A large font can be more easily read than a smaller one. Some fonts (e.g., Arial) are easier to read than others. Often, however, a designer will add decorative features such as images or pictures as background, multiple colours, different fonts and animation to make the interface more visually appealing. While these changes may attract more attention to the Web site, they also run the risk of making the Web site difficult to access and use.

The researcher should note that accessibility and usability are not interchangeable terms (Theofanos and Redish 2003). Using the root form of the words, usability refers to the ease of use, whereas accessibility refers to ability to access. Usability testing is often conducted at a variety of stages throughout the design process to ensure that a survey both meets the needs of the researchers and is efficient and perceivable with minimal errors. However, often 'the coding required for accessibility is only added during the final phases of implementation' (Murphy 2005 p. 3). Accessibility appears in many cases to be an after-thought at the end of the design process, with the goal being to meet the needs of the few users with disabilities, rather than being designed into the system from the beginning.

Universal design is the term used to describe design features that enable accessibility for all, designing so that all individuals can use the product equally and effectively. This term was first coined to define good practice in architectural design of buildings but is now applied across a wide range of settings to facilitate design of products that can be used by all members of society. There are seven over-arching principles that guide universal design (Conell et al. 1997); see Figure 5.3. These universal design principles were developed initially to ensure accessibility by all people with respect to manufactured products, but similar principles are important in interface usability (Figure 5.3) (Nielsen 1994; Molich and Nielsen 1990).

There are many considerations when designing an interface to ensure accessibility by all. The interface must be usable by all people equally and be flexible in methods of access, with a variety of input devices and modes. It should be both obvious and intuitive to the user as to how to respond. If the user responds in a manner that is

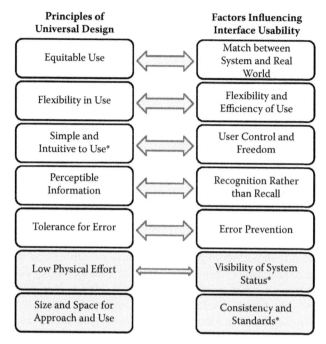

FIGURE 5.3 A comparison between Universal Design Principles and factors that influence interface usability (Nielsen, Jakob. 1994. Enhancing the explanatory power of usability heuristics. In *Proceedings of the SIGCHI conference on human factors in computing systems: celebrating interdependence.* Boston, MA: ACM) (Conell, B.R., M. Jones, R. Mace, J. Mueller, A. Mullick, E. Ostroff, J. Sanford, E. Steinfeld, M. Story, and G. Vanderheiden. 1997. *The principles of universal design.* Raleigh, NC: The Center for Universal Design, N.C. State University. http://www.design.ncsu.edu/cud/pubs_p/docs/UDPMD.pdf (accessed January 10, 2010).) The * indicates concepts that are similar but not represented in the mapping.

unexpected, there should be an option to try again (tolerance for error). It is important to integrate the aspects of accessibility at the early stages of the design process to (1) ensure full accessibility of all users and (2) enable usability testing to involve all individuals, rather than only those who have a specific form of access (Murphy 2005). Overall, the strategies applied to interface design are similar to those strategies used for product design, as they are integral to the successful design of any usable system.

In addition to the general guidelines of graphical interface design, there are specific requirements that apply to Web-based interfaces. The World Wide Web Consortium (www.w3c.org) has developed guidelines for Web page design known as Web Content Accessibility Guidelines (WCAG). These guidelines define the requirements for Web-based accessibility worldwide. Many governments have used these guidelines to develop their own legal standards for all government Web sites. For example, the United States has modified Section 508 of the Disability Act based on these standards (United States Congress 1998), and the New Zealand government has adopted WCAG 2.0 standards with cultural additions (Government Technology Services and Department of Internal Affairs 2009). Understanding these standards before undertaking the development and design of a Web-based survey is important to ensure accessibility by all.

WORLD WIDE WEB ACCESSIBILITY

The World Wide Web Consortium is an international community dedicated to leading the World Wide Web to its full potential (World Wide Web Consortium) with two key principles: (1) Web for all and (2) Web on everything. Generally this group seeks to enable equity of access to the Internet by everyone regardless of the type of input device (hardware, software, mobile phones or any form of assistive technology). The World Wide Web Consortium has developed comprehensive guidelines for developing Web sites to ensure equal access. These guidelines are continuously evolving as new computer languages become available and new standards are achieved. The main users of these guidelines are those individuals who are developing the Web-based interface (Web authors, tool developers and the technical contributors to the Web page), but it is important to be aware of these guidelines and have an understanding of the requirements when communicating with the survey developer.

The most recent version of the guidelines, WCAG 2.0, has four guiding principles for Web accessibility: perceivable (content is available to the senses — sight, hearing and touch), operable (interface forms, controls and navigation), understandable (content and interface) and robust (wide variety of user agents including assistive technologies) (Figure 5.4). Each of these main principles is defined more precisely to provide guidance in a specific area, under which more explicit guidelines (known as success criteria) are given to allow for conformance. For example, when referring to Guideline 1: Perceivable, the success criteria include (i) text alternatives, (ii) time-based media, (iii) adaptable (content should be presentable in various ways without loss of information), and (iv) distinguishable (make it easier to see and hear content by separating foreground and background). Each of these success criteria can be met by following the technical guidelines available on the WCAG 2.0 Web site (www.w3c.org 2010).

Within the success criteria for each principle, there are also three priorities identified for conformance with the guidelines. Level A conformance (sometimes called Priority 1) requires that basic requirements are met for accessibility by some groups. Level AA conformance (Priority 2) indicates better accessibility and the removal of barriers to accessing content. Level AAA conformance requires accessibility of the site to most individuals who may have a disability and is thus an attempt to ensure universal design to the fullest extent possible (World Wide Web Consortium).

An example of the stringency required to follow these standards for even small aspects of Web site design is presented in Table 5.1 (World Wide Web Consortium). The over-arching guideline, for which the requirements of Table 5.1 exist, is 'Guideline 1: Perceivable' (see Figure 5.4), under which the success criterion '1.2 Time-based media' exists. Within this heading, there are an additional nine requirements to ensure full accessibility in this area. These vary in priority level, depending on the information content on the site and the population to whom the Web site should be accessible. In most countries that have adopted WCAG guidelines, Level A priorities must be met such as the provision of captions and other means of access to pre-recorded video and audio. However, to ensure full accessibility, the Level

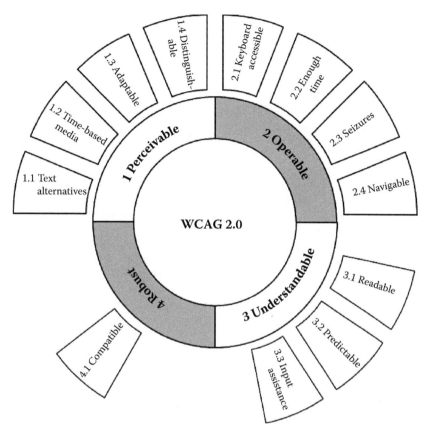

FIGURE 5.4 A diagram of the Web Content Accessibility Guidelines (WCAG) 2.0 put forth by the World Wide Web Consortium (www.w3c.org).

AAA priorities must also be met. For example, '1.2.6 Sign language (pre-recorded)' requires that for audio components of the media presented on the site, simultaneous sign language should be available. The Level AAA requirements are often not required by governments that have adopted these guidelines, but if a site is to be accessible for all, an attempt should be made to meet these priority levels as well.

In the United States, standards have been developed in the form of amendments to the U.S. Disability Act (United States Congress 1998) to ensure that Web pages for the U.S. Federal Government meet accessibility guidelines. These guidelines have been developed based on the first version of the WCAG standards, WCAG 1.0, and follow similar principles. Section 508: 1194.22 defines 16 items to ensure equal access for Web-based intranet and Internet information and applications. A general mapping of Section 508: 1194.22 to WCAG 2.0 can be found in Figure 5.5. While the two standards, WCAG and Section 508, have similar end goals, the specific language varies, allowing different interpretations of the standards. Although the WCAG standards are more comprehensive, if a Web-based survey is to be used by individuals in the United States, it is important to ensure that the standards of Section 508 are also met.

TABLE 5.1

Example of WCAG 2.0 Levels of Success Criteria for One Aspect of Guideline 1.0

Success Criteria			
	Level	Heading	Intent
1.2		Providing alternatives for time-based media	Provide access to time-based and synchronised media including audio-only, video-only, audio-video, and audio and/or video combined with interaction.
1.2.1	A	Audio only and video only (pre-recorded)	Pre-recorded audio: An alternative for time-based media is provided that presents equivalent information for pre-recorded audio-only content.
			Pre-recorded video: Either an alternative for time-based media or an audio track is provided that presents equivalent information for pre-recorded video-only content.
1.2.2	A	Captions (pre-recorded)	Captions are provided for all pre-recorded audio content in synchronised media, except when the media is a media alternative for text and is clearly labelled as such.
1.2.3	A	Audio description or media alternative (pre-recorded)	An alternative for time-based media or audio description of the pre-recorded video content is provided for synchronised media, except when the media is a media alternative for text and is clearly labelled as such.
1.2.4	AA	Captions (live)	Captions are provided for all audio content in synchronised media.
1.2.5	AA	Audio description (pre-recorded)	Audio description is provided for all pre-recorded video content in synchronised media.
1.2.6	AAA	Sign language (pre-recorded)	Sign language interpretation is provided for all pre-recorded audio content in synchronised media.
1.2.7	AAA	Extended audio description (pre-recorded)	Where pauses in foreground audio are insufficient to allow audio descriptions to convey the sense of the video, extended audio description is provided for all pre-recorded video content in synchronised media.
1.2.8	AAA	Media alternative (pre-recorded)	An alternative for time-based media is provided for all pre-recorded synchronised media and for all pre-recorded video-only media.
1.2.9	AAA	Audio-only (live)	An alternative for time-based media that presents equivalent information for live audio-only content is provided.

Information for table obtained from www.w3.org/TR/WCAG201. Copyright © 2008 W3C® (MIT, ERCIM, Keio). All rights reserved.

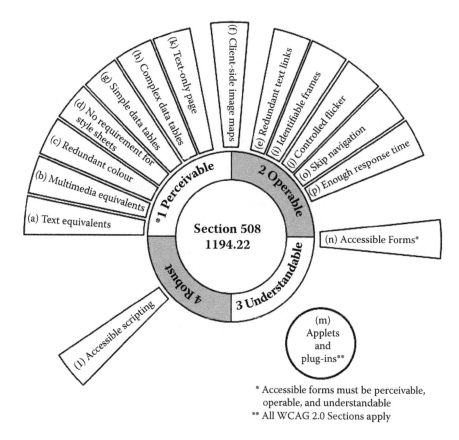

FIGURE 5.5 A mapping of the WCAG 2.0 (www.W3C.org) to Section 508: 1194.22 of the U.S. Disability Act (www.section508.gov).

Example: University of Auckland Faculty of Medical and Health Sciences (FMHS) Web Site

In New Zealand, the New Zealand Government Web Standards 2.0 (WCAG 2.0 including level A and level AA with additional guidelines) must be met by all public Web sites created by Public Service Departments, the New Zealand Police, the New Zealand Defence Force, the Parliamentary Counsel Office, and the New Zealand Security Intelligence Agency (Government Technology Services and Department of Internal Affairs 2009). Although schools and universities are not yet required to meet these guidelines, we recently reviewed several of the Faculty of Medical and Health Sciences Web pages at the University of Auckland to understand the extent to which university Web site designers have achieved voluntary compliance with these standards (University of Auckland 2010).

The main University of Auckland Web site has made attempts to provide accessibility options by providing a link (albeit a difficult link to find unless you are aware of its existence) that describes the steps to resize text and change colours, magnify pages and use shortcut keys. The same options are available on the Faculty of

Medical and Health Science Web pages, but there is no mention on the Faculty Web site about the existence of these tools.

There are several areas of Web site design in which the Faculty is successful in providing accessible information. The use of colour on Web pages is generally very effective, the change in font colour is not the only method of displaying important information and sufficient contrast is provided to allow the Web page to be viewed in a black-and-white format (WCAG 1.4). Style sheets are used as a template for all Web pages, but the document is always understandable if the style sheet is turned off (WCAG 1.3, WCAG 2.4). Also, most of the Web pages that were reviewed allowed the user to have control over modifying the Web page (WCAG 2.1). This enables individuals to use a screen reader or to change contrast colours when required.

Those areas of greatest concern require minimal changes to the current template and can increase efficiency of access by those with difficulty viewing the Web site. Navigational shortcuts are essential to allow the user to skip over lists of navigational menus when using devices such as a screen reader to audibly describe the information (WCAG 2.4). The requirement to listen to every list prior to moving to another part of the screen is a time-consuming endeavour especially when the same lists exist on each page.

Alternative text formats should exist for all images on the page (WCAG 1.1). While images may (or may not) add appeal to some users, for those who have difficulty viewing a page, these images can be a distraction. These images may convey important information, but a user who is functionally blind cannot access these images. Alternative text formats require the image to be described in a short, succinct manner to allow interpretation by those who cannot otherwise view them. Background images can exist, but to enable the user to understand that these do not convey important information, they should hold empty text boxes. When videos or audio segments are displayed, synchronised captions should also be provided (WCAG 1.2).

Unfortunately, there were Web pages that failed to achieve specific accessibility items. All Web pages failed to provide a text equivalent for every non-text element (WCAG 1.1). Every image is required to have a description that should appear when the 'Alt' button is pressed or a text description must be described in the adjacent text. These descriptions should be succinct and interpretable. Empty alt descriptions in which alt="" can be used to display decorative graphics that have no other function, but they must exist. Another area of concern is the lack of ability to effectively read forms on all Web pages. The forms themselves do not have labels associated with them, though they do have a text description beside them (WCAG 1.1, 1.3).

It is important to be aware of these requirements for conformance to accessibility standards and to design Web pages and Web-based surveys that meet these guidelines. Although these guidelines should be followed to enable access to those with permanent disability, there are also individuals who require access with temporary or short-term disabilities, for instance, a broken arm, recovering from laser eye surgery, etc. that must be considered in the design of all surveys. Access to all means being aware of these requirements and designing for everyone!

Legal Requirements of Meeting WCAG or Section 508 Standards

The legality of not meeting the Section 508 or WCAG standards is dependent on the country, but legal issues have the potential to cover more than one jurisdiction if the site is used (or is available, which is likely unless otherwise protected) abroad. Current precedence has governed that, in the United States, Web sites are required to meet these standards as required by the Disability Act. There are several cases in which human rights violations have resulted in cases brought against major private companies that perform Web-based services. A class-action lawsuit of the National Federation of the Blind (NFB) was brought against Target Corporation for lack of accessibility to their online Web site Target.com (*Class Settlement Agreement and Release: National Federation of the Blind, the National Federation of the Blind of California v. Target Corporation* 2008). While the case was settled out of court, Target did agree to a 3-year relationship in which the Web site would be made accessible to blind individuals requiring assistive technology and that usability testing would be conducted by the NFB.

In another case, Sam Latif, who was functionally blind and located in the United Kingdom, sought to be examined for the internationally recognised Project Management Professional qualification through the Project Management Institute (PMI) based in the United States. She requested the exam to be made available in a format that could be read with JAWS screen-reading software, but was denied and, instead, provided a reader of the exam. This action increased the time required for completion of the examination as her JAWS reader was typically programmed to read at a pace 60% faster than a person. The U.K. tribunal found that although PMI was a U.S.-based company, it was required to pay amends to Sam Latif. The tribunal chairperson (Richard Barrowclough) stated, 'The respondent has not established that it took all steps as were reasonable in order to prevent the claimant being put at a substantial disadvantage by their practice of exam questions being read by candidates in a test centre and thereafter recording their answers' (Out-law.com 2007). While most countries only require government agencies to comply with accessibility standards, legal and ethical issues surrounding human rights will eventually require compliance by all in both the private and public sectors.

GRAPHICAL USER INTERFACE DESIGN

In addition to meeting accessibility standards in Web page design, surveys also require that specific areas of the Web page be more easily targeted to enable the answering of questions. The International Standards Organization uses Fitts's law to make recommendations about the relative sizes of screen targets to enable efficient task precision. Fitts's law can be used to evaluate the trade-off between speed and accuracy while selecting specific targets (MacKenzie 1992). In addition, the Hick-Hyman law can provide information about the trade-offs between the number of targets on the screen and the ease of hitting one specific target. Ensuring that the interface design of the survey requires minimal precision may enable individuals with upper limb impairments and motor control problems to access the survey.

Fitts's Law

Fitts's law is used to model the act of pointing during human-computer interaction, either directly by physically touching an object (e.g., a touch-screen) or virtually by use of a pointing device (e.g., mouse or joystick) to manoeuvre a virtual cursor to an object on the screen (Fitts 1954; Fitts and Peterson 1964). The law describes a linear

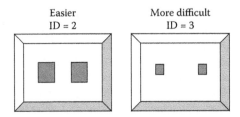

FIGURE 5.6   Icons that are smaller and farther apart are more difficult to target than those that are closer together.

relationship between the time taken to perform the movement (MT) and the ratio of distance between the centres of the targets (A) and size of target (W) as a logarithmic equation: $MT = a + b\log_2(2A/W)$, where a is the intercept and b is the slope of the regression line. Fitts's law predicts a trade-off between the speed and accuracy of visually guided movements, with the time taken to move to a target area being a function of both the size and distance of the target. Generally, the larger the target and the smaller the spacing between targets, the easier it is to select (Figure 5.6).

Fitts's law has been extensively used in the field of human-computer interaction to study aiming tasks (see Guiard and Beaudouin-Lafon 2004) and has been shown to apply across many different user groups [e.g., the elderly (Bakaev 2008), those with spastic hemiplegia (Smits-Engelsman 2007)], a variety of input devices [e.g., cross scanner, ASL mouse (Man and Wong 2007), joystick (Rao, Seliktar and Rahman 2000)], and different parts of the human body [e.g., brain (McFarland, Sarnacki and Wolpaw 2003), hand (Kabbash, Mackenzie, and Buxton 1993), and eyes (Zhang and MacKenzie 2007)]. Of interest, early work by Card, Engish and Burr (1978) using Fitts's law to assess the ease of use of different input devices is credited with influencing the choice of the mouse as the preferred input device by Xerox and then Apple (Card 2010). Since then, many studies of conventional mouse and touch pads using Fitts's law have been conducted (MacKenzie 1992; Mackenzie and Buxton 1994). Others have used Fitts's law to evaluate assistive technology. [For several studies that evaluate computer access using assistive technology by individuals with cerebral palsy, see Davies et al. (2009).]

Fitts's Law and Survey Interface Design

Understanding Fitts's law enables the interface designer to reduce physical load on the user. International Standards Organization Guidelines (ISO 9241-9 p. 30, the international standard for "Ergonomic Requirements for Office Work with Visual Display Terminals [VDTs] Part 9, 2000) have been developed to guide development of non-keyboard devices for computer access. The index of difficulty (ID) is defined as $ID = \log_2(2A/W)$, with the numerical value of the ID used as a guide to task precision. The task precision (ISO 9241-9 p. 30) 'is the measure of the accuracy required for pointing, selecting or dragging task primitive and (is) quantified by the index of difficulty'. Task primitives are those actions that can be evaluated independent of input device or disability and include 'pointing' or 'dragging' tasks rather

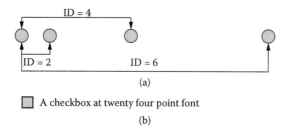

(a)

▨ A checkbox at twenty four point font

(b)

FIGURE 5.7   (a) The higher the index of difficulty between targets, the greater precision required. Those with an index of difficulty less than or equal to 4 require low precision, while those greater than 6 require high precision (ISO 9241). (b) A typical survey checkbox that is 24-point font will require high precision unless the default position of the cursor is close to the checkbox.

than 'word processing,' which is goal oriented and more difficult to evaluate (Cakir 2009). Interfaces that have an ID of 4 or less require only a low task precision. Those interfaces with an ID of 4 to 6 can be classed as requiring a moderate level of precision, and those with an interface with an ID over 6 require a high level of precision. Figure 5.7a shows the relative distances for a circle and the corresponding IDs to target one circle followed by the other. Most survey checkboxes and radio buttons are designed to complement the size of the accompanying text. Figure 5.7b shows the relative difference for a checkbox of 24-point font (twice the size of a typical font). Depending on the default position of the cursor, checkboxes or radio buttons are not easily targeted. This can be particularly difficult for those individuals with motor or sensory deficits in the upper limbs. Reducing the ID by increasing the size of the target area is a simple way to enable easier access for all people.

Hick-Hyman Law

In addition to Fitts's law, the Hick-Hyman law (Hick 1952; Hyman 1953) should also be considered. This law describes the linear relationship between the reaction time and the number of possible stimulus response alternatives (N) such that $RT = a + b\log_2 N$. The number of choices on a screen will affect the individual's time to respond. When completing a questionnaire, the individual must scan all possible alternatives seeking a particular response. Depending on the number of possible alternatives, the length of time to select a response can take considerably longer than if a series of questions with a smaller number of choices were available.

As an example, some surveys request information about the origin of one's family. The recent Youth2000 survey held in New Zealand asked the question: 'Which ethnic group do you belong to? (choose all that apply)' and gave a possible selection of 24 choices for this question (Youth2000 2010). Assuming a value of a = 0 (intercept) and b = 1 (slope) for Equation (5.2), then the reaction time would take 4.8 sec for the first selection. If, instead, a carefully thought out branched question were formed with four choices per page provided, only 2 sec would be required for each selection. The total time required to obtain the same result may be equivalent to scanning all 24 possible responses for the average user, but in combination with

Fitts's law, the survey can be designed to minimise the overall physical load for those with disabilities. The method of branching within the survey would depend on the end goal of the survey and what information was most important. In addition, the cognitive load of fewer possible responses is also likely to yield better results, especially for an individual with a visual impairment who would otherwise have to remember all the possible alternatives.

WEB-BASED SURVEY DESIGN

The key elements for interface design should be followed in the design of Web-based surveys. All pages in the survey should comply with the WCAG 2.0 standards (or Section 508) and the survey pages themselves should be designed to require minimal task precision as dictated by Fitts's law and the Hick-Hyman law.

SURVEY SOFTWARE

The easiest method to design a Web-based survey without employing a Web developer is by using online software (Gordon and McNew 2008). Easily modifiable survey software is available online (for example, SurveyMonkey http://www.survey-monkey.com or SurveyGizmo http://www.surveygizmo.com) that allows researchers to develop and test their survey for free. This can give the survey developer the chance to evaluate the survey and do preliminary usability studies before paying a service provider. To date, it appears that SurveyMonkey is the only survey software that advertises compliance with Section 508 and provides guidelines for designing accessible surveys. Based on these advertisements, Wentz and Lazar (2009) developed their survey on SurveyMonkey but, during usability studies, found that it was inaccessible using JAWS screen-reader software. This is clearly an issue of being accessible, but not usable! For the final survey, they opted to use SurveyGizmo, which they found was more compliant with JAWS screen-reader software. When using readily available software to design surveys, it is important to ensure that accessibility issues are addressed and the survey is tested through usability studies before the final online survey is released.

Many online surveys are designed to simulate the paper-and-pen type of survey with small radio buttons and fonts (an example can be found in Figure 5.8). This allows the same questions to be asked in the same format they would have been asked, but in an online version. However, this approach does not take advantage of the potential simplifications in Web-based questionnaire designs that can enable greater access than can be achieved using standard forms.

OTHER CONSIDERATIONS WHEN DESIGNING WEB-BASED SURVEYS

The design of the survey Web pages must follow WCAG standards to allow independent access and to ensure that a variety of devices can be enabled. The use of Fitts's law and Hick-Hyman's law allows determination of the size of targets to reduce physical load. Development of surveys following these guidelines can enable access when a user is in a home environment where he or she is using a personal computer.

Which ethnicity best describes you?
- ☐ European
- ☐ Maori
- ☐ Pacific peoples
- ☐ Asian
- ☐ Middle Eastern/Latin American/African
- ☐ Other Ethnicity

Which of the following best describes your current student status?
- ○ Undergraduate
- ○ Diploma
- ○ Postgraduate

FIGURE 5.8   Sample questions from a Web-based questionnaire showing checkboxes and radio buttons. Note the difficulty in targeting one answer over another.

When designing a stand-alone questionnaire or survey that may be accessed in a public area, there are other considerations that must not be overlooked. The operating system on most computers can simplify the design of the interface to enable access (ease of access in Windows Vista, Windows accessibility options in XP, Mac OS X or Mac OS X Leopard). Incorporating these accessibility options in design can minimise the cost of hiring a designer, while still enabling accessibility. The following subsections detail a few items to keep in mind in the design of the survey.

The Graphical User Interface

Cursor size. The size of the cursor can be adjusted easily on all computers. Increasing the size of the cursor and choosing a cursor shape that is more easily recognised is important in display design. For instance, cross hairs (+) are more difficult to see than an arrow (↖). The larger the cursor size, the easier it is to use. A study by Durfee and Billingsley (1999) showed that for one of their clients, an increased cursor size allowed for better precision than a touch screen, even though the client had used a touch screen instead of a mouse for 2 years prior to the evaluation.

Font size. Although most individuals who require it can increase the font size as desired, a Web site or survey is much easier to use if the default font is sufficient to enable all users to read it effectively. Use the full screen for each question and increase the font to fill the screen.

Colour. The use of colour can appeal to many users, while preventing others from access. Although it may not be as visually appealing to design with black on white or white on black, it is easier to view than words superimposed over background wallpaper.

Scanning. Scanning is a method used by individuals who can only access one or two switches. The cursor systematically moves across the icons in a chosen mode, such as automatic (clicking a switch), inverse (holding a switch down and releasing) and step scanning (successive clicking). A questionnaire should be designed to allow for a scanning mode in which the movement of the cursor travels from one potential response to another. The respondent can then self-select a response by pressing a button, reducing the need for precision during mouse movement.

Feedback. Once an item in a questionnaire is selected, it is very important for the user to ensure that the selection was the intended selection. This is often achieved by changing the colour, changing the size and bolding the response (also addressed in WCAG standards). In addition to visual cues, the selected response should also be made available in an auditory form so the individual with visual difficulties or literacy problems can be assured of the response.

Screen readers. A screen reader interprets the information on the screen and converts the data into a usable format. It can be used to provide auditory information using text to speech for those individuals who have visual impairment or literacy difficulties and can be converted into Braille format for individuals who read Braille. Ensuring that all surveys meet WCAG or Section 508 standards allows screen readers to effectively interpret the information on the screen and minimise errors and frustration by the users of this technology.

Auditory output. Although screen readers can be used when an individual is at home, if the survey is to be accessed at another location, it is useful to design the survey with auditory output. Audio clips can be inserted to make questions more accessible to those with visual impairments or reading difficulties. The question can be read aloud into earpieces or headphones. Each possible response should be read as well, pausing between each to allow the user to understand the different choices. There should also be the option to move the mouse over a specific alternative to have that alternative repeated. Once the user has made a selection, it is very important for the selection to be confirmed with auditory feedback to ensure that the individual has selected the intended response.

Default mouse position. When designing a survey, the default mouse position is often not considered. Those individuals who have difficulty seeing a mouse will expect the cursor location to be the same from one Web page to the next. Keeping a standard position for the mouse also ensures ease of movement when attempting to select a response to a question. Following Fitts's law, putting the mouse at a default location that allows for ease of access to all responses (e.g., the centre) minimises physical load.

Touch screen. Although not usually considered due to the cost of the device, touch screens are useful in situations where individuals are not familiar with a computer mouse. The spatial mappings required to move a mouse which then moves a cursor on the screen may be difficult for some. Touch screens are becoming less expensive and can provide access to those individuals who have never used a mouse before or who have difficulty using a mouse or other accessibility device.

The Web-Based Survey

Length. While gathering as much information as physically possible is a researcher's dream, the individual responding to the questionnaire may easily become bored and want to move onto something else. This has the potential to skew the responses. Also, the longer the questionnaire, the greater potential for a computer error in which the computer freezes or the Internet connection is lost. Keeping the survey short will increase the response rate and decrease the error rate.

Randomization of answers. While not always easy to do, changing the order of responses reduces the possibility of skewed responses. This is more important in a list-type survey as those nearest the top or bottom (primacy and recency effects)

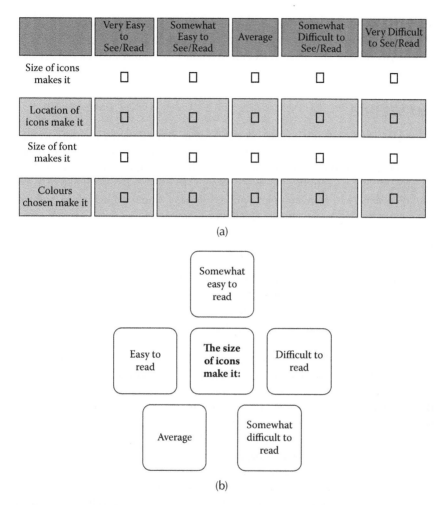

FIGURE 5.9   (a) Matrix question used to obtain a lot of information from one page of the survey. (b) A more accessible version of the matrix question requires that each question be asked on an independent Web page.

are more likely to be selected than other responses (Krosnick and Alwin 1987). If responses are spatially distributed around the question, this minimises skewed responses, but randomization may prevent it further.

Use simple questions rather than matrix questions. Matrix questions are those that ask a variety of questions with the same possible responses (Figure 5.9a). Simpler questions with the same responses from page to page are easier for an individual with accessibility problems to understand and to respond to (Figure 5.9b).

State the number of responses required; for example, 'select one' or 'select all that apply.' If individuals know how many responses they are supposed to be selecting, they can more easily prepare for the responses. For instance, for the question,

'Which accessibility options do you use most often? (Give one response),' an individual with a screen reader must listen to all responses and decide which one best fits, whereas if he or she must 'select all that apply,' the individual can select as the screen reader passes over each response.

CASE STUDIES

Accessibility and usability studies are essential in understanding the improvements that must be made to your own survey, but understanding the hurdles that other researchers have also had to overcome can simplify the design process as well. We now present four case studies that range from a simple survey distributed to a small population sample to more complex national surveys to understand where and when issues can arise during the survey development process.

PAPER-AND-PEN-BASED QUESTIONNAIRE OF ACCESS

Our research group recently conducted a pen-and-paper-based survey of computer access by youth with cerebral palsy. Our purpose was to determine how many individuals with cerebral palsy use computers, where they use computers, the type of assistive devices of which they are aware and how often they use assistive devices. We worked with several different researchers to develop the most concise questionnaire. This questionnaire was to be filled in by the caregiver, the individual and the researcher with the assistance of the individual. The end result, designed in New Zealand, was to fit on one A4 page. It was designed with 12-point font, but with little spacing between questions. For the researcher, and likely most parents, this questionnaire was relatively easy to fill in, but there were some issues, especially when the study was also conducted in Canada and the same questionnaire was to fit on one page, where the size of pages are 8.5 × 11 in. (shorter and wider). To get the same questionnaire on one page in Canada, it was necessary to decrease the font size, which made it more difficult to read. The resulting font size may have decreased response rate or accuracy of response by parents of youth with cerebral palsy as well as youth who were self-administering the questionnaire.

If instead of using a pen-and-paper-based survey, we had used an online Web-based version, the visual issues could have been easily addressed. Our branching diagram in Figure 5.2 can now be used to easily design the Web-based questionnaire. For each of the boxes, an individual Web page can be designed. This will result in a questionnaire that appears linear to the user, but changes dynamically depending on the answers. In total, there would be a maximum of 14 Web pages seen by the avid computer user who does not use a mouse but uses a variety of different assistive technologies (darkened boxes), or a minimum of 3 pages for those who have never used a computer and have no interest in doing so.

By using all the screen real estate, each question could be placed at the centre of the page with the default mouse position being in the question box and the possible responses around the outside (Figure 5.10). By using all the available space, the font size of the question and the responses could be maximised. Placing the response boxes around the question, the distance to a response is equal in all directions. According

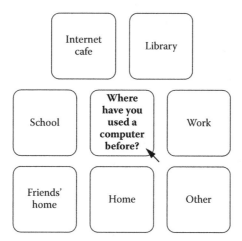

FIGURE 5.10   To make questions accessible, the font should be large and the objects well distributed. Placing the default cursor position at the centre of the screen allows for ease of targeting.

to Fitts's law and ISO standards, the ability to target any of the individual responses would require similar precision when using a mouse or a pointing device. Although some directions are more easily targeted than others (Radwin, Vanderheiden and Lin 1990; Davies, Stott and Ameratunga 2010), this approach attempts to minimise the physical load on the user as compared to a list. It provides minimal information on the screen so that a screen reader can easily read all options. Scanning software can simply and easily go from one response to another. By moving from a paper-and-pen-based survey to a Web-based survey, we allow accessibility by those individuals who cannot hold a pen, those with vision problems, those who rely on scanning and those who may have spastic movement. Rather than relying on a researcher or a parent/caregiver to respond on behalf of the individual, we can ask the questions directly to the individual themselves.

FMHS WEB SITE

An earlier example discussed the Faculty of Medical and Health Sciences Web site and the aspects in which it voluntarily conforms to WCAG accessibility standards. In addition to evaluating compliance with WCAG 2.0 (and New Zealand government) standards, we also surveyed students about usability and accessibility of the faculty and university Web sites. The main purposes of the survey were to determine usability of the FMHS Web site by students within the faculty and awareness of possible accessibility issues previously identified. We also sought to determine how many individuals were aware of accessibility controls as these students would be part of the healthcare community and should be aware of those options that may simplify the lives of individuals with access difficulties.

This survey was designed with SurveyGizmo (www.surveygizmo.com), a useful survey tool in this situation. Understanding the needs of the users is paramount in the design of Web-based surveys. We were seeking information from university students who required access to the Internet for online course selection. We are also aware of the biases against individuals with disabilities entering medicine and health sciences (Kailes and Shreve 2002; Manders 2006) and did not expect many (if any) to admit to having a disability. Based on this prior knowledge, we determined that SurveyGizmo would offer sufficient flexibility for our needs in this survey. This Web-based survey software had been used successfully by the faculty in the past for other surveys.

The Web-based survey itself took the form of a typical paper-and-pen-based survey with no dynamic branching. The narrator on Windows was able to read the responses and most questions within the survey, but there were some issues that were not considered in the planning stages. For example, for the question, 'What is/are the cause/s of your impairment?', the narrator reads 'What is slash are the cause slash "s" of your impairment?' An individual who can read the screen realises that the question is asking for the singular and the plural within the same statement, but the flow of the question is disrupted with the use of a screen reader. A better question might be, 'What is the cause of each of your impairments?' This allows the screen reader to maintain the flow of the question while allowing the responder to concentrate on the question without the requirement to further decipher what information is being requested.

Another important consideration is to keep the questions short and to the point. When requesting information about disabilities in our questionnaire, we described specific answers to questions in greater detail such as, 'Decreased agility (e.g., difficulty picking something up off the floor, difficulty dressing or using small objects like scissors, difficulty cutting up food, difficulty getting in and out of bed)'. While this information better describes the information requested, it also serves to cause difficulties. An individual using a screen reader must remember the first part of the answer and wait for the screen reader to pass over all the other parts of the answer. An individual using a magnifier must scan over the entire question as it cannot easily be seen in a given screen window. Ensuring that questions are kept short and easy to comprehend is important in questionnaire design.

The results of this survey showed that of those who responded, only 39% were aware of options within the operating system that enable access (ease of access in Windows Vista, Windows accessibility options in XP, Mac OS X or Mac OS X Leopard). Of those, 59% were aware of the onscreen keyboard, but only 16% were aware of serial keys or alternative input device options. As a starting point for ensuring accessibility of a new survey (before usability testing), the designer should ensure that access can be achieved using the various accessibility options within the operating system, for example, a narrator to read the text on the screen. These accessibility requirements should be addressed prior to the usability testing to ensure that the needs of all are paramount within the design.

YOUTH2000 AND YOUTH2007 SURVEYS

In New Zealand, population-based Youth surveys have been conducted using a Web-based format twice over the last 10 years to evaluate youths' perceptions of home life, school life, culture and ethnicity, injuries and violence, health and emotional health, food and activities, sexuality, substance use, neighbourhood and spirituality (Youth2000 2010). In 2001, the Youth2000 survey was conducted using standard desktops to collect data from students at schools across New Zealand. The number of individuals responding to this survey included 9699 youth in secondary schools. From the students' perspective, the benefits of a computer-assisted Web-based survey included privacy, enjoyment and honesty (Watson et al. 2001). From the perspective of the researchers, they were able to design a branched survey in which there were over 500 questions, but the students would only answer those that applied to them and would not see the other questions. This allowed the researchers to limit the participants' exposure to sensitive questions; participants were not presented with questions in areas where they had no experience (Watson et al. 2001). The dynamic nature of this survey catered to each individual, making the survey comprehensive yet personalized.

In 2007, the survey was upgraded to Nokia 770 tablets and 9107 youths participated. Many students preferred the Nokia tablets as compared to laptops because they perceived increased privacy and confidentiality, which enabled them to make more truthful responses (Denny et al. 2008). The Nokia 770 is a handheld device that is 5.5" × 3" and is activated by a stylus on a touch screen. The manual dexterity to hold the device while simultaneously clicking on icons is very difficult for an individual with upper limb impairment. A desktop version of the survey was available for those individuals who could not access the Nokia tablet, but no information has been reported with regard to the number of individuals who accessed the questionnaire with a desktop version. Of those who were invited to complete the survey but chose not to, 41 individuals were unable to do so due to lack of computer access or language barriers (Adolescent Health Research Group 2008), and no data were available about another 740 who chose not to participate. It is believed that individuals who do not respond to surveys often have worse health and well-being than those who do complete surveys (Adolescent Health Research Group 2008). Of the students who did complete the survey, 448 reported that they had a chronic disability but this was not broken down further to give an indication of how many might have upper limb difficulties or visual impairment.

In addition to the size of the tablet, there were several other aspects that influenced the design and possibly the response rate for this survey. One of the main barriers to completion for this survey was the amount of time to complete the survey. This Web-based questionnaire required a mean time of 70 to 80 min for completion, with some completing the survey in 20 to 30 min while others required 120 to 130 min. The time commitment required to complete the survey possibly decreased the number of potential participants in the survey.

The interface design on the survey went through several iterations and was generally very inclusive. Only one question was asked per page. If the question was not answered, another page indicated that the question had not been answered, but permitted the individual to continue to the next question if he or she did not wish to answer the question. Auditory output was given to those who required additional assistance with reading or needed information in addition to the visual cues.

However, some problems with accessibility did exist that, had they been addressed, might have enabled additional individuals to participate in the survey. First, a mouse (or input device) was required for completion of the questionnaire. Keyboard inputs and scanning could not be used. Second, the question always started at the top left corner of the page, but the button to move to the next question, the 'GO' button, was in the far right corner. This resulted in an ID of 6, which, from ISO guidelines, indicates a requirement for relatively high precision. For those with motor control issues, this is very difficult to achieve. Also, once a selection was made, a check was placed in the selection box and an auditory icon (click) indicated that a response had been selected. However, there was no auditory feedback about which response had been selected. When using the narrator on a Windows system, a response was deselected using the same auditory icon as was heard when selection occurred. As such, the individual would not be sure whether the icon was selected until he or she attempted to move to the next page. While considerable time and effort were taken to ensure usability (Watson et al. 2001) and some effort was made to ensure accessibility, the investigators did not discuss testing the interface with individuals with disabilities before the final survey was administered. It is possible that the investigators in the Youth2000 survey inadvertently excluded disabled participants by virtue of the survey design characteristics. A key lesson from this survey is that, to be truly representative of the population, population-based surveys must employ interface design that enables universal accessibility.

2010 CENSUS

As we have seen from the Youth2000 questionnaire, the ability to effectively design a survey that allows accessibility requires testing with many different populations. One of the largest surveys typically held is the census of population. Several countries have facilitated online reporting for census information, including Canada (Statistics Canada 2006), New Zealand (Statistics New Zealand 2006), Singapore and Australia (Castro 2008), but the United States is still not ready to do so (U.S. Census Bureau 2010). Other countries do not appear to report on the usability testing prior to implementation of these online census surveys, but the trials and tribulations associated with getting an effective, accessible online census in the United States have been documented. This last case study reflects the usability issues that became apparent during the 2000 U.S. census, which did allow for online responses and the further usability and accessibility testing efforts by the United States Bureau of the Census in the lead up to the 2010 census.

In the United States, a census is held every 10 years (Murphy, Malakhoff and Coon 2007) and has typically been reported through census takers or mailing a paper version. The Paperwork Reduction Act of 1995 (chapter 35 of title 44, United States Code) requires that efforts be made to work toward conducting these surveys online. In the year 2000, the census was available to some online, but as it was considered experimental, only a small portion of the population was able to complete it online (Whitworth 2001). Abandonment of the intended online version of the 2000 census in early 1998 and then its reinstatement in the fall of 1998 provided the single Web site developer minimal time to design and implement the online version (Whitworth 2001). As a result, the final version closely simulated the paper version, was only available for the short form of the survey and was only available in English. Accessibility in the form of WCAG standards (changes to Section 508 were not enacted at that time) was attempted in the design. Usability testing at the National Foundation for the Blind showed that screen readers were unable to effectively interpret the information on the census form (Murphy 2005). On the actual census day, 90,000 attempts were made to respond online, but a mere 66,163 were successful. The majority of errors reported included an inability to log in with the correct 22 digit ID code, which was placed in an obscure position (underneath a bar code) on the original census documentation, and attempts to use the system for the long form of the census (Whitworth 2001; Murphy 2005; Murphy, Malakhoff and Coon 2007).

Since then considerable efforts have been made in the development of an online version of the form to allow everyone the opportunity to report online. In preparation for the proposed online version of the 2010 census, it was identified that a requirements specification was needed that included usability and accessibility followed by iterative testing (Murphy 2005). One of these key requirements was to ensure adherence to the Section 508 requirements. Usability studies conducted by the Statistical Research Division of the U.S. Bureau of the Census have attempted to integrate accessibility into the design of the census from the initial design stages. This has included the procurement of software to test general compliance with Section 508 and enable corrections as well as a test facility with JAWS screen-reader software. The Statistical Research Division found, however, that certain aspects of Section 508 also have to be checked manually (e.g., HTML for all images must have appropriate alternative text ALT or Longdesc tags) (Murphy, Malakhoff and Coon 2007). An accessibility specialist separately verifies each of the fields with a screen reader, ensuring the ability to use up and down arrow keys, the ability to tab to each field both forward and backward, and match between the vocalization and the words on the form.

Through usability testing of the census, several recommendations have been suggested (Murphy, Malakhoff and Coon 2007). Although the census did conform to Section 508 when tested for accessibility, the interface was found not to be usable in certain situations. Suggestions based on usability testing included the provision of a separate 'help' window for each 'help topic' as a help window with scrolling text was found to be difficult to use. This would simplify the task both for individuals with visual impairments and for those with full vision who had difficulty figuring out where the information was within the help page. Another recommendation was the use of complete information in the alternative text (ALT text). Usability testing showed that 'MI' used to represent Middle Initial was difficult to understand and abbreviations should be spelled out. Other recommendations included ensuring that checkboxes were correctly labelled, and giving an indication of the amount of space available for answering an open text type (fill in the blank) question. These recommendations were a few of many given after the second round of usability testing of the census form (Murphy, Malakhoff and Coon 2007).

Based on the usability studies by the U.S. Bureau of the Census, one can understand the importance of designing for access prior to conducting usability studies.

Both usability issues and access issues can then be addressed, concurrently minimizing the need for additional testing.

While there is evidence that mixed surveys receive a greater response than do single-mode surveys (Greenlaw and Brown-Welty 2009), the 2010 census was still not available in an online format (U.S. Census Bureau 2010; Castro 2008). Although a large amount of testing went into the design of a possible 2010 online census, there are still concerns that response rate will not be increased and that costs will not be reduced (Castro 2008). For individuals who are unable to access the written census, an enumerator will be required to visit their home. While the argument may be made that they will be given the same opportunities as others to complete the census, they must do so in the presence of another individual who is not known to them. This decreases privacy and increases discomfort. Consideration must be given to these members of our society who are required to complete these forms, but cannot access the form as it is issued.

CONCLUSIONS

To design an effective Web-based survey, one must consider all aspects of the design. The questions themselves must be evaluated cognitively as they would in a paper-and-pen-based survey. The Web pages themselves must conform to the WCAG (or Section 508) standards to ensure accessibility. The interface must reduce physical load requirements as much as possible by minimizing both the required task precision in targeting the answers and the number of response alternatives. Once the design of the survey adheres to these accessibility guidelines, further usability testing must be undertaken by a subset of the group that will be surveyed. Changes to the survey design must be undertaken and both accessibility and usability testing repeated. The design of an effective survey is an iterative process that can ensure universal access. By moving from pen-and-paper-based surveys to Web-based surveys for youth with disabilities, we can increase response rate, allow all individuals to access the questionnaire by themselves and enable truthful responses.

REFERENCES

Adolescent Health Research Group. 2008. Youth'07: The health and wellbeing of secondary school students in New Zealand, Technical report. Auckland: The University of Auckland.

Angus Reid Global Monitor. www.angus-reid.com (accessed January 10, 2010).

Avery, R.J., W.K. Bryant, A. Mathios, H.J. Kang, and D. Bell. 2006. Electronic course evaluations: Does an online delivery system influence student evaluations? *Journal of Economic Education* 37(1):21–37.

Bakaev, M. 2008. Fitts' law for older adults: Considering a factor of age. In *Proceedings of the VIII Brazilian Symposium on Human Factors in Computing Systems*. Porto Alegre, RS, Brazil: Sociedade Brasileira de Computação. pp. 260–263.

Benyon, D., A. Crerar, and S. Wilkinson. 2000. Individual differences and inclusive design. In *User interfaces for all: Concepts, methods, and tools*, C. Stephanidis, Ed. Boca Raton, FL: CRC/Taylor and Francis.

Cakir, A.E. 2009. Accessibility in information technology. In *Industrial engineering and ergonomics*, C.M. Schlick, Ed. Berlin: Springer-Verlag.

Card, S.K., W.K. English, and B.J. Burr. 1978. Evaluation of mouse, rate-controlled isometric joystick, step keys, and text keys for text selection on a CRT. *Ergonomics* 21(8):601–613.

Card, S.K. 2010. User Interface Research. http://www2.parc.com/istl/projects/uir/people/stuart/stuart.htm (accessed January 10, 2010.)

Castro, D. 2008. e-Census unplugged: Why Americans should be able to complete the census online. http://www.itif.org/files/eCensusUnplugged.pdf. (Accessed August 13, 2010.)

Class Settlement Agreement and Release: *National Federation of the Blind, the National Federation of the Blind of California v. Target Corporation.* http://www.nfbtargetlawsuit.com/final-settlement-and-commerce-clause (accessed July 2010).

Clemence, T.G. 1985. Historical perspectives on the decennial census. *Government Information Quarterly* 2(4):355–368.

Conell, B.R., M. Jones, R. Mace, J. Mueller, A. Mullick, E. Ostroff, J. Sanford, E. Steinfeld, M. Story, and G. Vanderheiden. 1997. *The principles of universal design.* Raleigh, NC: The Center for Universal Design, N.C. State University. http://www.design.ncsu.edu/cud/pubs_p/docs/UDPMD.pdf (accessed January 10, 2010).

Converse, J.M., and S. Presser. 1986. *Survey questions: Handcrafting the standard questionnaire.* Newbury Park, CA: Sage Publications.

Copley, J., and J. Ziviani. 2004. Barriers to the use of assistive technology for children with multiple disabilities. *Occupational Therapy International* 11(4):229–243.

Davies, T.C., S. Mudge, S.N. Ameratunga, and N.S. Stott. 2010. Enabling self-directed computer use for individuals with cerebral palsy: A systematic review of assistive devices and technologies. *Developmental Medicine & Child Neurology* Published online January 5, 2010 (article online in advance of print).

Davies, T.C., N.S. Stott, and S.N. Ameratunga. 2010. How is cursor control related to MACS levels during computer use by youth with cerebral palsy? *Developmental Medicine & Child Neurology* 52(S2). p. 58.

Davis, R.E., M.P. Couper, N.K. Janz, C.H. Caldwell, and K. Resnicow. 2009. Interviewer effects in public health surveys. *Health Education Research* 25(1):14–26.

de Haan, J., M. Duimel, and P. Valkenburg. 2007. National Report for the Netherlands. Opportunities experienced by children online. http://www2.lse.ac.uk/media@/se/research/EUKidsOnline/EU9620Kids%201/Reports/wP3NationalReportNetherlands.pdf (Accessed August 13, 2010) 1:52.

de Leeuw, E.D. 2005. To mix or not to mix data collection modes in surveys. *Journal of Official Statistics* 21(2):233–255.

DeBell, M., and C. Chapman. 2006. Computer and Internet use by children and adolescents in 2003 [electronic resource] Washington, D.C.: Department of Education. U.S. National Center for Education Statistics.

Denny, S.J., T.L. Milfont, J. Utter, E.M. Robinson, S.N. Ameratunga, S.N. Merry, T.M. Fleming, and P.D. Watson. 2008. Hand-held Internet tablets for school-based data collection. *Biomedical Central Research Notes* 1(52).

Durfee, J.L., and F.F. Billingsley. 1999. A comparison of two computer input devices for uppercase letter matching. *The American Journal of Occupational Therapy* 53(2):214–220.

Edmonston, B., and C. Schultze, Eds. 1995. *Modernizing the U.S. Census.* Washington D.C.: National Academy Press.

Edwards, P.J., I. Roberts, M.J. Clarke, C. DiGuiseppi, R. Wentz, I. Kwan, R. Cooper, L.M. Felix, and S. Pratap. 2009. Methods to increase response to postal and electronic questionnaires. *Cochrane Database of Systematic Reviews* (3):MR000008.

Ellis, J.B. 2007. The digital divide in special education. *ISATT 2007 Conference Proceedings.* http://www.isatt.org/conference_proceedi.htm.

Fitts, P.M. 1954. The information capacity of the human motor system in controlling the amplitude of movement. *Journal of Experimental Psychology* 47(6):381–391.

Fitts, P.M., and J.R. Peterson. 1964. Information capacity of discrete motor responses. *Journal of Experimental Psychology* 67:103–112.

Gordon, J.S., and R. McNew. 2008. Developing the online survey. *Nursing Clinics of North America* 43(4):605–619.

Government Technology Services and Department of Internal Affairs. 2010. New Zealand Government Web Standards 2.0. http://www.webstandards.govt.nz/new-zealand-government-web-standards-2/ (accessed January 10 2010).

Grant, S., T.L. Milfont, R. Herd, and S. Denny. 2010. Health and well being of a diverse student population: The Youth2000 surveys of New Zealand secondary school students and their implications for educators. In *Delving into diversity: An international exploration of issues of diversity in education.* V. Green and S. Cherrington, Eds. New York: Nova Science Publishers, Inc. pp. 185–193.

Greenlaw, C., and S. Brown-Welty. 2009. A comparison of web-based and paper-based survey methods testing assumptions of survey mode and response cost. *Evaluation Review* 33(5):464–480.

Guiard, Y., and M. Beaudouin-Lafon. 2004. Fitts' law 50 years later: Applications and contributions from human-computer interaction — Preface. *International Journal of Human-Computer Studies* 61(6):747–750.

Hick, W.E. 1952. On the rate of gain of information. *Quarterly Journal of Experimental Psychology* 4:11–26.

Holbrook, A.L., J.A. Krosnick, and A. Pfent. 2007. The causes and consequences of response rates in surveys by the news media and government contractor survey research firms. In *Advances in telephone survey methodology*, J.M. Lepkowski, C. Tucker, J.M. Brick, E.D. de Leeuw, L. Japec, P.J. Lavrakas, M.W. Link, and R.L. Sangster, Eds. New York: John Wiley & Sons.

Hyman, R. 1953. Stimulus information as a determinant of reaction time. *Journal of Experimental Psychology* 45(3):188–196.

International Telecommunications Union. 2008. Free statistics, by country. ICT Eye. http://www.itu.int/ITU-D/icteye/Reporting/ShowReportFrame.aspx?ReportName=/WTI/InformationTechnologyPublic&RP_intYear=2008&RP_intLanguageID=1 (accessed January 10, 2010).

Jobe, J.B. 2003. Cognitive psychology and self-reports: Models and methods. *Quality of Life Research* 12(3):219–227.

Kabbash, P., I.S. Mackenzie, and W. Buxton. 1993. Human performance using computer input devices in the preferred and non-preferred hands. *Proceedings of INTERCHI'93 Conference on Human Factors in Computing Systems* 474–481 Amsterdam, The Netherlands.

Kaczmirek, L., and K.G. Wolff. 2007. Survey design for visually impaired and blind people. Universal access in human computer interaction: Coping with diversity, Part 1, HCII 2007, *Lecture Notes in Computer Science* 4554:374–381

Kailes, J.I., and M. Shreve. 2002. Thomas E. Strax, MD, Doctor, Physiatrist, Administrator, Executive. http://www.westernu.edu/xp/edu/cdihp/cdihp-resources-profiles-strax.xml (accessed January 10, 2010).

Keeter, S., C. Kennedy, M. Dimock, J. Best, and P. Craighill. 2006. Gauging the impact of growing nonresponse on estimates from a national RDD telephone survey. *Public Opinion Quarterly* 70(5):759–779.

Kellerman, S.E., and J. Herold. 2001. Physician response to surveys — A review of the literature. *American Journal of Preventive Medicine* 20(1):61–67.

Krosnick, J.A., and D.F. Alwin. 1987. An evaluation of a cognitive theory of response-order effects in survey measurement. *Public Opinion Quarterly* 51(2):201–219.

Lathouwers, K., J. de Moor, and R. Didden. 2009. Access to and use of Internet by adolescents who have a physical disability: A comparative study. *Research in Developmental Disabilities* 30(4):702–711.

Layne, B.H., J.R. DeCristoforo, and D. McGinty. 1999. Electronic versus traditional student ratings of instruction. *Research in Higher Education* 40(2):221–232.

Link, M.W., and A.H. Mokdad. 2005a. Alternative modes for health surveillance surveys: An experiment with web, mail, and telephone. *Epidemiology* 16(5):701–704.

Link, M.W., and A.H. Mokdad. 2005b. Effects of survey mode on self-reports of adult alcohol consumption: A comparison of mail, web and telephone approaches. *Journal of Studies on Alcohol and Drugs* 66(2):239–245.

Mackenzie, I.S., and W. Buxton. 1994. Prediction of pointing and dragging times in graphical user interfaces. *Interacting with Computers* 6(2):213–227.

MacKenzie, I.S. 1992. Fitts' law as a research and design tool in human-computer interaction. *Human-Computer Interaction* 7:91–139.

Man, D.W.K., and M.S.L. Wong. 2007. Evaluation of computer-access solutions for students with quadriplegic athetoid cerebral palsy. *American Journal of Occupational Therapy* 61(3):355–364.

Manders, K. 2006. Disabled medicine. *Canadian Medical Association Journal* 174(11): 1585–1586.

McFarland, D.J., W.A. Sarnacki, and J.R. Wolpaw. 2003. Brain-computer interface (BCI) operation: Optimizing information transfer rates. *Biological Psychology* 63(3):237–251.

Media Awareness Network. 2009. *Young Canadians in wired world.* http://www.media-awareness.ca/english/research/ycww/phaseII/key_findings.cfm (accessed January 10, 2010).

Michaels, C., F. Prezant, S.M. Morabito, and K. Jackson. 2002. Assistive and instructional technology for students with disabilities: A national snapshot of postsecondary service providers. *Journal of Special Education Technology* 17(1):8.

Molich, R., and J. Nielsen. 1990. Improving a human-computer dialogue. *Communications of the ACM* 33(3):338–348.

Murphy, E. 2005. Steps toward integrating accessibility into development of an Internet option for the 2010 U.S. census. Washington D.C.: Statistical Research Division, U.S. Bureau of the Census.

Murphy, E., L. Malakhoff, and D. Coon. 2007. Evaluating the usability and accessibility of an online form for census data collection. In *Universal usability: Designing computer interfaces for diverse user populations*, J. Lazar, Ed. Chichester, England: John Wiley & Sons, Ltd.

Nielsen, J. 1994. Enhancing the explanatory power of usability heuristics. In *Proceedings of the SIGCHI conference on human factors in computing systems: Celebrating interdependence.* Boston, MA: ACM.

Norris, M.L. 2007. HEADSS up: Adolescents and the Internet. *Paediatrics & Child Health* 12(3):211–216.

Out-law.com. 2007. Computer-based exam discriminated against blind candidate: US company found liable under UK law. http://www.theregister.co.uk/2007/01/25/computer_based_exam_discriminated_against_blind_candidate/page3.html (accessed January 10, 2010).

Pealer, L.N., R.M. Weiler, R.M. Pigg, Jr., D. Miller, and S.M. Dorman. 2001. The feasibility of a Web-based surveillance system to collect health risk behavior data from college students. *Health Education & Behavior* 28(5):547–559.

Radwin, R.G., G.C. Vanderheiden, and M.L. Lin. 1990. A method for evaluating head-controlled computer input devices using Fitts' law. *Human Factors* 32(4):423–438.

Rao, R.S., R. Seliktar, and T. Rahman. 2000. Evaluation of an isometric and a position joystick in a target acquisition task for individuals with cerebral palsy. *IEEE Transactions on Rehabilitation Engineering* 8(1):118–125.

Rew, L., S.D. Horner, L. Riesch, and R. Cauvin. 2004. Computer-assisted survey interviewing of school-age children. *ANS Advances in Nursing Science* 27(2):129–137.

Rhodes, S.D., D.A. Bowie, and K.C. Hergenrather. 2003. Collecting behavioural data using the World Wide Web: Considerations for researchers. *Journal of Epidemiological Community Health* 57(1):68–73.

Schmidt, W.C. 1997. World Wide Web survey research: Benefits, potential problems, and solutions. *Behavior Research Methods Instruments & Computers* 29(2):274–279.

Smits-Engelsman, B.C.M., E.A.A. Rameckers, and J. Duysens. 2007. Children with congenital spastic hemiplegia obey Fitts' law in a visually guided tapping task. *Experimental Brain Research* 177(4):431–439.

Statistics Canada. 2006. Nearly one in five households completed their census questionnaire online. http://www12.statcan.ca/census-recensement/2006/ref/info/online-en_ligne-eng.cfm (accessed January 10, 2010).

Statistics New Zealand. 2006. New Zealand Census – 2006 and looking forward. *11th Meeting of the Heads of National Statistical Offices of East Asian Countries.* Tokyo, Japan.

Survey Gizmo. 2005. www.surveygizmo.com (accessed January 10, 2010).

Survey Monkey. 1999. www.surveymonkey.com (accessed January 10, 2010).

Sutter, E., and J.D. Klein. 2007. Internet surveys with adolescents: Promising methods and methodologic challenges. *Adolescent Medicine: State of the Art Reviews* 18(2):293–304.

Theofanos, M.F., and J. Redish. 2003. Bridging the gap: Between accessibility and usability. *Interactions* 10(6):36–51.

U.S. Census Bureau. 2010. *United States Census 2010: It's in our hands.* http://2010.census.gov/2010census/how/questions.php (accessed January 10, 2010).

United States Congress. 1998. Section 508 (29 U.S.C. ' 794d), Subpart 1194.22: Web-based intranet and Internet information and application. www.section508.gov (accessed January 10, 2010).

University of Auckland. 2010. Faculty of Medical and Health Sciences. http://www.fmhs.auckland.ac.nz/ (accessed January 10, 2010).

Watson, P.D., S.J. Denny, V. Adair, S.N. Ameratunga, T.C. Clark, S.M. Crengle, R.S. Dixon, M. Fa'asisila, S.N. Merry, E.M. Robinson, and A.A. Sporle. 2001. Adolescents' perceptions of a health survey using multimedia computer-assisted self-administered interview. *Australian and New Zealand Journal of Public Health* 25(6):520–524.

Webb, P.M., G.D. Zimet, J.D. Fortenberry, and M.J. Blythe. 1999. Comparability of a computer-assisted versus written method for collecting health behavior information from adolescent patients. *Journal of Adolescent Health* 24(6):383–388.

Wells, J., L. Lewis, and B. Greene. 2006. Internet access in U.S. public schools and classrooms: 1994–2005. U.S. Department of Education National Center for Education Statistics.

Wentz, B., and J. Lazar. 2009. Email accessibility and social networking. *Online Communities and Social Computing, Proceedings* 5621:134–140.

Whitworth, E. 2001. Implementation and results of the Internet response mode for Census 2000. Paper read at *Annual Meeting of the American Statistical Association,* Montreal, Quebec.

Williams, J.A. 1968. Interviewer role performance — further note on bias in information interview. *Public Opinion Quarterly* 32(2):287–294.

World Wide Web Consortium. 2010. *Web Content Accessibility Guidelines (WCAG) 2.0.* http://www.w3.org/TR/WCAG/ (accessed January 10, 2010).

Young, N.L., J.W. Varni, L. Snider, A. McCormick, B. Sawatzky, M. Scott, G. King, R. Hetherington, E. Sears, and D. Nicholas. 2009. The Internet is valid and reliable for child-report: An example using the Activities Scale for Kids (ASK) and the Pediatric Quality of Life Inventory (PedsQL). *Journal of Clinical Epidemiology* 62(3):314–320.

Youth2000. 2010. http://www.youth2000.ac.nz/survey-tools-1106.htm (accessed January 10, 2010).

Zhang, X.A., and I.S. MacKenzie. 2007. Evaluating eye tracking with ISO 9241 — Part 9. *Human-Computer Interaction, Pt 3, Proceedings* 4552:779–788.

6 Paediatric Seating

Eric Tam

CONTENTS

INTRODUCTION

Sitting is the most common posture adopted in daily living. At around 4 months of age, healthy infants achieve their first sitting experience and, by 7 months, a child gains stability and is able to sit unsupported in an upright posture (Knobloch and Pasamanick 1975). This position allows the child to explore the environment and progress in other areas of gross motor development. For children with neurological deficits and musculoskeletal dysfunctions, proper sitting becomes challenging. Physical limitations including joint instability, muscle weakness and tonal abnormalities affect postural control and movement. These limitations also lead to many other secondary complications such as skeletal deformities, contractures, pressure ulcers and back pain (Pope 2002). The complications not only can impact sitting comfort, but may also affect the functional performance of the child, including his or her ability to communicate with others. Furthermore, severe skeletal deformities can affect cardiopulmonary function, which can be life threatening if not properly managed (Stewart 1991).

Sitting balance is controlled through a complex neuromuscular system. To assist individuals with neuromuscular deficits to maintain a functional sitting position, combinations of external postural support devices (PSDs) and/or orthoses can be used. Depending on the severity of the impairment, these PSDs and/or orthoses are used to provide corrective forces to restore skeletal alignment, to prevent structural deformities and facilitate body movements, or to accommodate body deformities to preserve skin integrity. Proper positioning can also increase sitting comfort, reduce dependence, prevent or delay progressive deformities, and improve physiological performance, communication, education and self-esteem (Trefler et al. 1993). Furthermore, the care of children with seating needs is made easier when they are safely positioned.

The goals of seating for children vary depending on their disability and stage of development (i.e., infancy, juvenility and adolescence). The most common paediatric populations requiring special/adaptive seating are those suffering from cerebral palsy, other neuromuscular diseases and spinal disorders. Specific objectives and considerations can be identified to meet the needs of each of these groups. Moreover, among all the seating objectives that are identified by a seating team, it is important that the child's needs are prioritised. The success of special/adaptive seating interventions requires input from many disciplines. A team approach is usually adopted by seating clinics around the world, to address the specific concerns of each client. This seating team typically consists of a combination of specialists that may include a paediatric orthopaedic surgeon, an occupational therapist, a physiotherapist, an orthotist, a rehabilitation engineer, a rehabilitation nurse, a social worker, a caregiver and the client's family members (Barlow et al. 2009; Peischl et al. 2005). The process of prescribing and fitting a paediatric user with a seating system is continuous. The needs of children change as they grow and so body support components must be adjusted, modified and replaced to meet these ever-changing demands until the child reaches skeletal maturity.

This chapter aims to provide the reader with an overview of seating principles for children with disabilities, with a focus on the rehabilitation engineering perspectives to consider in the design and implementation of special/adaptive seating systems. The overall organization of the chapter is depicted schematically in Figure 6.1. Following a brief introduction to the origins of special/adaptive seating, key seating principles are discussed. The seating challenges presented by children with neuromotor deficits are described, typical seating goals are identified, and some basic biomechanics of body support are presented. Next, the procedures for seating assessment are detailed, and important considerations for the design of special/adaptive

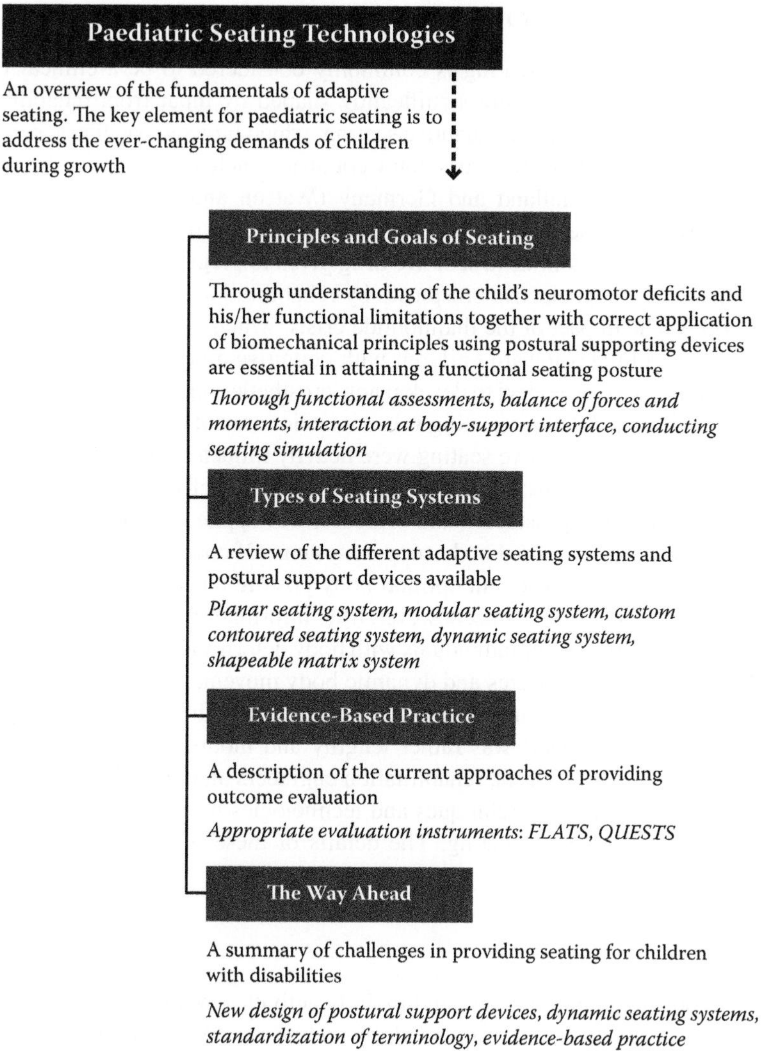

Paediatric Seating Technologies

An overview of the fundamentals of adaptive
seating. The key element for paediatric seating is to
address the ever-changing demands of children
during growth

Principles and Goals of Seating

Through understanding of the child's neuromotor deficits and
his/her functional limitations together with correct application
of biomechanical principles using postural supporting devices
are essential in attaining a functional seating posture

*Thorough functional assessments, balance of forces and
moments, interaction at body-support interface, conducting
seating simulation*

Types of Seating Systems

A review of the different adaptive seating systems and
postural support devices available

*Planar seating system, modular seating system, custom
contoured seating system, dynamic seating system,
shapeable matrix system*

Evidence-Based Practice

A description of the current approaches of providing
outcome evaluation

Appropriate evaluation instruments: FLATS, QUESTS

The Way Ahead

A summary of challenges in providing seating for children
with disabilities

*New design of postural support devices, dynamic seating systems,
standardization of terminology, evidence-based practice*

FIGURE 6.1   A roadmap depicting the organization of this chapter.

seating are discussed. Specific areas pertaining to seating designs for which there
are gaps in the literature are emphasised herein. The reader is then introduced to the
different types of seating systems available, and some of the strengths and weaknesses of these designs. As the chapter nears its end, the steps of service delivery and
challenges in this area are presented, followed by a review of outcome measures that
have been used to assess special/adaptive seating. In closing, the trends and on-going
developments in paediatric seating are summarised, and recommendations are made
for further improvement in the field.

EARLY DEVELOPMENT OF SPECIAL/ADAPTIVE SEATING

Although special/adaptive seating is commonly considered to be a clinical issue, its origin and development were significantly shaped by input from rehabilitation engineers. The original work in adaptive seating, which targeted paediatric services, started almost simultaneously across many countries, including Canada, the United States, Great Britain, Holland and Germany (Watson and Woods 2005). In the 1960s, a drastic increase of children with severe congenital limb deficiencies, due to the side effects of thalidomide (a sedative drug given to pregnant women), expedited the development of myoelectric prostheses by rehabilitation engineers (Watson and Woods 2005). The impact of the thalidomide crisis, which increased awareness and changed social attitudes toward children with cognitive and physical impairments, also triggered service providers to develop non-prosthetic solutions to meet the needs of affected children. Adaptive seating was one major area of development.

The early works of adaptive seating were heavily influenced by the field of prosthetics and orthotics (Watson and Woods 2005). Plaster-of-Paris, used to capture body shape for making prostheses and orthoses, was applied to create the required cast for fabricating a contoured body support system. Of course, to successfully create a suitable seat for the user, an optimal body posture must be established before capturing body shape. At the time, however, little information was available concerning the correct positioning of individuals with body deformities and tonal abnormalities. Moreover, postural reflexes and dynamic body movements further complicated the process of establishing an optimal sitting posture. The time required to fabricate a contoured seating support was rather lengthy and modification of the cast was not easy. Over the past decades, rehabilitation engineers and therapists have worked together to develop various techniques and technologies for assessment, simulation and fabrication of adaptive seating. The details of these innovations will be discussed later in the chapter.

PRINCIPLES OF SEATING

Sitting is a posture commonly adopted in daily activities. Many of us spend a great deal of time sitting during learning, working and leisure. While sitting may be misunderstood as a static posture, it is in fact rather dynamic. Braton (1966) points out that a seated individual is 'not merely an inert bag of bones, dumped for a time in the seat, but a live organism in a dynamic state of continuous activity.' Sitting in a fixed posture causes muscle fatigue and limits the body's ability to perform functional tasks (Zacharkow 1988). Instead, postural changes in sitting are frequently made to prevent tissue distress. Linder-Ganz (2005) conducted a study on healthy adults to examine the frequency and extent of spontaneous motion to relieve tissue loads during sitting. They found that average weight shifting occurs every 6 to 9 min. There is also evidence to suggest that postural responses to sitting could be gender-based and that the choices of interventions to prevent fatigue and injury during prolonged sitting should be carefully considered (Dunk and Callaghan 2005). Specifically, seating individuals with disabilities should be considered from two perspectives: clinical and technological. Clinically, in addition to ergonomic considerations, deformities and muscle weaknesses as well as changes in postural alignment and abnormal movement patterns resulting from tonal and reflex abnormalities all need to be considered. Technologically, the availability of suitable PSDs that can be used and integrated into a seating system, to hold the body in a balanced and functional posture, is also essential.

Children who cannot ambulate effectively due to injury or disease should be considered for a proper seat and mobility base as soon after diagnosis as possible. The earlier the seating intervention, the higher the chances that further skeletal deformities (e.g., scoliosis, hip dislocations, joint contractures, etc.) may be prevented or minimised (Alexander et al. 2006). To guide the development of this intervention, a thorough physical assessment is needed to identify each child's unique conditions and limitations. An overview of the steps to follow in conducting such a seating assessment is provided later in this chapter. Finally, given that children grow rapidly, even after the implementation of an adaptive seating intervention, it is important that a child's postures and prescribed supports be reviewed regularly to ensure that effective treatment is maintained.

NEUROMOTOR SYMPTOMS

Children with seating needs often present with neuromotor symptoms including tone and muscle imbalance, abnormal reflexes, deformities, impaired sitting balance and uncoordinated movements (Trefler et al. 1993). Muscle tone refers to the resistance of muscles to passive elongation or stretch. Proper muscle tone helps to maintain posture. However, when tone is abnormal, it affects seating, positioning and movement. Abnormal muscle tone may be the result of injury to, or dysfunction of, motor pathways of the brain or spinal cord (Ham et al. 1998). Muscle tone can be classified as flaccid (absence of tone), hypotonic (decreased tone), normal, hypertonic (increased tone) and rigid (stiff/no movement) (Brooks 1986). Hypotonia, which presents as 'floppiness,' is commonly seen in clients with lower motor neuron lesions such as spina bifida, low-level spinal cord injury and amyotrophic lateral sclerosis (ALS). Hypertonia is commonly seen with cerebral palsy (CP), stroke (CVA), traumatic brain injury (TBI) and spinal cord injury (SCI). In these latter patient populations, an increase in muscle tone in the extremities and low muscle tone in the trunk makes voluntary movement of the limbs difficult. There are different kinds of hypertonia: spasticity, dystonia and rigidity (Sanger et al. 2003). Spasticity is the velocity-dependent increase in resistance of a muscle to stretching and can vary depending on external stimuli and an individual's state of alertness, posture and activity. Dystonia refers to involuntary muscle spasm, which presents with abnormal postures, twisting and repetitive movements (Sanger et al. 2003). The characteristic postures of dystonia include, for example, elbow and wrist flexion with the hand near the body, turning of the neck, inversion at the ankle and facial contortions (Tarsy and Simon 2006). Rigidity refers to a condition in which muscle on both sides of the joint is activated simultaneously, causing a stiff extended limb.

Healthy newborn babies have primitive reflexes (e.g., grasp, crawl, step and tonic neck reflexes) that disappear at different stages of infancy (Knobloch and Pasamanick

1975). A reflex is an involuntary movement response to a stimulus. The presence of abnormal reflexes can alter movement patterns and cause abnormal posture. Children with CP often display asymmetric tonic neck reflex (ATNR), symmetric tonic neck reflex (STNR), tonic labyrinthine reflex-supine (TLRS) and tonic labyrinthine reflex-prone (TLRP). ATNR is elicited when the head is laterally rotated. The limbs go into extension on the face side and flexion on the skull side. There is lateral pelvic obliquity (down on the skull side) and flexion of the trunk (convex on the skull side) (Trefler et al. 1993). STNR is elicited with flexion or extension of the neck. When the neck is flexed, the upper extremities go into flexion and the lower extremities go into extension. The pelvis is tilted posteriorly and the trunk adopts a kyphotic posture. In contrast, when the head is extended, the upper extremities go into extension and the lower extremities go into flexion. In most of these cases, the pelvis remains posteriorly tilted and the trunk stays in a kyphotic posture (Trefler et al. 1993). TLRS and TLRP are elicited when the head is posteriorly or anteriorly tilted from the upright position. During sitting, an individual experiences extension of all extremities when the head is tilted posteriorly to 90 degrees. Conversely, flexor tone dominates when the head is tilted anteriorly to 90 degrees.

Deformities can result from the improper positioning of the body for a prolonged period of time under the influence of tonal abnormalities. In seating, hip dislocation and pelvic obliquity are the most common deformities affecting children with disabilities. As the body tends to compensate for alignment changes resulting from abnormal muscle pulls, further skeletal deformities may result. Scoliosis is one example of this phenomenon.

To attain sitting balance, the function of vision and of the vestibular organs is important to consider. For individuals presenting with the neuromotor symptoms just discussed, maintaining the head properly in space can facilitate controlled movements and functional vision, improving the opportunity for learning and interaction.

GOALS OF SEATING

As is apparent from the literature related to adaptive seating, the goal of seating interventions is typically to improve function (Bergen et al. 1990). However, in dealing with individual clients, specific objectives that address user needs should also be considered. Table 6.1 lists some of the possible goals of a seating intervention.

In general, the seating needs of children with disabilities vary according to their stage of physical development. Infants with physical disabilities do not require adaptive seating systems before the age of 6 to 8 months, at which point commercially available seating devices are usually adequate for use. At this early stage of development, stable sitting allows the infant to explore the world. As the non-ambulatory child grows older (18 to 36 months), however, skeletal deformities may start to develop due to rapid body growth (Letts et al. 1984). The development of the acetabular is of particular concern. Poor interlink between the acetabular and the head of the femur can result in subluxation or even dislocation at the joint. To avoid this, the child's affected thigh(s) should be positioned in abduction (Bergen et al. 1990).

For service providers, juvenile seating (3 to 12 years) is the most challenging to provide. During this developmental stage, the body build of children changes rapidly

---

TABLE 6.1
Goals of Seating

To improve posture	• to prevent deformities
	• to correct deformities
	• to accommodate deformities
	• to promote symmetrical postures
To improve physical function	• to increase mobility
	• to normalise muscle tone
	• to decrease reflexive movements
	• to promote proximal stability and functional distal movement
	• to improve feeding and swallowing
	• to improve chest function
To improve comfort and security	• to increase sitting tolerance
	• to decrease sliding out
	• to relieve pressure
	• to relieve pain

To prevent decubitus ulcers
To meet caregiver goals
To meet transportation/vocational/school needs
To allow for growth/weight gain
To increase visual/perceptual abilities
To enhance communication
To improve personal appearance/increase self-esteem

---

and deformities become permanent, affecting many daily activities as well as sitting comfort. The primary goal of juvenile seating is to ensure that the child has full access to his or her environment, allowing social interaction as well as opportunities for learning. The specific aims of adaptive seating include maintaining a neutral head position, retaining proper lumbar lordosis, controlling sitting stability with proper selection of seat supports, maintaining leg abduction to prevent hip subluxation and providing arm and foot support (Letts 1991). To facilitate feeding and pressure relief, it is advantageous for the seating system to incorporate a tilt-in-space mechanism. Further, whenever possible, the seating system should restrict the child as little as possible to give maximum freedom of motion. Instead of relying solely on PSDs, foot-ankle as well as spinal orthoses should be considered. Orthotic devices are particularly effective in controlling deformity (Bowker et al. 1993). However, good device fit is necessary to avoid pressure problems and ensure user tolerance over the long term. It should also be noted that, during juvenility, surgical procedures may be conducted to correct muscle tightness and deformities. The aims of seating interventions should be modified to complement these changes accordingly.

When a child reaches adolescence, most of the problems associated with fixed skeletal deformities requiring surgical interventions should have been dealt with. At this stage, the concentration of the seating team focuses on two main goals: maintaining good body support in response to rapid body growth and providing a seating system that can ensure functionality and comfort. Weight increases during adolescence and prolonged seating time can put the user at risk of developing pressure ulcers (Elsner and Gefen 2008). Therefore, selection of compliant materials for the tissue-support interface is important. Another concern for the adolescent involves progressing deformities of the spine. Scoliosis must be carefully handled with PSDs and orthotic intervention and, in more severe cases, surgical interventions may be required.

BIOMECHANICS OF BODY SUPPORT

The body is composed of many segments (i.e., head, trunk, pelvis, thighs and feet) that are linked together to form a highly flexible structure. An understanding of the forces acting on the body is crucial in order to provide clients with effective seating. To achieve a stable posture, balance of forces and moments in all planes (sagittal, coronal and transverse) is essential. This situation is termed static equilibrium (i.e., the sum of all forces and moments acting on the system is zero). In biomechanics, a free-body diagram is commonly used to analyze the forces and moments acting on the human body. In sitting, these forces originate from within the body (muscular action), outside the body (resistance applied to body segments by external structures) and from gravity. Body weight during sitting is transferred through the buttocks, the thighs, the feet, the forearms and the back.

Stability of body posture is established through the precise control of muscular actions among different joints. However, spasticity and hypotonicity can prevent individuals from sitting properly. Imbalance of sitting forces also predisposes an individual to skeletal deformities, aggravates physiological conditions and limits his or her functional performance (Schmeler et al. 2007). To supplement a lack of muscular force, PSDs can be used to alter the line of gravitational action or provide external corrective forces to attain a state of static equilibrium in sitting. PSDs can be classified into primary postural support devices (PPSDs) (i.e., seat and back supports) and secondary postural support devices (SPSDs) (i.e., lateral supports, headrests, pelvic positioning belts, leg harnesses, etc.). The correct implementation of these devices requires careful consideration of the biomechanical principles involved.

A balanced sitting posture starts with a stable sitting base. Proper positioning of the pelvis, which balances on the ischial tuberosities, is the key. The orientation of the pelvis during sitting creates considerably higher lumbar disc pressure as compared with standing (Andersson et al. 1974). This is due to a shift of the line of gravity anterior to the lumbar spine, creating a larger moment arm. Similarly, the magnitude of disc pressure is highest during anterior sitting (i.e., sitting in a functional task position) and lowers during posterior sitting (i.e., sitting in a slumped posture). From a biomechanical perspective, taking the hip joint as the fulcrum, the force of gravity applies a torque (rotational force) on one side of the hip joint that has to be counteracted by a muscle force pulling on the other side in order to maintain static equilibrium. In anterior sitting, the forward shift of the line of gravity creates a larger moment arm that in turn needs to be counteracted by a larger spinal muscle force. This increases spinal disc pressure. Zacharkow (1988) suggested that a neutral pelvic posture should be adopted for sitting, as it requires minimum muscle effort to gain maximum stability.

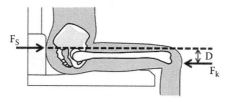

FIGURE 6.2   Application of external forces to control the pelvis (F_s is the force acting on the sacrum and F_k is the force acting on the knee. $F_k \times D$ is the restoring torque on the pelvis to resist posterior tilting).

To hold the pelvis in a neutral position (as in the case of erect sitting), external forces may be required for some individuals. For example, to control posterior pelvic tilt, a counteractive moment needs to be generated using PSDs. Unfortunately, the seat upholstery of manual wheelchairs is inadequate for use as a PPSD. Therefore, a rigid seat pan should be used. Furthermore, SPSDs including knee blocks, sacral pads, anti-thrust blocks and sub-ASIS bars are commonly used to generate the required turning moment about the hip joint. Figure 6.2 shows the line of force action required in these designs.

In some instances, to control the movement about a skeletal joint, more than one external force may be required. For example, in the specific case of windswept hip (one hip positioned in abduction and the other in adduction), four external forces are required. Figure 6.3 shows the desired force application by PSDs on the body. The two forces acting on the pelvis immobilise its rotational motion and the forces acting on the femora correct the windswept positioning.

The positions of the femora also affect the orientation of the pelvis during seating. Ideally, the femora should be positioned in parallel with the seating surface. Tilting of the anterior end of the femora will tend to pull on the hip and promote posterior pelvic rotation. Similarly, if the femora are lifted at the distal end, the body's weight will be shifted toward the ischial tuberosities, causing a localised concentration of

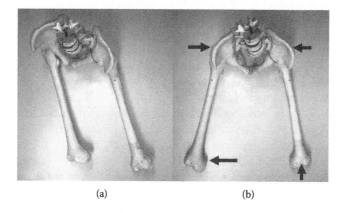

(a)   (b)

FIGURE 6.3   (a) Windswept hip positioning. (b) Location of force application for the correction of windswept hip (arrows indicate the line of force action).

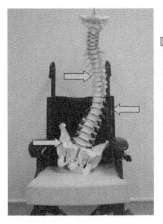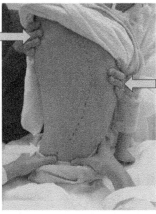

FIGURE 6.4   (See color insert following page 240.) The three-point force system for the correction of S-curve scoliosis.

interfacial stresses on the tissues overlying the bony prominences. Finally, to ensure that excess loading is not exerted on the seat pan, adequate support should be provided to the feet. PSDs, such as ankle and toe straps, are commonly used to control foot position. However, for effective control of pronation and supination, use of ankle-foot orthoses is recommended.

After pelvic movement has been controlled, trunk stability should be considered next. Although an upright midline posture is desired, individuals with weakened trunk control often have spinal deformities. Hyperlordosis, kyphosis, scoliosis or a combination of these deformities is common. To support the collapsing structure in the case of a simple S-curve scoliosis, for example, external forces can be applied at three different points: usually at the apex on the convex side of the spine, under the axilla and on the lateral side of the pelvis. Figure 6.4 shows this three-point support system. As trunk rotation is often associated with scoliosis, the direction of corrective force application needs to be carefully aligned. In addition, it should be noted that these external forces are actually applied at the tissue-support interface, which is some distance away from the skeletal structure. The effectiveness of correcting spinal deformity in this way is still not clear. In some cases, PSDs including chest straps and shoulder retractors are also used to control trunk posture. However, these PSDs limit the functional movement of the user.

One of the challenges in adaptive seating is to support the head in a functional position. Weak musculature of the neck and neck hyperextension, lateral flexion and rotation all contribute to improper head alignment. By reclining the back support of a seating system, gravity can help to stabilise the head in a supported posture to facilitate communication and learning. However, this solution is far from ideal. A tilted sitting posture forces an individual's line of eyesight upward, limiting his or her awareness of the environment. As a preferred alternative, head and neck PSDs (i.e., head and facial supports, occipital pads and forehead straps) can be used to balance the forces acting on the head and achieve static equilibrium.

SEATING ASSESSMENT

It is essential to understand the body's capacities and limitations in order to implement a successful seating intervention. In general, a seating assessment will examine a client's physical and motor performance (Bergen and Presperin 1990). The seating assessment starts with the examination of resting sitting posture, including a general observation of body alignment, sitting balance, postural control and stability. This examination can be performed with the client sitting on his or her own chair or on a rigid surface with his or her legs supported.

Since the pelvis provides the foundation of support in sitting (Letts 1991), assessment should start with the pelvis. With the client in a seated posture, it should be determined whether the pelvis is neutral, posteriorly or anteriorly tilted, rotated or tilted to one side (oblique). The presence of extensor thrust will prohibit the client from sitting. In these cases, pelvic control can be revealed by asking the client to adopt different pelvic postures. To assess hip flexibility, it should be determined whether the hip is neutral, internally or externally rotated, adducted or abducted, windswept or constantly moving. Next, the posture and control of the trunk should be assessed. From the sagittal plane, trunk alignment should be observed to determine if it is neutral, kyphotic or extended. From the frontal plane, spinal alignment should be examined and described in terms of spinal curvature (e.g., S- or C-shaped curve). From the transverse plane, it should be determined if trunk rotation is present. For the knees, knee angle should be observed and described as neutral (i.e., 90 degrees), flexed or extended. For the ankle and foot, the position is described as neutral, dorsi-flexed, planar-flexed, inverted or everted. When describing head and neck posture and control, the head position is said to be in extension (pushes or falls back), flexion (protrudes or falls forward), side flexion or rotation. For the shoulder girdles, the posture can be neutral, elevated, protracted with internal rotation or retracted with external rotation. Arm control is also important for functional task performance. Thus, it is important to assess whether the client has active control of his or her arm. Moreover, the influence of tone and reflexes during sitting should also be noted, as well as the levels of postural control that the individual can achieve. If the client can maintain an erect trunk position without using his or her hands for support, the client is said to be a hands-free sitter. On the contrary, if one or both hands are needed to maintain sitting balance, he or she is described as a hands-dependent sitter. Finally, if the individual is unable to sit independently, he or she is a propped sitter.

After achieving a basic understanding of the client's postural control, a mat assessment can be conducted. Mat assessments can be divided into two stages: (1) supine evaluation and (2) sitting evaluation. Supine evaluation is performed to determine joint flexibility and range of motion, whereas sitting evaluation determines how the body should be supported to restore a functional posture and accommodate deformities.

To examine the flexibility of the pelvis, the client should adopt a supine position. Movement of the pelvis can then be assessed by gripping the anterior superior iliac spine (ASIS) and checking if the pelvis is confined in a fixed position or if it can be moved into anterior or posterior tilt. If it can be moved, the pelvis is flexible. To check for pelvic obliquity and rotation, depicted in Figure 6.5, the client should sit upright. Pelvic obliquity refers to the angulations of the pelvis from horizontal and is

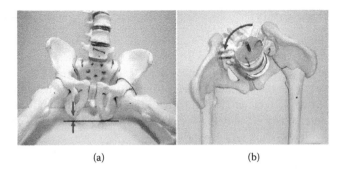

(a)   (b)

FIGURE 6.5   (See color insert following page 240.) Views of (a) oblique and (b) rotated pelvic orientations.

best viewed in the frontal plane. Pelvic rotation, which occurs when one side of the pelvis is forward of the other side, can be best observed in the transverse plane.

The flexibility of the hip joint and its surrounding muscles play an important role in determining whether a person can be positioned in a sitting posture. Any tightness or contractures of the tissue surrounding the joint will affect pelvic alignment. To assess potential sitting limitations, five hip postures should be considered with the client in a supine position: flexion (i.e., bilateral and unilateral limitations), adduction, abduction, and internal and external rotation. To examine the movement of each hip, the pelvis should be held in a neutral position while moving the thigh and feeling the resistance from the surrounding tissues of the hip joint. Also, knee extension should be examined, with the hip positioned at 90 degrees, to reveal any tightness of the hamstring. Similarly, foot and ankle flexibility should be checked to assess range of motion limitations in dorsiflexion, planarflexion, invertion and eversion.

In assessing trunk posture, an initial check for spinal alignment should be performed while the client is in a supine position. Then, to feel the allowable movement of the trunk, the client should be seated in an upright posture with his or her hips and knees flexed, and feet resting flat on the support surface. For this evaluation, the pelvis should be held in its neutral posture. Maintenance of this pelvic alignment can be facilitated by sitting behind the client and gripping his or her pelvis with one's thighs. This technique also allows the examiner to use both hands in order to determine the necessary trunk support. Typical postures of the trunk, such as kyphosis, hyperlordosis, rotation and scoliosis can also be revealed during upright sitting. However, scoliosis, a three-dimensional spinal deformity characterised by a 'rib-hump' (i.e., ribs stick out on one side), can be best observed with the client bent forward (i.e., using the forward bend test).

The head and neck complex is very sensitive and difficult to assess. It is best to perform this assessment, if possible, with the client in an upright sitting position. Head balance and active control should be checked by observing whether the client is able to hold his or her head up and turn it to both sides. This control is important in order for the client to explore the environment and perform functional tasks like eating and watching television.

As mentioned, the goal of a seating assessment is to determine what type of support the body requires in order to restore a functional posture. Therefore, it is essential to fully understand the functional tasks that the client needs to perform during sitting. Before fully implementing a new seating system, a simulation is always advantageous. This allows the seating team to assess the functional performance of the user under the influence of PSDs and to fine-tune the supports to achieve an optimal sitting posture. However, sufficient time (half a day) must be allowed for both the assessment and the simulation.

SEATING SIMULATION

Seating simulation is an important step in seating assessment and should occur prior to product prescription. Simulation can be best performed with the use of a positioning chair (Saftler et al. 1988). This 'positioning chair,' herein referred to as a 'seating simulator,' is a multi-adjustable chair that can be altered, in terms of its dimensions (seat depth, back height, foot support) and angulations (seat-back angle, tilt in space), to accommodate different body sizes. PSDs can also be added to the simulator frame and adjusted to fit client needs. In addition, a seating simulator allows for the installation of bead bags to provide total body contoured support to the client. Most simulators currently on the market have a wheeled base. Figure 6.6 shows a planar and a contoured seating simulator.

DESIGN CONSIDERATIONS

ANTHROPOMETRIC DATA

Although paediatric seating has been found to be important for the prevention of deformities and maintenance of function throughout a person's lifespan, paediatric seating systems are usually produced as a scaled-down version of adult products.

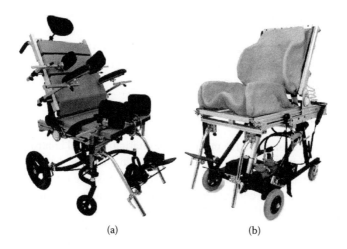

(a)   (b)

FIGURE 6.6   (See color insert following page 240.) (a) A planar seating simulator and (b) a contoured seating simulator. (Courtesy of Prairie Seating Corporation.)

There is little information available in the literature concerning the design of seating systems for children. From infancy to adolescence, the body undergoes many physical changes. Body dimension, segmental proportion and weight change drastically over the development period. Anthropometric information is essential for appropriate design of seating and mobility systems of the target population. Unfortunately, anthropometric data available in the literature are usually focused on the non-disabled population and are somewhat outdated. Recently, Paquet and Feathers (2004) reported on an anthropometric study aiming to provide an updated database of structural characteristics of manual and power wheelchair users. However, the target population was, once again, adults.

Compared to what was found decades ago, general observations of today's children have identified noticeable changes to growth rate during childhood and increases in the weight and length of newborns. These changes in body size can greatly influence the design of seating systems. Of the anthropometric studies available in the literature, most are outdated, while sampling methods and means of age categorization were not standardised in the few more recent ones (Kroemer 2006). Furthermore, in considering the use of the available anthropometric data for the design of adaptive seating systems, it is important to recognise that body dimensions of children with physical, neurological and/or developmental disabilities may be very different from the typical population. Such data, while available in most seating clinics, has not been published. These data are essential for designers and manufacturers to develop suitable seating systems for children with disabilities.

User Strength

Body strength is another parameter that is commonly considered in ergonomics. For example, handgrip and grasp forces have been measured by Owings et al. (1975) and Haeger-Ross et al. (2002). For children with abnormal tone, body strength information can be important for the development of suitable PSDs. Exceptionally high forces (500 kg) can be generated during an extensor thrust, putting high stresses on PSDs (Zeltwanger et al. 2001). These forces can break the supports or injure the user. Information on body strength would aid engineers in the development of more durable PSDs and seating systems.

Seat Orientation

The use of gravity is an effective means of facilitating postural control as it helps to attain balance and stability (Kreutz 1997). The tilt-in-space mechanism is an important innovation in adaptive seating (Fields 1991). Tilt-in-space refers to the ability to rotate a specific seat-back configuration around a fixed axis. The orientation of the seat-back complex is usually set at 90 degrees. The tilt-in-space mechanism has demonstrated some potential and advantages for prolonged seating, including improved head and postural control, respiratory function, pressure relief and ease of transfer (Sprigle et al. 1997; Lacoste et al. 2003; Dewey et al. 2004). To maintain stability of the seating system, among the different tilt-in-space mechanisms tested (Fields 1991) the floating pivot and centre pivot designs were found to be the safest as the centre of gravity of these seating systems were independent of the degree of tilting.

Gravity can also help to normalise tone and facilitate postural control, particularly for children with CP (Bwaobi et al. 1983, 1986). In this population, spasticity was found to be reduced when the body centre of gravity was anterior to the hip joint (i.e., in a forward leaning posture). In contrast, when the hip joint angle opened up, the centre of gravity moved behind the hip joint and spasticity increased (Myhr and vonWendt 1990, 1991, 1993, 1995). A long-term follow-up of children positioned with their centre of gravity anterior to their ischial tuberosities (i.e., in a forward leaning posture with legs abducted) showed improved motor control over a 5-year period (Myhr et al. 1995). Despite the effect of a reclining posture on individuals with CP, some clients do rely on a reclining feature for pressure relief (Angelico 1995).

Repetitive changes in seat-back or seat-foot orientations can upset the predetermined sitting balance posture, causing the body to slide out of the chair or creating interfacial shear stresses leading to pressure ulcers. Warren et al. (1982) reported the extent of back displacement of a typical reclining wheelchair. Using a four-bar linkage mechanism, Warren demonstrated a significant reduction in body-chair displacement over the reclining range. Thereafter, engineers have developed seating systems that almost completely eliminate relative sliding. The mechanism used is designed to allow the seat-back support to translate and follow the path of body movement during postural changes. Such a design is called a 'non-shear system' or a 'zero-shear system' (Cooper 1998).

MANAGEMENT OF THE BODY-SUPPORT INTERFACE

Improved comfort and the prevention of tissue distress due to prolonged sitting are major concerns requiring careful consideration when using PSDs to attain sitting stability. Comfort is difficult to quantify. As mentioned, sitting is never static and changes in body posture and habitual movements are expected. Excess use of PSDs can restrict movement and lead to discomfort. Furthermore, corrective forces applied by PSDs can cause high interfacial pressures (Holmes et al. 2003). Prolonged tissue compression is known to be an etiological factor in the onset of pressure ulcers (Dinsdale 1974). This situation is of particular concern for individuals who have hypotonia or reduced sensation. Reswick and Rogers (1976) reported a parabolic relationship between magnitude of pressure and duration of loading. They found that, even with relatively low interface pressure, if loading was prolonged, pressure ulcers could result. Therefore, the design and application of PSDs should be carefully considered. In general, materials used for the contact interface of PSDs should be somewhat compliant. The choice of materials for use in seating systems is discussed in the section that follows.

In addition to pressure, shear stresses that arise at the body-support interface can cause distortion and other physiological complications. An early study by Bennett (1974) demonstrated the effect of shear on blood circulation in the skin. Blood flow terminated at low interface pressure magnitude when higher shear force was applied as compared to lower shear force. In adaptive seating, shear forces can be generated at the support interface during postural changes. Tangential forces develop at weight-bearing areas, and frictional forces can abrade the dermis and distort tissues at subcutaneous and muscle layers. This can interrupt blood perfusion, causing cellular damage and pre-disposing tissue to pressure ulcer formation (Bennett et al. 1979; Gawlitta et al. 2007).

As most individuals requiring adaptive seating for postural support are confined to body-support systems for a prolonged period of time, the interface microenviron-ment also threatens tissue breakdown. The microclimate (temperature and mois-ture) is frequently overlooked when considering the suitability of a seating system. Moist tissue is mechanically weaker than dry tissue (Park et al. 1972) and moisture increases the coefficient of friction of the tissue-support interface (Elsner et al. 1990). In the presence of bacteria, moisture can also increase microbiological activities (Hartmann 1983) and cause tissue breakdown. In considering temperature, it is known that increases in skin temperature cause higher metabolic demands on cells, leading to an increase in oxygen consumption (Ruch and Patton 1965; Krouskop 1983). Thus, to maintain thermal equilibrium between heat generated through metabolism and heat lost to the environment, the temperature at the tissue-support interface needs to be regulated. PSD cover materials influence thermal regulation and must there-fore effectively dissipate heat and moisture away from the tissue-support interface. Ideally, temperature at the interface should be stable, with temperature fluctuating by no more than a few degrees. The humidity should be between 40% and 65% relative humidity (Cochran and Palmieri 1980). In general, foam cushioning increases inter-face temperature while gel cushioning increases humidity. Furthermore, one should remember that there are actually two layers of fabric at the tissue-support interface. These fabrics include the cushion cover and the clothing that the user wears.

MATERIALS

Ensuring durability and suitability of materials for use in a seating system is the task of a rehabilitation engineer. In addition to the high loads exerted due to abnormal tone, impact loads resulting from collision with environmental objects, during transportation and traffic accidents, also need to be taken into consideration. Nowadays, in addition to the use of metals (i.e., stainless steel or aluminium) for construction of the seating system, plastic materials are commonly used for the seat-back chassis to reduce weight. Other materials such as carbon fibre and honeycomb board are also available for use.

Cushion and cushion cover materials must also be carefully selected. There are a variety of cushioning materials available on the market (e.g., foam and gel), as well as different densities and stiffness from which to choose. When selecting cushion cov-ers, surface characteristics are important to consider. Interfacial friction and shear properties, temperature and humidity control, pressure redistribution characteris-tics, infection control capability, flammability and life expectancy all contributed to the efficiency of the PSD. To test the microclimate at the tissue-support interface, a buttock-shaped temperature and humidity measurement system, as reported by the International Organization for Standardization (ISO) in Standard 16840-2 (ISO 2007), can be used for evaluation (Ferguson-Pell et al. 2009).

In order for seating systems to be used safely in motor vehicles, PSDs must be tested to ensure that they conform to ISO Standard 16840-4 (ISO 2009). However, this standard only puts forth requirements for adult seating systems. Currently, no standards specifically address seating system safety requirements for motor vehicle use for children with disabilities.

TYPES OF SEATING SYSTEMS

ADAPTIVE SEATING SYSTEMS

Adaptive seating systems can be classified into three major categories: planar, modular and custom contoured (Figure 6.7). Engineers have made significant contributions to the design of these devices including, for example, innovations in body-shape sensing techniques and custom contour-cushion fabrication methods.

Planar Seating Systems

In planar seating systems, a rigid, flat surface is used to support the body. These systems were originally designed for individuals who required only minimal assistance with upright sitting. However, the support offered by planar seating systems has improved since, with conventional seat and back upholsteries that provided little body support having been replaced with plywood support, padded with foam cushioning (1 to 1.5 in. thick). A planar seating system is usually prefabricated and can be fit onto the user's chair almost immediately after assessment is performed. Drop hooks are commonly used to anchor the support surface to the chair frame. Common PSDs that are used in planar systems include drop seats (Figure 6.8a), adductors and abductors, hip pads, trunk laterals and headrests (see Figure 6.7). To account for different body builds among users, PSD mounting brackets are designed to allow some degree of dimensional adjustment. Furthermore, to accommodate greater changes in body width, the 'I'-back design (Figure 6.8b) is commonly used. Since a good fit of the PSDs used is essential for the success of postural positioning, caregivers usually find that the tightly fitted PSDs make it difficult to position the child's body within the supports. To overcome this, engineers have developed various quick release mechanisms for use with PSDs, thereby facilitating body repositioning after

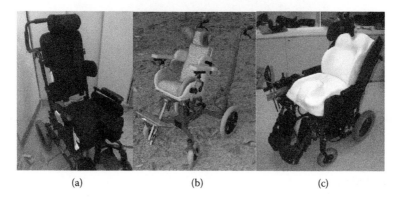

(a)   (b)   (c)

FIGURE 6.7   (See color insert following page 240.) (a) A planar seating system with flat postural support surfaces (courtesy of Adaptive Engineering Lab, Inc.), (b) a modular seating system and (c) a custom contoured seating system.

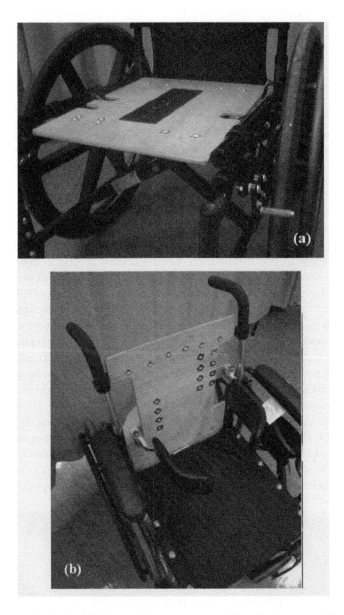

FIGURE 6.8 Two planar seating system components: (a) a drop seat and (b) an I-back. (Courtesy of Adaptive Engineering Lab, Inc.)

transfer. Figure 6.9 shows different designs of quick release mechanisms that are used with PSDs.

Modular Seating Systems

Modular seating systems utilise PSDs that are adjustable and easy to attach and detach to and from the chair. In this way, these seating systems can be modified to

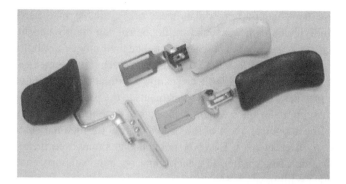

FIGURE 6.9   Different postural support device quick-release mechanisms.

effectively accommodate body growth. Seat and back chassis are available in different dimensions covering various body sizes from infant to adolescent and typically these components have some degree of adjustability built in. For example, the x:panda™ system (Snug Seat Inc., USA) is available in three different sizes and within each size, seat depth and width have 10 cm of adjustability.

Modular seating systems can also improve sitting compliance through the use of contoured PSDs. Pre-shaped contour cushions are available in many forms. Although generally made from cellular materials with various support characteristics, air and gel are also commonly used as the support medium. The effect of pre-shaped contour cushions on pressure relief has been found to be significant (Sprigle et al. 1990). Among the different contour cushion designs available, the Stimulite® cushion (Supracor Inc., USA) is particularly interesting. Its honeycomb structure, depicted in Figure 6.10, conforms well to the body and provides good permeability to air and moisture. Thus, although it may be less effective for pressure relief compared to other products, the open cell matrix design allows for better air circulation, which can be advantageous when moisture prevention is a primary concern.

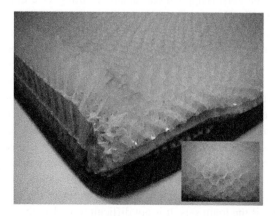

FIGURE 6.10   The Stimulite® (Supracor Inc., USA) honeycomb cushion. (Courtesy of Supracor, Inc.)

To improve trunk support, modular backs are available in different contours and depths. Individuals with weakened trunk control can greatly benefit from these designs, which can be selected to best accommodate their unique disability. Examples of modular back supports include the Jay® Modular Back (Sunrisemedical, USA) and ProContour back cushions (Otto Bock, Germany). Modular back cushions usually also allow service providers to make minor adjustments to the padding, including the addition of lumbar supports or the creation of cut-outs to accommodate bony protrusions.

In terms of head control, most of the head supports for modular seating systems are available in different sizes. However, some designs may even incorporate more complex PSDs, including cradle pads, neck rings, occipital supports, facial pads and forehead straps (Whitmeyer, USA).

Custom Contoured Seating Systems

It is generally agreed that total contact provides the best pressure distribution and support to the body (Hertzberg 1972). The goal of custom contoured seating systems is to achieve exactly that. To fabricate custom contoured PSDs, traditional freehand shaping techniques can be used. Foam blocks with different densities provide the required support characteristics. These blocks are shaped by a skilled technician with an artistic mind to replicate the user's body contour as closely as possible. In the case of more complicated contours, such as seat cushions and back supports, freehand shaping may not be able to achieve a good match and total body support may not be achieved.

In view of the demand for custom contoured seating systems, development in the area has focused on new techniques to speed up the fabrication process. Hobson and co-workers (1984), at the University of Tennessee, pioneered the creation of a novel custom contoured support system for severely involved children with CP. Their design, the Bead Seat system, consists of a thin-film elastic plastic bag filled with polystyrene beads. Using a vacuum consolidation technique, the bead-filled bag is shaped to the body to create a supportive contour. An adhesive binder is then added to the beads to harden the cushion in the desired shape. To finish off the cushion surface, a two-way stretchable vinyl is applied via vacuum forming. Overall, the bead seating fabrication technique has been well received as it can greatly reduce fabrication time. However, one drawback of this technique is that the seating specialist has limited working time (45 min) to re-capture the desired posture before the adhesive sets.

Foam-in-place is another fabrication technique used to create custom contoured cushions directly (Hobson 1978). The polyurethane foam used for this method is usually manufactured by mixing liquid foam and a hardener together. To form directly to the client's body shape, a moulding bag is first inserted at the interface between the seat and the back support. Then, before the foaming process is started, the seating specialist must once again ensure that the client is positioned with the best postural alignment that he or she is able to attain. While the seating specialist holds the client in this 'optimal' posture, an assistant mixes the liquid foam with its hardener and then pours the mixture into the moulding bag. The client is held in the desired posture until the foam sets. It is not difficult to realise the limitations of this process as most clients requiring custom contoured seating have tonal abnormalities and severe deformities, making it difficult for them to attain quiet sitting.

Due to difficulties encountered in shape capturing and forming during seating simulation, researchers began to explore new techniques in which the body contour could be digitised, allowing for automated systems to be used to fabricate the desired cushion. A number of works (Chung 1987; Brienza et al. 1988; McGovern et al. 1988) conducted in this area contributed to the development and use of Computer Aided Design-Computer Aided Manufacturing (CAD-CAM) for custom seating. This process utilises a CAD-CAM system to digitally capture a patient's body contour and store the data to a computer where any necessary modifications can then be made. The electronic file can then be sent to a computer-controlled carver to fabricate the desired contour cushion automatically. This type of seating is discussed in detail in the next section.

CAD-CAM Seating

Body shape capturing can be achieved by direct or indirect means. In the practice of prosthetics and orthotics, plaster-of-Paris has been used to replicate the body contour and make moulds for fabricating the desired prosthetic socket or spinal brace. This technique has also been used in adaptive seating. Patrick (1980) used bead bags to capture the three-dimensional body contours of patients and then transferred these body shapes by creating plaster-of-Paris moulds that could be used in a foaming process to fabricate custom cushions. However, this technique is cumbersome, expensive and time consuming. Seeking improvement, Chung (1987) developed a buttock contour gauge to capture the buttock shape and digitise the information onto a computer for subsequent computer-controlled cushion fabrication. The Silhouette® (Pindot, USA) was developed from Chung's work. Kwiatkowski and Inigo (1993) further enhanced Chung's system by incorporating 128 electronically actuated force-sensing probes controlled by stepper-motors. With this system, based on the specific support characteristics (foam stiffness, interface pressure, etc.) determined by the operator, the computer-controlled actuators automatically adjust to attain the desired support characteristics. As the system is under closed-loop control, the process continues until the desired characteristic is met. However, depending on the specification made, the time required to attain the ultimate seating condition may be lengthy or even endless (Wang et al. 2000).

Building on the bead bag approach, McGovern et al. (1988) developed a linear array digitiser based on linear variable differential transformers (LVDTs). Using this approach, after capturing body shape using bead bags, a mechanical digitiser is moved across the support surface at a fixed distance to automatically digitise the contour. After a software program reconstructs the contour surface, the data can be sent to a computer manufacturing machine for cushion fabrication. A similar technique that utilises a magnetic digitiser (Otto Bock, USA) can also be used. The advantage of having contour information in digital format is that minor modifications to the contour surface can be made easily after the digitizing process. This is particularly important to the seating specialist if additional supports or pressure relief must be incorporated prior to cushion fabrication.

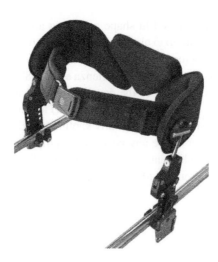

FIGURE 6.11   The Hip Grip™ (Bodypoint Inc., USA). (Courtesy of Bodypoint Inc.)

DYNAMIC SEATING SYSTEMS

High-tone extensor thrust, commonly experienced by children with CP, can generate powerful muscle forces that can throw a client's body out of their seating system. The traditional approach to handle this unwanted motion is to strap the body down using restraints or seatbelts. However, this approach has not been very successful as the tension in the restraints can cause tissue injury and the forces generated can damage the PSDs. Over the years, there has been some development of moveable PSDs that give way or change shape when involuntary muscle contractions occur. Examples include the Activeline Traveling Seat (Markwald 1998) and the seat assembly designed by Farricielli (1997) for a portable wheelchair. These systems utilised springs and actuators to dissipate energy during an extensor thrust. Using a similar concept, it is possible to make a very basic dynamic seating system simply by adding dampers to the footrest to dissipate unwanted energy.

Maintaining control of the pelvis is essential to the stability of seating. Conventional methods of locking the pelvis in position using PSDs limit the movement of the user. Noon et al. (1998) developed a pelvic stabilization system to provide continuous stability support to the pelvis while allowing some degree of pelvic movement during wheelchair activities. The device, called Hip Grip™ (Bodypoint Inc., USA), aims to improve the functional reach capacity of the user while maintaining pelvic stability for proper sitting. The Hip Grip™ assembly, shown in Figure 6.11, consists of a sacral pad, a pair of 'T' bars attached on each side to pivot brackets, and a padded-belt system across the front to provide a secure grip at the iliac crests. Although it allows some movement of the pelvis, the Hip Grip™ system also provides resistance, generating counteractive forces that help to return the pelvis to its original (neutral) position. Clinical evaluations of the Hip Grip™ with 23 wheelchair users showed that the device could improve posture; forward, backward and lateral lean; user performance and satisfaction (Axelson et al. 2004).

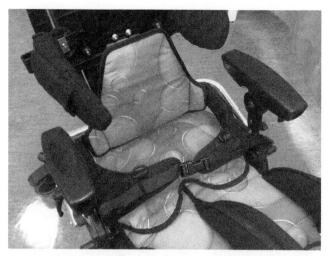

FIGURE 6.12 (See color insert following page 240.) The Mygo pelvic stabilisation system (Leckey, UK), including a pelvic positioning harness and flexible sacral support. (Courtesy of Leckey, UK.)

Another new PSD design that can effectively control the pelvis is the pelvic positioning harness and flexible sacral support that is incorporated in the Mygo system (Leckey, UK) and depicted in Figure 6.12. The components of this support system can be adjusted to fit different pelvic orientations by adjusting the tension in the pelvic straps.

THE SHAPEABLE MATRIX SEATING SYSTEM

The Matrix seating system, shown in Figure 6.13, was originally designed in the 1970s by a group of engineers from the University of London (Trail and Calasko 1990). The system consists of many interlocking modules (Figure 6.13a) attached to a specific mounting frame and integrated onto a mobility base. Each module has a central locking screw and four ball-and-socket joints on each side; tightening the central screw locks the four joints simultaneously. Using an array of the interlocking modules, seat and back support surfaces can be created, shaped to the client's body contour, and then tightened in position. The average seating system requires over 100 interlocking modules such that tightening the central screw of each module often requires tedious effort. Nonetheless, the system is versatile and is able to fit almost every body contour, regardless of the deformities that may be present. In addition, the tremendous adjustability of the Matrix system allows it to 'grow' with the user.

According to an evaluation conducted by Trail and Galasko (1990), the Matrix seating system did not cause significant pressure sores to develop and over 80% of the participants were satisfied with the system, with the primary reason for dislike being due to appearance. The authors recommended the system, but noted that it was not able to prevent hip dislocation or the deterioration of scoliosis. Although the Matrix system is not commonly applied in clinical situations, perhaps due to the

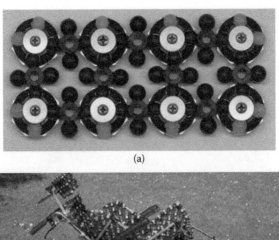

(a)

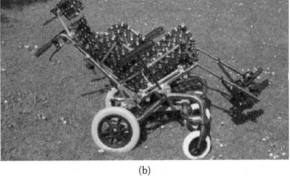

(b)

FIGURE 6.13   (See color insert following page 240.) (a) An array of interlocking plastic modules that comprise the Matrix seating system and (b) the Matrix seating system mounted on a mobility base. (Courtesy of Southwest Seating & Rehab Ltd., UK.)

demands it places on technical support for installation and follow-up adjustments whenever resting posture changes, it has been found to successfully seat and position children with severe disabilities (Cousins et al. 2005).

SERVICE DELIVERY

Providing adaptive seating interventions to children with disabilities is a lengthy process. Dimensional changes in these children preclude the possibility of having a prescribed seating system that can serve the child until skeletal maturity. Rather, the seating system must be constantly reviewed and renewed during the growth period to ensure that all necessary PSDs are provided at the right time to prevent, control or delay the onset of skeletal deformities.

The implementation of an effective and timely adaptive seating intervention can be difficult to accomplish. The complete process, including prescription, funding application, order and delivery, can easily take from weeks to many months. During this long waiting period, the child may outgrow the prescribed seating system before it is even obtained. Although some seating and mobility systems on the market claim to grow with the child, they typically only accommodate minor changes in body size. Furthermore, most seating systems have insufficient adjustability to accommodate possible postural changes due to skeletal deformities or muscle tone. Due to these limitations, the need to frequently change or upgrade seating systems during childhood places a significant financial burden on the end user and his or her family. Further, when replacing a seating system, some of the PSDs from the old system may no longer be useable or needed, although still in good condition. Unfortunately, if there is no channel for recycling, these components are usually discarded.

One seating service model that has been successfully demonstrated in Hong Kong (the seating clinic and wheelchair bank, Hong Kong) to ease the financial burden imposed on the families of children requiring adaptive seating involves the establishment of a service, like a library service, that owns a collection of adaptive seating systems and PSDs. This approach offers several unique advantages over traditional service delivery practices. First, it allows associated seating service providers to capitalise on the available equipment so that they are able to provide seating services to children in a timely manner. When a child outgrows a particular system, it can be replaced easily with another one that is more suitable and the old system can be recycled for use by another child. Furthermore, the availability of a library of PSDs allows seating specialists to test different PSD designs in order to ensure that the best possible clinical outcomes are achieved. Finally, in terms of cost, the project in Hong Kong found that, with recycling, cost savings could be more than 50% (Lau et al. 2009).

In order to gain a better understanding of the seating needs of children throughout childhood, a comprehensive and accessible informational database is required. As discussed earlier, children with disabilities often have unique needs at each stage of their development. A detailed understanding of postural support and postural control requirements can enhance the effectiveness and efficacy of service delivery. Clinical data can help to reveal the effectiveness of a particular intervention, and monitoring of physical changes can provide valuable information for the development of future seating systems that can best serve a particular patient group. Information regarding the types of PSDs most commonly used for intervention and recommendations on how to address PSD limitations would also be beneficial. When conducting clinical research involving children who use seating systems, such an informational database may be of great importance (e.g., for longitudinal studies). Individual seating clinics may already use similar types of databases for management purposes.

To properly position the body in a functional posture, appropriate PSDs are needed, which can be expensive. Unfortunately, funding for such devices can be difficult to obtain due to a "chicken and egg" type of scenario. To obtain funding, the service provider needs to demonstrate the effectiveness of the intervention, while to obtain the necessary PSDs, funding is required. Therefore, adaptive seating service delivery needs to be evidence-based. To most efficiently address this requirement, instead of conducting single-subject studies with pre- and post-evaluations, it has been suggested that outcome research could be conducted using objective measures to reveal the effect of specific methods on the seating goals of a particular client group (Ferguson-Pell 1995). However, in research design, the study group needs to be homogenous and individuals with adaptive seating needs are typically rather unique. The clinical manifestations of CP, for example, can be very different among individuals and can thus have different effects on the outcome of the intervention (Chung et al. 2008). In addition, assessing new seating interventions can be difficult as there are ethical issues associated with study designs that might deplete a client's condition from what is believed to be attainable using the best intervention available at the time.

OUTCOME MEASURES

Adaptive seating interventions have been in practice in clinical settings for over three decades (Watson and Woods 2005). Successful experiences have been reported mainly in conference presentations and proceedings or as case studies published in related magazines. Little information related to outcome measures can be found in peer-reviewed journals. A lack of appropriate evaluation instruments and method-ologies may be one obstacle contributing to this gap in the literature. In rehabilitation settings, a number of instruments have been developed to measure the functional improvement of individuals in terms of, for example, activities of daily living, com-munication, cognitive function and psychosocial adjustment [e.g., the Barthel Index (Mahoney and Barthel 1965) and the Functional Independence Measures (Uniform Data System for Medical Rehabilitation 1997)]. However, these instruments do not specifically reveal the changes occurring due to technological intervention.

Typically, the success of an assistive technology intervention is evaluated based on effectiveness, efficacy, availability and efficiency of the product or the related deliv-ery process (Sackett 1980). In adaptive seating, the primary concerns of the inter-vention outcome are effectiveness (i.e., does the intervention work?) and efficiency (i.e., is it worth intervening?) (DeRuyter 2002). User satisfaction is also an important assessment parameter. The Quebec User Evaluation of Satisfaction with Assistive Technology (QUEST) (Demers et al. 1996) is one instrument that addresses this lat-ter consideration. QUEST is a two-part questionnaire consisting of 18 open-ended questions covering user characteristics, context for use and characteristics of the technology (part 1) and 27 questions, scored on a 6-point scale, assessing factors that are most likely to affect user satisfaction (part 2). Weiss-Lambrou et al. (1999) used QUEST to evaluate consumer satisfaction of modular seating devices. Although the results revealed that seating comfort was rated as the least satisfactory, this feedback should be considered in a positive light as it provides equipment designers and ser-vice providers an opportunity to significantly improve the situation. One drawback of implementing outcome measure questionnaires like QUEST is that the user needs to be able to comprehend the questions and communicate his or her answers to the researcher. In reality, many special seat users are unable to communicate at this level and so the sample size for such studies is usually limited. In fact, only 24 subjects participated in Weiss-Lambrou's study.

To overcome the limitations of questionnaire-based outcome assessments, McDonald et al. (2008) recently reported on a new measurement technique designed to objectively evaluate body posture and movement. Thirty-one subjects were included in the study. Accelerometry, actigraphy, pressure mapping and manual goniometry were used, as objective measures, to compare the differences between a ramped con-toured cushion and a flat seat cushion. In addition, McDonald and co-workers used the Non-communicating Children's Pain Checklist – Revised (NCCPC-R) (Breau et al. 2004) to measure seat comfort and a portion of the Seated Postural Control

Measure (Fife et al. 1991) supplemented with four hand- or head-activated switch activities to assess function while seated. The results of the objective measures used in the study were promising, while the measures of comfort and function needed refinement.

Instead of gathering feedback from the user directly, which is sometimes very difficult if not impossible, outcome measures can be conducted with input from the caregiver or family members. Recently, Ryan et al. (2009) explored the impact of PSDs on the lives of young children with CP (aged 2 to 7) and their families. Outcome measures were conducted using the Family Impact of Assistive Technology Scale (FLATS) (Ryan et al. 2006, 2007) and the Impact on Family Scale (IFS). The FLATS measures the impact of the following domains: autonomy of the child, caregiver relief, child contentment, child function, caregiver effort, family and social interaction, caregiver supervision and safety. The IFS was included to assess the psychological and social burden on the parent of having a child with disabilities. The FLATS scores showed that adaptive seating interventions had a positive impact on family life while removal of PSDs showed negative impact. In contrast, no effect was shown from the IFS regarding the psychological and social consequences of having a child requiring adaptive seating support. This could have been due to the fact that IFS was not designed to measure technological intervention specifically (Ryan et al. 2009).

It is important to note that the design and sensitivity of outcome measurement tools can greatly affect the results of the evaluation. This is particularly important to technological interventions. Unfortunately, most of the currently available outcome measures may not be specific enough to reveal the true effects of an intervention. Chung et al. (2008) recently conducted a literature review concerning the effectiveness of adaptive seating on sitting posture or postural control in children with CP. Considering literature published between January 1980 and July 2007, only 14 articles met the inclusion criteria, reporting outcomes related to sitting posture or postural control for non-ambulatory children under the age of 20 that received intervention related to adaptive seating. These articles included interventions using various seating components and systems. The conclusion of the review was that no single intervention was more effective in providing better sitting posture or postural control. The ultimate goal of the reviewed studies, to improve functional abilities through postural interventions, was weakly supported. Nonetheless, although literature support may be limited as evidenced by Chung's review, the use of adaptive seating in clinical settings has demonstrated that seating systems can greatly improve the functional status of the user if correctly implemented. The challenge ahead is to identify suitable instruments that can provide objective evaluation of the effect of this technological intervention.

THE WAY AHEAD

Adaptive seating service delivery is limited by the availability of PSDs on the market. Despite the fact that sitting is always dynamic, available seating systems for individuals with disabilities are still largely designed to restrict movement. However, the recent development of dynamic seating components that accommodate body movements during tonal reflex has started a new era of development in adaptive seating. Future PSDs should be designed to be dynamic; they should provide continuous support during postural changes as required for various daily tasks, but should subsequently be able to restore a child's desired resting posture. Powered exoskeletons, devices developed to provide additional strength to body extremities for military applications, offer great potential for assisting a child with muscle weakness to gain postural control. This technology has already influenced the development of novel prosthetics and orthotics (Herr 2009) and it likely will not be long before adaptive seating is impacted by this technology as well.

Another challenge in the field of adaptive seating is that most systems currently on the market are not developed specifically for children. Many seating systems are simply down-sized versions of systems designed for adults. A child with seating needs should not be fitted to an adaptive seat, but rather, an adaptive seat should match the needs of the child. As anthropometric data for children with disabilities is essential for the development of new paediatric seating systems, data collection and reporting is required. Such measurements should be taken across the paediatric age spectrum and should include information on functional reach during dynamic sitting tasks.

Currently, there is only limited information available on the load transfer characteristics between PSDs and the body. Namely, the pressure distribution at the cushion-support interface can be determined using existing methods. However, given that PSDs are designed to exert supportive or corrective forces to attain postural alignment, knowledge of additional load transfer characteristics at the tissue-support interface is of practical importance. Both the properties of the materials and the contour of the support surface are important factors to consider. It is likely that new knowledge in this area would greatly facilitate the development of a novel generation of PSDs for use in adaptive seating.

Standardisation of seating terminology and definitions is also important for effective service to be provided. Recent development of the wheelchair seating posture standard, ISO 16840-1 (ISO 2006), has provided researchers, clinicians and manufacturers with common definitions of critical postural terminology related to the person and the person's orientation and dimensions within his or her seating system. With such a standard now in place, the next step is to adopt these definitions and terms for use in practice. The benefit of having and utilizing this standardised terminology is that it not only facilitates information exchange and clinical decision-making, but it also provides the foundation for evidence-based outcome evaluation.

Evidence-based practice in adaptive seating has been advocated by many researchers and clinicians for more than a decade (Minkel 1998). Over these years, new instruments have been developed to assess the effectiveness of adaptive seating interventions. This work needs to continue. Furthermore, given that the ultimate goal of adaptive seating is to improve function, investigation into the effect of seating postures on functional performance is needed. Should the person be positioned in an erect seating posture? Is symmetrical seating a must? What is the so-called optimal posture that one should strive to attain? Many of these questions still require the attention of researchers.

CONCLUSION

This chapter has provided an overview of the fundamentals of adaptive seating and introduced the reader to various types of seating systems. Although seating system technology has come a long way, there is still much room for improvement. Overall, the design of adaptive seating systems for children with disabilities should be child-centred, dimensionally correct, clinically sound, easy to use, lightweight, durable, innovative, recyclable and reusable. Furthermore, given that the specific seating needs of the paediatric population are ever-changing, the design of adaptive seating must continue to evolve as well.

REFERENCES

Alexander, G., L. McNamara, L. Neville, A. Porter-Armstrong, J. Quigg, and W. Wrifht. 2006. Postural management and early intervention in seating: What's the evidence. *Proceedings of the 22nd International Seating Symposium*. Vancouver, Canada. 91–94.

Angelico, M. 1995. Seeking comfort. *TeamRehab Report* 6(7):14–16.

Axelson, P.W., D.Y. Axelson, A.M. Hayes, S.L. Hurley, J.H. Noon, and A.R. Siekman. 2004. HipGrip pelvic stabilization device for wheelchair users — Phase II final report. http://www.beneficialdesigns.com/wcseating/118%20Ph2%20Final%20Report-WEB.pdf (accessed March 2010).

Barlow, I.G., L. Liu, and A. Sekulic. 2009. Wheelchair seating assessment and intervention: A comparison between telerehabilitation and face-to-face service. *International Journal of Telerehabilitation* 1(1):17–27.

Bennett L., D. Kavner, B.K. Lee, and F.A. Trainor. 1979. Shear vs. pressure as causative factors in skin blood flow occlusion. *Archive of Physical Medicine and Rehabilitation* 60:309–314.

Bergen, A.F., J. Presperin, and T. Tallman. 1990. *Positioning for function: Wheelchairs and other assistive technologies*. Valhalla, NY: Valhalla Rehabilitation Publications.

Bowker, P., D.N. Condie, D.L. Bader, and D.J. Pratt. 1993. *Biomechanical basis of orthotic management*. Oxford, UK: Butterworth-Heinemann.

Breau, L.M., P.J. McGrath, C.S. Camfield, and G.A. Finley. 2004. Non-communicating Children's Pain Checklist – Revised (NCCPC-R). http://www.aboutkidshealth.ca/Shared/PDFs/AKH_Breau_everyday.pdf (accessed March 2010).

Brienza, D.M., K.C. Chung, and R.M. Inigo. 1988. Design of a computer aided manufacturing system for custom contoured wheelchair cushions. *Proceedings of the International Conference of the Association for the Advancement of Rehabilitation Technology* 312–313.

Brooks, V.B. 1986. *The neural basis of motor control*. New York: Oxford University Press.

Chung, J., J. Evans, C. Lee, J. Lee, Y. Rabbani, L. Roxborough, and S. Harris. 2008. Effectiveness of adaptive seating on sitting posture and postural control in children with cerebral palsy. *Pediatric Physical Therapy* 20(4):303–317.

Chung, K.C. 1987. Tissue contour and interface pressure on wheelchair cushion. PhD Dissertation, University of Virginia.

Cochran, G., and V. Palmieri. 1980. Development of test methods for evaluation of wheelchair cushions. *Bulletin of Prosthetics Research* 17(1):9–30.

Cooper, R.A. 1998. *Wheelchair selection and configuration*. New York: Demos Medical Publishing, Inc.

Cousins, S., D. May, and R. Clarke. 2005. Custom body support using the 2nd generation matrix system. *21st International Seating Symposium* 175.

DeRuyter, F. 2002. Outcomes and performance monitoring. In *Clinician's guide to assistive technology*, D.A. Olson and F. DeRuyter, Eds. St. Louis: Mosby Inc.

Dewey, A., M. Rice-Oxley, and T. Dean. 2004. A qualitative study comparing the experiences of tilt-in-space wheelchair use and conventional wheelchair use by clients severely disabled by multiple sclerosis. *British Journal of Occupational Therapy* 67:65–74.

Dinsdale, S.M. 1974. Decubitus ulcers: Role of pressure and friction in causation. *Archives of Physical Medicine and Rehabilitation* 55:147–152.

Dunk, N.M., and J.P. Callaghan. 2005. Gender-based differences in postural responses to seated exposures. *Clinical Biomechanics* 20:1101–1110.

Elsner, P., D. Wilhelm, and H.I. Maibach. 1990. Frictional properties of human forearm and vulvar skin: Influence of age and correlation with transepidermal water loss and capacitance. *Dermatologica* 181:88–91.

Elsner, J., and Gefen, A. 2008. Is obesity a risk factor for deep tissue injury in patients with spinal cord injury? *Journal of Biomechanics* 41:3322–3331.

Holmes, K.J., S.M. Michael, S.L. Thorpe, and S.E. Solomonidis. 2003. Management of scoliosis with special seating for the non-ambulant spastic cerebral palsy population — a biomechanical study. *Clinical Biomechanics* 18(6):480–487.

Farricielli, S. 1997. Ergonomically designed seat assembly for portable wheelchair. U.S. Patent 5,904,398.

Ferguson-Pell, M., H. Hirose, G. Nicholson, and E. Call. 2009. Thermodynamic rigid cushion loading indenter: A buttock-shaped temperature and humidity measurement system for cushioning surfaces under anatomical compression conditions. *Journal of Rehabilitation Research & Development* 46(7):945–956.

Fields, C.D. 1991. Getting centered with tilt-in-space. *TeamRehab Report* 2(5):22–27.

Fields, C.D. 1992. Living with tilt-in-space. *TeamRehab Report* 3(4):25–27.

Fife, S.E., L.A. Roxborough et al. 1991. Development of a clinical measure of postural control for assessment of adaptive seating in children with neuromotor disabilities. *Physical Therapy* 71(12): 981–993.

Gawlitta, D., W. Li, C.W. Oomens, F.P. Baaijens, D.L. Bader, and C.V. Bouten. 2007. The relative contributions of compression and hypoxia to development of muscle tissue damage: An in vitro study. *Annals of Biomedical Engineering* 35(2):273–284.

Knobloch, H., and B. Pasamanick. 1975. *Gesell and Amatruda's developmental diagnosis; the evaluation and management of normal and abnormal neuropsychologic development in infancy and early childhood.* Hagerstown, MD: Harper & Row.

Ham, R., P. Aldersea, and D. Porter. 1998. *Wheelchair users and postural seating: A clinical approach.* New York: Churchill Livingstone.

Hartmann, A.A. 1983. Effect of occlusion on resident flora, skin moisture and skin pH. *Archives of Dermatological Research* 275:251–254.

Herr, H. 2009. Exoskeletons and orthoses: Classification, design challenges and future directions. *Journal of Neuroengineering & Rehabilitation* 6:21.

Hertzberg, H.T.E. 1972. The human buttocks in sitting: Pressures, patterns and palliatives. *Society of Automotive Engineers* Technical Paper no. 720005.

Hobson, D.A. 1978. Foam-in-place seating for the severely disabled. *5th Annual Conference on Systems and Devices for the Disabled.* Houston, TX: Texas Institute of Rehabilitation and Research, 154.

Hunt, A. 2003. Paediatric Pain Profile. London: University College London/Institute of Child Health and Royal College of Nursing Institute. www.ppprofile.org.uk (accessed March 2010).

International Organization for Standardization [ISO]. 2006. Wheelchair seating — Part 1: Vocabulary, reference axis convention and measures for body segments, posture and postural support surfaces. ISO 16840-1.

International Organization for Standardization [ISO]. 2007. Wheelchair seating – Part 2: Determination of physical and mechanical characteristics of devices intended to manage tissue integrity – Seat cushions. ISO 16840-2.

International Organization for Standardization [ISO]. 2009. Wheelchair seating – Part 4: Seating systems for use in motor vehicles. ISO 16840-4.

Kangas, K.M. 2004. Why current pediatric seating systems configured to "support growth" are not working. In *Proceedings of 20th International Seating Symposium,* Vancouver, Canada, 36–39.

Kreutz, D. 1997. Power tilt, recline or both. *TeamRehab Report* 8(3):31–33.

Kroemer, K.H.E. 2006. *"Extra-ordinary" ergonomics: How to accommodate small and big persons, the disabled and elderly, expectant mothers and children.* Boca Raton, FL: Taylor & Francis.

Krouskop, T.A. 1983. A synthesis of the factors that contribute to pressure sore formation. *Medical Hypotheses* 11:255–267.

Kwitatkowski, R.J., and R.M. Inigo. 1993. A closed loop automated seating system. *Journal of Rehabilitation Research & Development* 30(4):393–404.

Lacoste, M., R. Weiss-Lambrou, M. Allard, and J. Dansereau. 2003. Powered tilt/recline systems: Why and how are they used? *Assistive Technology* 15:58–68.

Lau, H., E.W. Tam, and J.C. Cheng. 2008. An experience on wheelchair bank management. *Disability and Rehabilitation — Assistive Technology* 3(6):302–308.

Letts, K., L. Shapiro, D. Mulder, and O. Klassen. 1984. The Windblown Hip Syndrome in total body cerebral palsy. *Journal of Pediatrics Orthopedica* 4:55–60.

Letts, R.M. 1991. *Principles of seating the disabled.* Boca Raton, FL: CRC Press.

Linder-Ganz, E., M. Scheinowitz, Z. Yizhar, S.S. Margulies, and A. Gefen. 2005. Frequency and extent of spontaneous motion to relief tissue loads in normal individuals seated in a wheelchair. *2005 Summer Bioengineering Conference of the ASME Bioengineering Division,* Vail, CO, June 22–26.

Mahoney, R.I., and D.W. Barthel. 1965. Functional evaluation: The Barthel Index. *Maryland State Medical Journal* 14:61–65.

Markwald, M. 1998. Traveling seat. U.S. Patent 6,488,332.

McDonald, R., A. Richardson, and A. Jackel. 2008. Contoured and flat seat cushions for children. *Proceedings of ARATA Conference 2008,* Adelaide, Australia. www.arata.ovau/arataconfowheeledmobilityseating.html (Accessed 11/8/).

McGovern, T.F., S.I. Reger, E.N. Snyder, and B.L. Sauer. 1988. A new technique for custom contoured body supports. In *Proceedings of the International Conference of the Association for the Advancement of Rehabilitation Technology.* Montreal, 306–307.

Minkel, J.L. 1998. Evidence based practice: A foundation. Paper presented at the *14th International Seating Symposium,* Vancouver, BC, Canada.

Myhr, U., and L. vonWendt. 1990. Reducing spasticity and enhancing postural control for the creation of a functional sitting position in children with cerebral palsy: A pilot study. *Physiotherapy Theory and Practice* 6:65–76.

Myhr, U., and L. vonWendt. 1991. Improvement of functional sitting position for children with cerebral palsy. *Developmental Medicine and Child Neurology* 33:246–256.

Myhr, U., and L. vonWendt. 1993. Influence of different sitting positions and abduction orthosis on leg muscle activity in children with cerebral palsy. *Developmental Medicine and Child Neurology* 35:870–880.

Myhr, U., L. vonWendt, S. Norrlin, and U. Radell. 1995. A 5-year follow-up of a functional sitting position in children with cerebral palsy. *Developmental Medicine and Child Neurology* 37:587–596.

Noon, J.H., D.A. Chesney, and P.W. Axelson. 1998. Development of a dynamic pelvic stabilization system. In *Proceedings of the Annual Conference of Rehabilitation Engineering and Assistive Technology of North America, RESNA* 98:209–211.

Nwaobi, O.M. 1986. Effects of body orientation in space on tonic muscle activity of patients with cerebral palsy. *Developmental Medicine and Child Neurology* 28:41–44.

Nwaobi, O.M., C.E. Brubacker, B. Cosich, and M.D. Sussman. 1983. Electromyographic investigation of extensor activity in cerebral palsied children in different seating positions. *Developmental Medicine and Child Neurology* 25:175–183.

Park, A.C., and C.B. Baddiel. 1972. Rheology of stratum corneum. I: A molecular interpretation of the stress strain curve. *J Soc Cosmet Chen* 23:3012.

Patrick, J.H. 1980. Seating orthoses for severely paralyzed patients. *Physiotherapy* 66:195.

Pedersen, J.P., M.L. Lange, and C. Griehel. 2002. Seating intervention and postural control. In *Clinician's guide to assistive technology*, D.A. Olson and F. DeRuyter, Eds. St. Louis: Mosby.

Peischl, D., L. Koczur, and C. Strine. 2005. Seating systems. In *Cerebral palsy*, F. Miller, Ed. New York: Springer, 821–828.

Pope, P.M. 2002. Posture management and special seating. In *Neurological physiotherapy*, S. Edwards, Ed. London: Churchill Livingstone.

Reswick, J.B., and J. Rogers. 1976. Experience at Rancho Los Amigo Hospital with devices and techniques to prevent pressure sores. In *Bedsore biomechanics*, R.M. Kenedi, J.M. Cowden, and J.T. Scales, Eds. London: McMillan, 301–310.

Ruch, R.C., and H.D. Patton. 1965. *Physiology and biophysics*. Philadelphia: Saunders.

Ryan, S., K.A. Campbell, P. Rigby, B. Germon, B. Chan, and D. Hubley. 2006. Development of the new Family Impact of Assistive Technology Scale. *International Journal of Rehabilitation Research* 29(3):195–200.

Ryan, S.E., K.A. Campbell, P.J. Rigby, B. Fishbein-Germon, D. Hubley, and B. Chan. 2009. The impact of adaptive seating devices on the lives of young children with cerebral palsy and their families. *Archives of Physical Medicine and Rehabilitation* 90(1):27–33.

Ryan S.E., K.A. Campbell, and P.J. Rigby. 2007. Reliability of the family impact of assistive technology scale for families of young children with cerebral palsy. *Archives of Physical Medicine and Rehabilitation* 88(11):1436–1440.

Sackett, D.J. 1980. Evaluation of health services. In *Mosley-Rosenau's public health and preventive medicine*, J.M. Last, Ed. New York: Appleton-Century-Crofts.

Saftler, F., J. Winter, and M.A. Kelly. 1988. Use of a positioning chair in conjunction with proper seating principles for a seating evaluation. In *Proceedings of the International Conference of the Association for the Advancement of Rehabilitation Technology*. Montreal, 250–251.

Sanger, T.D., M.R. Delgado, D. Gaebler-Spira, M. Hallett, and J.W. Mink. 2003. Classification and definition of disorders causing hypertonia in childhood. *Pediatrics* 111:e89–e97.

Schmeler, M., B. Engstrom, B. Crane, and R. Cooper. 2007. Seating biomechanics and systems. In *An Introduction to Rehabilitation Engineering*, Cooper, R.A. et al., Eds. Boca Raton, FL: Taylor & Francis, pp. 101–115.

Sprigle, S., K.C. Chung, and C.E. Brubaker. 1990. Reduction of sitting pressure with custom contour cushions. *Journal of Rehabilitation Research & Development* 27(2):135–140.

Sprigle, S., and B. Sposato. 1997. Physiologic effects and design considerations of tilt and recline wheelchairs. *Orthopaedic Physical Therapy Clinics of North America* 6(1):99–122.

Stewart, C.P.U. 1991. Physiological considerations in seating. *Prosthetics and Orthotics International* 15:193–198.

Tarsy, D., and D.K. Simon. 2006. Dystonia. *The New England Journal of Medicine* 355(8):818–830.

Trail, I.A., and C.S. Galasko. 1990. The Matrix seating system. *Journal of Bone and Joint Surgery -British Volume* 72-B(4):666–669.

Trefler E., D.A. Hobson, S.J. Taylor, L. Monahan, and G. Shaw. 1993. *Seating and mobility for persons with physical disabilities.* Tucson, AZ: Therapy Skill Builders.

Uniform Data System for Medical Rehabilitation, Functional Independence Measure, version 5.1. 1997. Buffalo General Hospital, State University of New York.

Wang J., D.M. Brienza, Y. Yuan, P. Karg, and Q. Xue. 2000. A compound sensor for biomechanical analyses of buttock soft tissue in vivo. *Journal of Rehabilitation Research & Development* 37(4):433–443.

Warren, C.G., M. Ko, C. Smith, and J.V. Imre. 1982. Reducing back displacement in the powered reclining wheelchair. *Archives of Physical Medicine and Rehabilitation* 63:447–449.

Watson, N., and B. Woods. 2005. The origins and early developments of special/adaptive wheelchair seating. *Social History of Medicine* 18(3): 459–474.

Yang, T.S., R.C. Chan, T.T. Wong, W.N. Bair, C.C. Kao, T.Y. Chuang, and T.C. Hsu. 1996. Quantitative measurement of improvement in sitting balance in children with spastic cerebral palsy after selective posterior rhizotomy. *American Journal of Physical Medicine & Rehabilitation* 75:348–352.

Zeltwanger, A.P., D. Brown, and G. Bertocci. 2001. Utilizing computer modeling in the development of a dynamic seating system. In *Proceedings of the 24th RESNA Annual Meeting.* Reno, NV. http://www.rercwm.pitt.edu/RERCWM_Res/RERC_Res_DDT/ RERC_Res_DDT_D5/DDT_D5_RESNA2001.html (accessed March 2010).

Upper and Lower Extremity Prosthetics for Children and Youth

Elaine Biddiss and Jan Andrysek

CONTENTS

OVERVIEW OF REHAB ENGINEERING IN PAEDIATRIC PROSTHETICS

Rehabilitation engineering in prosthetics relates to the design, development, evaluation and application of technologies to decrease the impairment severity associated with limb loss. In limb prosthetics, these main components of rehabilitation include amputation surgery, application of prosthetic technologies, and training or physical therapy programs. A multidisciplinary approach is vital to cover the full spectrum of an individual's rehabilitation and habilitation needs so as to facilitate successful outcomes. Moreover, one may extend the role of rehabilitation engineering to further include, for example, the design and evaluation of techniques or approaches used to evaluate prosthetic interventions. For instance, engineering has contributed to the development and evaluation of instrumentation with which we can more effectively measure and quantify human movement. In turn, these 'instruments' have played a vital role in the assessment of the performance of prosthetic interventions. As such, the main goal of this chapter is to provide a comprehensive overview of the direct and indirect roles of engineering sciences in the rehabilitation of children with limb differences. In this chapter, the terminology 'absence,' 'loss,' and 'amputation' are used interchangeably irrespective of origin of limb difference (i.e., congenital or acquired). It is important to note that appropriate and sensitive usage of these terms depends largely on the individual perceptions, experiences and preferences of each child and his or her family. Likewise, the terms 'rehabilitation' and 'habilitation' are also interchanged, although the former, strictly speaking, refers to *restoring* previous abilities and functions (i.e., following an amputation), while the latter refers to attaining new abilities and functions (i.e., during development with a congenital limb difference). In both cases, the ultimate goal is the same: to provide individuals with the means to achieve their functional goals.

CHAPTER ROADMAP

In the spirit of user-centred design, this chapter begins with an introduction to the child with limb differences and a discussion of demographics, developmental physiology and psychosocial characteristics that define user needs. Following this, we trace a typical journey through paediatric prosthetics rehabilitation from amputation surgery and prosthetic design, through prosthesis fitting/training, to evaluation of outcomes. We conclude with a discussion of the latest research in this field and future directions for the advancement of paediatric prosthetics. A roadmap depicting the overall organization of this chapter is shown in Figure 7.1.

PROFILE OF THE CHILD WITH LIMB DIFFERENCES

Successful design, selection and fitting of limb prostheses depend largely on how well the devices meet with each individual's established needs (Biddiss and Chau 2008a). To provide consumer-friendly prostheses, it is important to first understand the needs, wants and limitations of the people who use them, in line with the philosophy of user-centred design (Norman 1988). The physical, psychological and social needs of children differ largely from those of adults and, as such, paediatric prosthetic rehabilitation offers a very unique set of challenges to overcome.

DEMOGRAPHICS

The occurrence of congenital limb defects is estimated to be between 0.3 and 1.0 per 1000 live births, of which the proportion of lower limb deficiencies is marginally less than upper limb deficiencies (McGuirk et al. 2001; Dillingham et al. 2002; Foster and Baird 1993; Kallen et al. 1984). The most common congenital difference is at the trans-radial level of the left limb, which occurs in 40% of upper limb cases (Nelson et al. 2006). Most prevalent lower limb anomalies are associated with the toes (30%), foot (24%), femur (24%) and tibia or fibula (22%) (Fisk and Smith, 2004, 773–778; Froster and Baird 1993) The aetiology of congenital limb deficiencies is poorly established, although genetic and environmental factors, complications in pregnancies and maternal diseases are attributed in the minority of cases (McGuirk et al. 2001; Sener et al. 1999).

Congenital limb absence is the most common cause of limb differences in children under the age of 10 years (Jain 1996). As the population ages, a greater proportion of limb absences are due to (in order of prevalence) trauma, disease, malignant tumours, vascular and neurological disorders, and other (Dormans et al. 2004; Krebs et al. 1991; Vannah et al. 1999). In developed countries, over 90% of lower limb amputations are performed in the latter stages of life and primarily to treat peripheral vascular disease (Nielsen 2007). In contrast, lower limb amputation in children comprises a niche of approximately 5% of all lower limb amputations (Pitkin 1997). As the population ages, the gender distribution also changes as males, historically, are associated with greater risk for traumatic amputations (Ziegler-Graham et al. 2008).

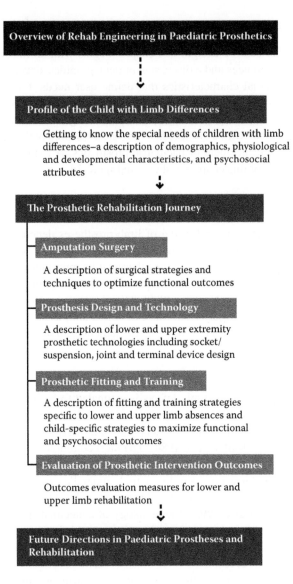

FIGURE 7.1   Roadmap.

It is important to note that the physical and psychological experiences and needs of a child who is born with a limb difference may be quite distinct from those of a child or adolescent who has undergone an amputation. A child with congenital limb absence typically learns to use a prosthetic limb at an earlier age, experiences no residual cortical motor mappings associated with the missing limb, reports a lower incidence of pain, and is less likely to feel a sense of loss for the missing limb as compared to an individual with acquired limb absence (Biddiss and Chau 2007). Likewise, level of limb absence is also definitive of many of the experiences and needs of the child. For example, the prosthetic options and extent of impairment is very different for an individual with partial hand loss as compared to a shoulder disarticulation (Biddiss and Chau 2007, 2008a).

PHYSIOLOGICAL AND DEVELOPMENTAL CHARACTERISTICS

Children are in a dynamic state of development and growth involving not only their size and strength, but also their manual dexterity, mobility, and motor and cognitive skills. With maturity comes changing needs and interests; with adolescence, the processes of self-actualization and transition to independence. The primary purpose of rehabilitation programs for children with limb differences is to facilitate the typical developmental sequence and prevent onset of secondary impairments and functional limitations.

In children with upper limb differences, motor learning largely follows the expected progression, although crawling and walking may be slightly delayed due to body imbalance (Nelson et al. 2006). Prosthetic options expand as the child grows in physical and cognitive abilities. At an early age, prostheses may aid in body balance and functional activities of play. Conversely, encasement of the residual limb is sometimes seen to interfere with sensory feedback needed for exploration and discovery (Jain 1996). With maturity, there is often a shift in functional needs from motor to cognitive skills as the child moves from the occupation of play to that of education (Postema et al. 1999). These transitional periods are frequently paralleled by a re-evaluation of needs and the ability of a prosthesis, or set of prostheses, to meet these needs. Prosthesis selection and maintenance must dynamically adapt to and anticipate developmental growth throughout infancy, childhood and adolescence.

As children with upper limb differences can generally perform most tasks with or without the aid of a prosthesis and find creative adaptations to achieve their goals (Nelson et al. 2006), prosthesis acceptance and use is more variable than for children with lower limb absence. Upon the completion of the rehabilitative process, children with lower extremity amputations are typically expected to perform satisfactorily in physical activities involving the lower limbs. Between 85% and 95% of children with limb loss become functional walkers and between 62% and 93% partake in physical education programs at school or in recreation with their peers (Vannah et al. 1999; Boonstra et al. 2000).

PSYCHOSOCIAL ATTRIBUTES

Children are legally and economically reliant on their parents to provide for many of their emotional and physical needs. It is therefore not surprising that the emotional health of a child with limb absence is inexorably tied to the attitudes and beliefs of his or her guardians (Postema et al. 1999; Varni et al. 1991). This emphasises the importance of caring for both the child and his or her family throughout the rehabilitation process. In fact, the very first activity of a successful paediatric prosthetics program often is to foster bonding between the child and parent and to mitigate negative response to what, in most cases, is an unanticipated breach of expectations (Hubbard et al. 2004a). A child's acceptance of prostheses often mirrors that of his or her parents (Postema et al. 1999). Consistent and realistic expectations for its use are essential and should be informed by healthcare providers.

In general, research suggests that socially, children with limb differences adjust better than do adults with limb differences and are largely well accepted by their peers (Hermansson et al. 2005; Tyc 1992). Varni and colleagues have written extensively on this subject and the importance of a strong social network of friends, family and teachers to the psychosocial health of the child (Varni et al. 1991a, 1991b, 1992). Not surprisingly, higher levels of social support are associated with positive self-esteem and lowered risk of depression in children with limb differences (Varni et al. 1991a, 1991b, 1992; Tyc 1992; Hermansson et al. 2005).

AMPUTATION SURGERY

In broad terms, amputation refers to the loss of a body part. When the limb is not transected through the bone, but rather at a joint between two adjoining bones, this is termed a disarticulation. Amputation surgery involves severing bone, nerve, muscle and skin tissues, the latter of which are typically reconstructed to provide anatomical attributes that are capable of transmitting and cushioning the interfacial loads between the prosthesis and residuum. Typically, the goals of amputation surgery are first to remove the traumatised, diseased, infected or, in the case of congenital deficiencies, malformed and dysfunctional portions of the limb. A secondary goal is to reconstruct the residuum to promote healing and provide a functional interface for the prosthesis. It is essential to consider not only surgical principles, but also the post-operative implications of the surgery on prosthetic intervention. As such, decision-making should be made by an interdisciplinary team including the surgeon, physician, prosthetist, physical therapist, patient and, in the case of a child, his or her parents. Decisions made at the time of surgery require a thorough understanding of the different characteristics of the anatomy, and their ensuing post-operative functions, which will undoubtedly affect prosthetic rehabilitation. Distinctions in surgical interventions and techniques are made in consideration of numerous factors including the diagnosis, aetiology, functional potential, patient age and other factors. A general overview is provided here and a more detailed one elsewhere (Lusardi and Nielsen 2000).

The residual limbs of children with severe congenital limb anomalies are frequently modified to allow or improve the outcome of prosthetic fitting. Limb deficiencies are generally categorised as longitudinal (i.e., occurs along the axis of the limb) and radial (i.e., the limb is absent across its longitudinal axis such as in a wrist disarticulation). Lower limb deficiencies are typically characterised as being fibular, tibial, femoral, or of the foot complex, while upper limb deficiencies can be broadly categorised as phalangeal, carpal, radial, humeral, or interscapulothoracic/forequarter (Froster and Baird 1993). These deficiencies commonly present various osseous and soft tissue deformities that can result in a shortening of the limb. Other aspects of the anatomy, such as the hip joint in the case of longitudinal deficiency of the femur-partial (LDFP), previously referred to as proximal femoral focal deficiency (PFFD), may also be affected or absent. Surgical procedures in general include fusing and reconstructing or removing dysfunctional osseous and soft tissues of the affected limb segments (Lambert 1972).

In some cases, amputation can be avoided using limb salvage techniques including limb lengthening and limb reconstruction. Although limb salvage techniques are known to improve functional outcomes (Aksnes et al. 2008), these interventions typically require on-going procedures such as surgical revisions over many years, an important consideration for the patient and the family involved (Walker et al. 2009). Furthermore, evidence suggests that complications occur more frequently with limb salvage procedures than with amputation (Sewell et al. 2009) and, although limb salvage is slightly favoured for increased physical functioning (Aksnes et al. 2008), the long-term outcomes are not profoundly different, compared with amputation, in regard to quality of life (Nagarajan et al. 2002).

Lastly, it is beneficial to preserve joint function as much as possible, as is evidenced by the higher levels of functionality of below-knee amputees over above-knee amputees (Waters and Mulroy 1999) and of below-elbow amputees compared to above-elbow amputees (Biddiss and Chau 2007a). Rotationplasty is another unique orthopaedic limb salvage technique in which the child's limb is amputated above the knee and the lower limb is rotated 180° and reattached. In this way, the ankle joint functions in place of the knee joint, enabling the use of a below-knee prosthesis. Compared to amputation, which would require an above-knee prosthesis, or issues with limb-salvage surgeries using endoprosthesis, this procedure is favoured not only due to the increased function it affords, but also because it relieves patients of phantom pain, and avoids limb length discrepancy and loosening of an endoprosthesis (Sawamura et al. 2008). A primary disadvantage of rotationplasty is poorer cosmesis due to the unusual appearance of the limb following this procedure.

In summary, the following general principles of childhood amputation surgery should be considered for attaining optimal functional results: preservation of limb length, joints, growth plates and muscle mass; performing disarticulation rather than transosseous amputation where possible; and stabilizing and normalizing the proximal portions of the limb (Krajbich 1998; Lambert 1972). These procedures aim to optimise the characteristics of the prosthesis and residual limb interface (weight-bearing capacity, residual limb length for improved control, stability and sensation in the case of the upper limb, and proximal limb stability) and limit complications due to bone overgrowth.

PROSTHESIS DESIGN AND TECHNOLOGY

The design of products and processes is an integral part of developing and improving components of the rehabilitation process. This includes the development of prosthetic components and fabrication methods (e.g., new socket casting techniques) or new physical therapy regimes. In addition, design plays a role in the development of research instruments and techniques that enable us, for example, to better measure prosthetic gait.

The design process, as shown in Figure 7.2, starts with the recognition of a societal or patient need, which is then formalised into a set of functional requirements (FRs), or 'things' that we want the new design to accomplish (Cummings 1996). Once the FRs have been defined in adequate detail, the next step is to map them

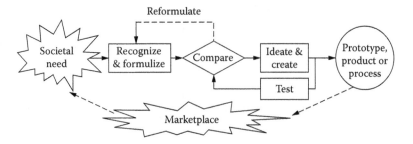

FIGURE 7.2 The design process. (Adapted from Wilson, D.R. 1980. An exploratory study of complexity in axiomatic design, PhD Thesis, with permission from the Massachusetts Institute of Technology.)

in the physical domain or, in other words, to find ways in which the FRs can be satisfied (Suh 1990; Bossert 1991; International Organization for Standardization 1996; Revelle et al. 1998). This is where the creative and inventive part of the design process occurs, as the designer tries to ideate and create the basis of the new design. At this point in the design process, many ideas may appear feasible and promising, but as these ideas are formulated in greater detail, a filtering process occurs. In the design of prosthetic components, three-dimensional computer-aided design (CAD) models, computer-aided engineering techniques such as finite element stress analyses, and biomechanical models simulating function can be invaluable.

The next step in the design process includes the construction of a prototype for testing. For prosthetic components, functional and structural tests, often in accordance with standards [e.g., ISO standard for lower limbs (Cummings 2004)], typically precede clinical testing to ensure patient safety. During this testing process, various tools can be applied to help determine whether the FRs have been adequately satisfied. The testing protocol will depend on a number of factors such as the resources that are available, timelines, and the nature of the design. Design is an iterative process requiring that FRs be reformulated or that ideas be re-synthesized many times. As a design becomes more refined through this process, it becomes imperative to perform more extensive evaluations, for example, in the form of field trials, and to develop a well-rounded understanding of the design's impact on the rehabilitation process.

TECHNOLOGIES COMMON TO UPPER AND LOWER EXTREMITY PROSTHESES

Sockets and Suspension

Both upper and lower limb prostheses share a common element, and that is the socket that is used to interface the rest of the prosthesis with the residual limb. The socket is essentially a container that restrains the residuum. The design and fabrication of this 'container' require careful consideration of a multitude of factors such that the pressures caused by loads being transmitted from the prosthesis to the biological limb are distributed to parts of the limb that are most able to deal with them and such that range of joint motion is not restricted. Sockets should also be designed to match the anatomical limb in shape, size and length as much as possible in order to optimise cosmesis and body balance. For upper limb prosthetics, the socket must also enable secure and consistent placement for electrodes and cables, while providing an avenue for kinesthesia and proprioception. A number of different socket designs exist and they are selected on the basis of the amputee's anatomy, activity level, level of amputation and personal preference (Kapp 2000).

The means for attaching the socket to the residual limb is referred to as suspension. Suspension plays a primary role in countering the effects of gravity and other forces, in order to keep the prosthesis securely attached to the limb. One of the primary goals of suspension is to minimise the effect of residual limb movement within the socket. In the case of lower limb prostheses, this commonly occurs during transitions between weight-bearing and non-weight-bearing movement, and is referred to as pistoning.

Common socket attachment techniques are loosely categorised as anatomical suspensions, strap suspensions and suction sockets. Anatomical suspension is achieved via a mechanical mating of the limb and socket. For example, for transtibial amputees, the socket walls are designed to come over and encompass the medial and lateral femoral condyles (Michael 2004). Applying anatomical suspension may involve the use of fenestrations, hidden panels, and expandable inner walls. The effect of friction between the prosthesis and residual limb, preventing the prosthesis from moving and slipping off, is an important aspect of this approach. In upper limb prosthetics, a common example of a self-suspending socket is the Muenster design (Sauter et al. 1986). Advantages of anatomical suspensions, such as the Muenster, include the lack of a harness, while disadvantages are the reduced joint mobility and skin irritation caused by the tight-fitting socket (Sauter et al. 1986). Suspension using straps, as implied by the name, refers to the process of attaching a strap to part of the body, such as the waist, to secure the prosthesis. In atmospheric pressure or suction socket suspension, a vacuum is developed between the socket and limb causing the prosthesis to remain attached using suction or negative pressure. The air seal needed to accomplish this may be achieved simply by using the soft tissue of the limb and the brim of the socket. Variations of these techniques, utilizing flexible liners and sleeves, possibly in combination with friction or mechanical locking pins (between the liner and socket), are typically applied to both upper and lower limb prostheses. Donning and doffing of the prosthesis is achieved by opening a valve at the distal end of the socket to control air pressures (Kapp 1999, 2000).

Specific to paediatric prosthetics, the challenges of socket fit are exacerbated by the child's continual growth. Significant changes in the shape and size of the residual limb require a new socket to be fabricated, sometimes within months. The use of socks, flexible and re-formable sockets, gel liners and slip sockets is helpful in postponing the need for a new socket (Cummings 2004). As with adults, suction-type prosthetic suspension systems offer substantial advantages to active young amputees in terms of improved comfort, function and appearance (Madigan and Fullauer 1991; Fishman et al. 1987).

Lower Extremity Prosthetic Technologies

Prosthetic technologies have played, and continue to play, a key role in the rehabilitation of children and youth with lower limb amputations. Upon the appropriation of surgical, prosthetic and physical therapy-based interventions, it is the functional symbiosis of the biological (human) and artificial systems (prostheses) that facilitates a successful rehabilitative outcome. Despite their various technical and performance limitations, lower limb prostheses are highly utilised, with 99% of fitted children using their prosthetic limbs to some degree, and 90% of children using their prosthetic limbs for more than 9 hours per day (Vannah et al. 1999; Boonstra et al. 2000). As children develop physically and intellectually, they become candidates for more advanced and effective prosthetic components, such as energy storing feet, articulating prosthetic knee joints and suction socket technologies, thus further facilitating their biopsychosocial development.

A typical lower limb prosthesis is comprised of a socket and suspension as a means for interfacing the prosthesis to the residual limb, a knee joint (in the case of an above-knee prosthesis) and a foot component, assembled (in the case of typical endoskeletal modular systems) using pylons and connectors (Figure 7.3). The consolidation of these components contributes toward a well-functioning prosthesis. Socket fit and suspension influence load-bearing capability, comfort, proprioception,

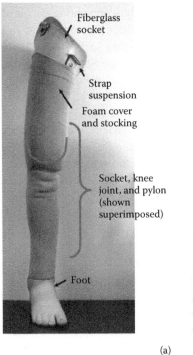
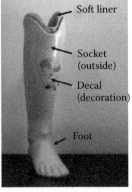

(a)

FIGURE 7.3 (See color insert following page 240.) (a) Paediatric lower-limb prostheses: modular above-knee prosthesis (left); and below-knee prosthesis (right).   *(Continued)*

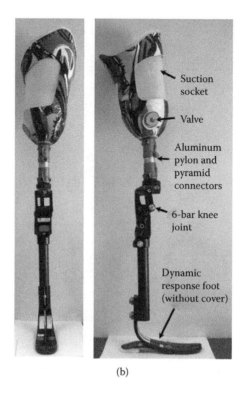

Suction
socket

Valve

Aluminum
pylon and
pyramid
connectors

6-bar knee
joint

Dynamic
response foot
(without cover)

(b)

FIGURE 7.3 (See color insert following page 240.) (Continued) (b) Modern modular above-knee prosthesis for adults showing suction socket, polycentric knee joint and dynamic response foot. A cosmetic foot cover would typically be used. A foam cosmetic cover may also be provided over the rest of the structure. *(Continued)*

and the control of the prosthetic limb (Kapp 2000). The prosthetic knee joint mechanism provides controlled articulation to enable tasks such as sitting and to allow the knee to swing during walking, and plays an important role toward achieving weight-bearing stability (Michael 1999; Cummings 1997). Prosthetic foot components also influence stability, as well as rollover characteristics, the progression of the shank, and overall comfort (Graham et al. 2007; Colborne et al. 2007). In summary, it is the interaction of these components with the human body, and within the environment, that will influence the outcome of prosthetic rehabilitation.

Prosthetic Feet and Ankles

The foot has the primary interaction with the environment through contact with the ground. During weight bearing, effects of ground contact at the plantar surface of the foot, which results in external loading of the limb, can be characterised by a single equivalent ground reaction force vector (GRFV), as shown in Figure 7.4, having an origin at the centre of pressure (between the foot and ground), and an orientation that is predominantly vertical. The dynamic interaction of the GRFV, the prosthetic system, and the human body is an important factor affecting functional mobility. The human foot is a complex biological system comprised of a plurality of joints, muscles and nerves that

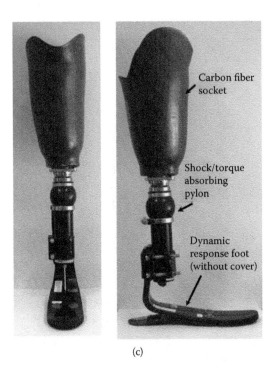

(c)

FIGURE 7.3   (See color insert following page 240.) (Continued) (c) Modern modular below-knee prosthesis for adults showing a shock/torque absorbing pylon and dynamic response foot. Cosmetic finishes are not shown.

allow the lower limb to effectively respond to various loading patterns to provide stability, propulsion and shock absorption during gait, thus facilitating functional mobility. The goal of modern prosthetic feet is to replace these basic aspects of mobility.

Prosthetic foot/ankle designs are generally categorised as single-axis (providing plantar/dorsiflexion), solid ankle-cushion heel or SACH (providing early stance-stability), multi-axial (providing inversion/eversion and/or internal/external rotation), flexible keel (allowing easy roll-over) and dynamic response (providing energy storage and return) (Michael 2004). Often, the features of different feet can be competing. For instance, providing dynamic push-off requires the forefoot to be relatively stiff, which makes roll-over* more demanding at slower walking speeds and during slope ascents. In addition to functional differences, the trade-offs between foot components include the costs associated with implementation and maintenance, and component weight. A constraint for foot prescription includes build height, which precludes the use of some foot components in the case of transtibial amputees with long residual limbs. Typically, in children, these component attributes are not only important considerations from a clinical perspective, specifically during the fitting

---

* Roll-over refers to the interaction of the foot with the ground in stance phase. Typically this involves the function of the heel, ankle and forefoot rockers, which are highly dependent on the mechanical properties of the specific prosthetic foot. Roll-over can be characterised by the progression of the centre of pressure on the plantar surface of the foot, and the kinematics of the lower leg.

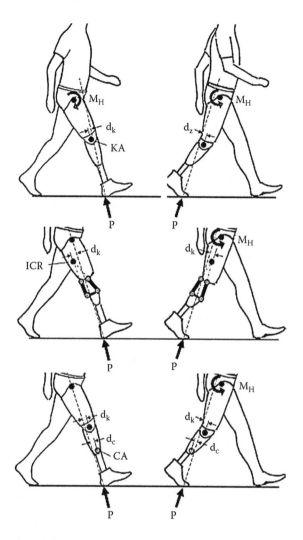

FIGURE 7.4 Sagittal-plane ground reaction force vector (GRFV), P, shown in initial stance phase (left) and late stance phase of gait (right). Initial contact typically occurs with the heel of the foot, and progresses to the forefoot. Exemplified, is an above-knee prosthesis with a single-axis knee joint (top), a four-bar knee joint (middle), and a knee joint using a 'control' axis (bottom). For the single-axis knee, the individual must generate a hip extension moment using hip musculature, M_H, to stabilize the knee joint and in effect cause a knee extension moment, in initial stance. Otherwise, the knee joint will buckle. M_H brings the P anterior of the knee axis, KA, resulting in a knee stabilizing moment that is equal to $P \times d_k$. In late stance, knee flexion initiation is achieved by producing a hip flexion moment (top right). A four-bar knee, with an instantaneous centre of rotation, ICR, that is posterior and proximal of the anatomical knee centre, can help to stabilize the knee joint without the need for a hip extension moment (middle left), and without increasing the effort (hip flexion moment) to initiate flexion in late stance (middle right). Alternatively, a control axis (CA) can be used to impose control at the knee axis. For example, in early stance, when P is behind the control axis, this imposes 'braking' at the knee axis, thus keeping the knee stable (bottom left). When P is anterior to the control axis, the braking is disengaged (bottom right).

of prostheses, but also for researchers, engineers and designers involved in the design and development of new prosthetic components.

Biomechanical and functional studies have elucidated some of the performance differences between the various prosthetic foot component technologies. The summative findings of these studies suggest that high-end dynamic prosthetic feet may be of little benefit in high-activity transfemoral amputees, but that they are likely to benefit transtibial amputees by increasing walking speed and improving gait on inclined surfaces (Hofstad et al. 2004). For children with transtibial amputations, dynamic feet may help to decrease metabolic demands, increase walking speed and improve certain gait characteristics (Schneider et al. 1993; Colborne et al. 1992). It is important to remember, however, that these performance differences are typically measured under ideal laboratory conditions, and that real-world situations (i.e., alternate activities and environmental conditions) may yield different results. Hence, ecologically relevant studies in the form of field trials should always be considered in the later stages of research and development activities.

Prosthetic Knees

The knee is the largest and one of the most complex joints in the human body, and a key facilitator of mobility. Replacing its function using artificial systems is proving very difficult at present and, therefore, whenever possible, great effort is taken during amputation surgery to preserve the anatomical knee joint (Krajbich 1998). Where this is not possible, the patient will ultimately need to depend on an artificial substitute.

The primary goal of prosthetic knee joint function is to provide controlled articulation. During weight acceptance and mid-stance of gait, the knee mechanism should mimic the function of the quadriceps in resisting knee flexion, and preventing collapse at the knee. Resistance (of a lesser magnitude) at the knee is also desirable during the swing phase, in mid-swing phase to control the amount of knee flexion and in late-swing phase to slow the extension of the shank prior to full knee extension. Prosthetic knee joint control is conventionally achieved using passive systems such as dampers, brakes, locks and linkage mechanisms. This approach is highly effective during level and downhill walking, but mainly due to the absence of active knee flexion and extension torque, it impedes activities such as standing up, running and walking up inclines and stairs. In recent years, an artificial knee joint capable of generating active knee torque has become available to adult amputees. Although improvements are continually being made, the utility of this POWER KNEE™, by Össur, is limited in part by its heaviness and also by the electrical power requirements requiring frequent battery recharging.

During weight-bearing (i.e., the stance phase of gait), the resistance to knee flexion acts in response to some prosthetic loading condition. The simplest approach involves the posterior placement of the knee axis so that in early and mid-stance phase it is behind the GRFV, thus generating a knee extension moment. Prosthetic component properties, setup and alignment of the prosthesis, and the ability of the child to apply control using his or her residual musculature (mainly at the hip) will in large part dictate the effectiveness of this approach. The application of polycentric mechanisms in the form of four-, five- and six-bar linkages (see Figures 7.3 and 7.4) is an effective approach for enhancing stance phase control, making the knee joint more stable in early to mid-stance, but allowing it to be voluntarily flexed in late stance phase prior to swing phase.

Alternatively, when a braking or damping mechanism is used to resist stance phase flexion, the strategy is to have a sensing point on the knee joint that determines whether the knee is being loaded, and whether the load is in flexion or extension as a result of the GRFV. This, in turn, provides the appropriate signal to increase or decrease resistance in the brake or damper at the knee joint axis. This can be achieved in a purely mechanical fashion or by using electromechanical systems. The latter represents a relatively new breed of prostheses that utilise on-board microprocessors to enhance knee control under a broader range of mobility conditions. The adaptability of these dampers is further extended to control the swinging characteristics, thus allowing individuals to achieve smoother and more kinematically and temporally symmetrical movements of the limb. Where funding is available to cover the high cost of these microprocessor-based technologies, they are quickly becoming the prescription norm for active adults with above-knee amputations. Microprocessor knee joints have been shown to promote more normal gait characteristics (Segal et al. 2006), lower energy expenditure (Datta et al. 2005; Buckley et al. 1997) and cognitive demand during walking (Heller et al. 2000) and decrease falls (Kahle et al. 2008).

Prosthetic knee joint technologies for children are substantially less sophisticated than those prescribed for adults. Most utilise either single-axis configurations or four-bar linkage mechanisms, and swing phase control is typically friction based (Andrysek et al. 2004). Only a handful of studies have looked at the biomechanical performance of paediatric prosthetic knee joints, establishing the importance of fitting children with articulating knee joints at an early age (Wilk et al. 1999), exposing the limitations of friction-based swing phase control (Hicks et al. 1985), and examining the outcomes of different surgical and prosthetic technology options (Loder and Herring 1987; Andrysek et al. 2007). More advanced function in paediatric prosthetic knee joints is being achieved using a six-bar knee mechanism (total knee) and a unique automatic stance phase lock (Cumming 1997; Andrysek et al. 2004, 2005; Andrysek 2007). Aside from providing good stance phase control, both of these technologies also allow for stance phase flexion, which has been shown to provide shock absorption and more natural gait (Gard and Childress 1999). However, only one paediatric prosthetic component provides hydraulic swing phase control (3R65 by Otto Bock) and that is at the expense of less functional stance phase control.

The degree of disability increases with more proximal levels of amputation and especially with the loss of major joints. As such, the gait of individuals with above-knee prostheses is slower, more energy expending, and presents more gait deviations and compensations when compared to the gait of transtibial amputees (Waters and Mulroy 1999; Mensch and Ellis 1986; Nolan 2003). Biomechanical deviations associated with unstable joints, inadequate joint musculature, limb rotations and limb length differences exacerbate the functional limitations of children with congenital limb deficiencies.

UPPER EXTREMITY PROSTHETIC TECHNOLOGIES

The following describes the state-of-the-art in paediatric upper limb prostheses. Upper limb prostheses can generally be subdivided by control system (i.e., passive, body-powered, electric, hybrid and activity-specific) and by terminal device (i.e., hook or hand). *Passive prostheses* do not incorporate an active control mechanism by which to control prehension grip, although some devices do include spring-loaded linkages to enable a basic grasp of objects introduced to the hand. *Body-powered prostheses* rely on gross body movements (e.g., of the shoulder, upper arm or chest) that are transferred via a cable and harness system to control opening or closing of the terminal device or movement of the elbow. *Electric prostheses* incorporate small motors that can be activated by a variety of means including muscle signals and touch pads or strain sensors. *Hybrid devices* combine elements of both body-powered and electric control. *Activity-specific prostheses* are designed to enable participation in activities (e.g., swimming, fishing, cycling or golf) that are not conducive to any of the standard prosthesis types. A final prosthetic option of importance to this topic is the decision not to wear a prosthesis at all. Prosthesis rejection is far more common for children with upper limb absence than for lower limb absence, and is therefore included in the pursuant discussion in order to better understand current satisfaction with, and limitations of, prosthetic devices. For a detailed guide of commonly used and commercially available prosthetic components, several excellent handbooks are available to the interested reader (Lusardi and Nielsen 2000; Carroll and Edelstein 2006). Manufacturers of paediatric prosthetic components include OttoBock, RSL Steeper, the Fillauer Companies (Hosmer Dorrance, Motion Control, Centri) and TRS Inc.

Passive Prostheses

Passive devices are often prescribed at a very early age to acclimatise the child to prosthesis use and to aid in support and balance. The initial device is likely a passive baby mitt or crawling prosthesis to aid the child in attaining developmental milestones. The passive prosthesis is often followed by an active device once the child is physically and functionally able to benefit from, and emotionally ready to embrace, its use. Several passive devices are commercially available, some with limited gripping functionality. The Wilmer Hand (Plettenburg 2009), as depicted in Figure 7.5, is an example of a passive hand designed specifically for children from 1 to 5 years

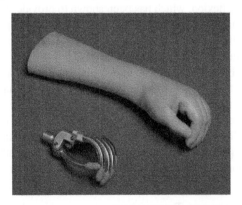

FIGURE 7.5 The Wilmer Hand is a passive hand designed specifically for children from 1 to 5 years of age that enables some gripping function through a mechanical linkage and spring system. Picture is courtesy of Dr. Dick Plettenburg (2006a).

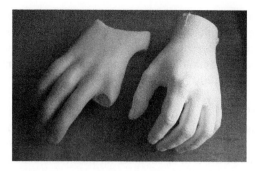

FIGURE 7.6 A customized and life-like silicone cosmetic hand (right) alongside a plaster mould of the contralateral hand (left). Picture is courtesy of prosthetic artist, Mr. James Vanderkleyn.

of age. The device opens when an object is pressed against the fingertips by means of a four-bar mechanical linkage and spring system that mechanically couples the movement of the fingers to that of the thumb. The principle backing this design is that, for children with unilateral deficiencies, the intact hand is generally used to hold the object and present it to the prosthesis. The Easy Feed Hand, developed at Rancho Los Amigos National Rehabilitation Center, is another example of this design approach (Landsberger et al. 1998).

Given their simple design, passive prostheses are generally quite resistant to dirt, sand and water. This durability is of particular importance in paediatrics, but does not always extend to the cosmetic covering that is applied to the terminal device. Prosthetic gloves are usually fabricated from economical and durable polyvinylchloride (PVC) or from more life-like and expensive silicone elastomers. Figure 7.6 depicts a silicone elastomer cosmetic glove designed for a partial hand prosthesis. For active, growing children, the cost of life-like silicone elastomer coverings can be prohibitive given that frequent replacements are often needed.

Passive prostheses are most often used functionally for steadying and support, and can offer aesthetic appeal in a comparably light package. Passive prosthetic hands, for example, can weigh as little as 39 g for small sizes (e.g., Alpha Infant Hand, TRS Inc.), while a body-powered hook or hand might be on the order of 49 or 74 g, respectively (e.g., Lite Touch Hand or Adept Prehensor, TRS Inc.). Electric hands are typically the heaviest and might start at 86 g (e.g., Electrohand 2000, Otto Bock). In general, the weight of prosthetic systems can vary greatly depending on the level of limb absence and the prosthetic components required (e.g., wrist or elbow, hook or hand, active or passive control mechanism). Weight, and its distribution, is one of the most important parameters in prosthesis design with direct implications for the comfort and acceptance of a device.

Very few studies have evaluated the use of passive devices in children with the exception of Crandall who reported a 62% acceptance rate of passive hands (Crandall et al. 2002). Passive wear of active prostheses has been reported in various studies with reported prevalence ranging from 20% (Mendez et al. 1985) to 47% (Reid et al. 1987). A consumer survey of 96 parents and children identified a number of important design priorities specifically for the improvement of passive devices. These included more life-like appearance (e.g., size, shape and colour) and improved dexterity, ease of cleaning (particularly with respect to gloves) and heat dissipation. For methodological details of this study, the interested reader is referred to Biddiss et al. (2007).

Body-Powered Prostheses

Body-powered prostheses offer the facility for active prehension and are typically considered lighter and less noisy than electric devices. The harness and cable system transfers movements of the arm or shoulder for prosthesis control (e.g., opening or closing of the hook or hand). Body-powered control systems can be configured either as voluntary-opening (most common) or voluntary-closing. The terminal device of a voluntary-opening prosthesis remains closed until activated by the user. Conversely, a voluntary-closing prosthesis remains open until tension in the cable pulls the terminal device closed. The pinch or grip strength of the terminal device depends on the force inputted by the user and the gripping mechanism, which is composed of elastic elements and springs. An important design goal of body-powered prostheses is to optimise the mechanical efficiency of the control mechanism, such that the preponderance of force inputted by the user is translated to the output of the prosthesis (i.e., the pinch or grip strength). TRS Inc. claims the most efficient mechanical hand on the market (i.e., the Lite Touch Hand), which ranges in size and weight (74 to 207 g) for children from age 2 years to young adults.

The literature suggests variable rates of acceptance for body-powered devices ranging from 34% (Kruger et al. 1993) to 68% (Scotland et al. 1983) in children. The type of terminal device (i.e., hook or hand) appears to be a critical factor in device abandonment. Hands have a more anatomically realistic appearance, which may be appealing to many children. However, historically, body-powered hands are associated with higher rates of rejection than are hooks (Biddiss and Chau 2007b). In general, hooks are considered to be lighter, enable a stronger grip (i.e., higher mechanical efficiency) and offer good visibility of the object being held for precise manipulation.

The absence of electrical components makes body-powered devices particularly appropriate for play activities involving sand, mud or water. Conversely, harness discomfort is a common consumer concern (Biddiss et al. 2007; Atkins et al. 1996). When asked, consumers of paediatric body-powered devices indicated a number of important areas for design improvements (Biddiss et al. 2007). Weight was the predominant issue, followed by general concerns with overall function, comfort and appearance. With respect to the latter, one product line of hooks (Plettenburg 2006) directed toward children offers devices with vibrant colours to generate interest and appeal. Hilhorst philosophises on the value of this design approach, which breaks from conformity and 'sameness,' and offers an opportunity to celebrate identity and the unique experience of the individual (Hilhorst 2005). At some rehabilitation clinics, children can bring in a favourite picture or pattern that can be laminated onto the prosthetic socket. This approach to aesthetics is clearly an option that will be amenable for some children and not for others. It is, however, a valuable addition to the paediatric prosthetics toolbox.

Electric Prostheses

Electric prostheses are most commonly controlled via electrical activity generated by voluntarily contracting muscles in the residuum. These signals are referred to as myoelectric signals. Small contractions elicit activity from a small number of fibres deep within the muscle. As the strength of contraction increases, more superficial muscle fibres are activated and the rate at which they contract increases. As a result, the myoelectric signal that is observed on the surface of the skin varies with the strength of the contraction and is a summation of the contractions of these individual muscle fibres. The degree of summation depends on the size and sensitivity of the surface electrodes. The tissue layer separating the muscle and the skin attenuates the signal to amplitudes that range from 10 μV to 10 mV (Lovely 2004) and the signal appears largely as noise. It is the magnitude of this noise that is used as an indicator of the signal strength. The strength and number of sites from which distinct myoelectric signals can be generated and detected varies depending on the physiology of the limb difference and the child's neuromuscular control. The myoelectric signals must be amplified, rectified and filtered for practical use and are largely processed using power detection techniques.

Electrodes for detecting myoelectric activity are configured as differential amplifiers to account for the frequency overlap of the myoelectric signal and the voltage that appears on the skin's surface as a result of the body's capacitive coupling with the environment. As such, sensors for detection of myoelectric activity are composed of two electrodes to measure and eliminate this common voltage, in addition to the reference electrode. Electrodes are precisely located and must be maintained in close contact with the skin to reduce motion artefacts introduced by movements of the electrode relative to the skin. The electrodes are generally embedded in the prosthetic socket or sleeve to maintain this contact. A good-fitting socket is essential to the reliable control of myoelectric prostheses. For a detailed review of the information summarised herein on myoelectric electrodes, signals and processing, the interested reader is directed to Lovely (2004).

While electrodes detect the myoelectric signal, a controller is used to interpret it and activate the appropriate response. The control strategy will vary from individual to individual and typically increases in complexity as the child grows. The type of control strategy depends on the number of available myoelectric sites and may employ amplitude coding (i.e., threshold levels to control prosthetic functions), or rate coding (i.e., speed of contraction to control prosthetic functions). The control strategy can be optimised to the client by changing various parameters, for example, the input signal amplification and threshold, the differential gain, and the output voltages and currents, to name a few. Young children often start out with the 'cookie crusher' strategy (Hubbard et al. 2004a), which uses a single threshold value above which the prosthesis opens and below which the prosthesis is closed. (Note: paediatric terminal devices are typically equipped with a child-release function to enable a parent to manually release the grasp if needed.) This kind of configuration is termed voluntary opening. When the young child is first fitted with the device, it can be helpful to set the threshold of detection at a very low value to draw attention to the device and encourage the child to try to open the hand (Hubbard et al. 2004b).

Young children quickly learn through self-discovery the cause-and-effect nature of the operation at which point the electrode sensitivity can be reduced. As children grow they may graduate from one to two myoelectric sites and may be capable of more complex control strategies (e.g., two function control, proportional control or mode selection). For a comprehensive review of control strategies, the interested reader is referred to Hubbard et al. (2004a).

The advantages offered by electric devices include increased pinch strength and the elimination of harnessing. Conversely, they tend to be heavier than body-powered or passive devices, partially owing to the need for a power supply. Advances in battery technologies have greatly reduced the weight of electric prostheses over the years. Typically, batteries can be contained within the prosthesis to enable a more streamlined, cosmetic appearance, or the prosthesis may be designed to enable easy access to the battery for charging and interchanging with a backup battery. Where weight or space are of great concern, batteries may be worn non-locally (e.g., in a waist pouch). Electric hands are often viewed as a good mixture of cosmesis and function. At present, paediatric electric hands are not equipped with multi-articulated fingers, but offer a pinch-like grasp.

A large number of studies have explored the acceptance of electric prostheses, likely in justification of their high costs, typically $15,000 US (Galiano et al. 2007). The mean rate of acceptance based on 12 studies is 68 ± 19% as reported in Biddiss and Chau (2007b). For paediatric electric prosthesis wearers, weight was by far the most frequently reported and most highly rated design priority. Heat dissipation, glove durability and lack of sensory feedback were also issues noted by consumers in the design of electric prostheses (Biddiss et al. 2007). Commercially, the only device offering sensory feedback is provided by the Otto Bock Sensor hand, which integrates slip detection and adjustment capabilities into the hand and controller. This prosthesis is directed toward adult populations. Caldwell and Lovely (2004) provide a review of commercial product lines and hardware for the implementation of an electric prosthetic system (Caldwell and Lovely 2004). Recent introductions include Otto Bock's Electrohand 2000, which was designed specifically for children and offers a more natural appearance with a light-weight aluminium construction and miniaturised drive system.

Hybrid Prostheses

Hybrid prostheses make use of both body-powered and electric systems to provide multi-functional control of prosthetic components (e.g., elbow, wrist, shoulder and terminal device) and are typically used by individuals with high-level limb absence. At this point, a few notes on the different prosthetic joints available in paediatric prostheses are warranted. Wrist units are generally passive friction (i.e., manually repositioned) or electric devices that most frequently offer rotation, and in some cases flexion/extension and/or radio-ulnar deviation (Kestner 2006). Passive friction wrists are most common in paediatrics, although electric wrists are recommended for children with high-level limb absence, particularly if bilateral (Hubbard et al. 1997). Wrist devices that offer quick release disconnect can be advantageous for easy interchange of terminal devices. Very little research is available on use, utility and satisfaction with wrist units in adult populations, with even less directed toward paediatrics. A study by Kestner (2006) found that although performance was not strongly dependent on prosthetic wrist function in a number of tasks performed in a clinic environment, participants' qualitative reports indicated that the extra degrees of freedom were in fact useful for a range of activities of daily living (Kestner 2006). Consumers also identified wrist dexterity as a primary design priority for the improvement of upper limb prostheses in a study by Atkins (1996). Even less research has focused on prosthetic elbows, which are available in passive friction, mechanical locking and electrical configurations. A passive friction elbow is often selected for young children with high-level limb absence (Hubbard et al. 1997). Elbow joints are also sometimes used as shoulder joints to meet the size constraints of small children. At present, there are no powered shoulder joints on the market. Each additional degree of freedom adds complexity to the prosthetic system and its control. As the child matures both physically and cognitively, more complex control schemes may be adopted to provide greater functionality. Special consideration with regard to weight and size of prosthetic joint components is needed in their selection and design, particularly for children and youth. The combined weight of a hybrid prosthetic system that incorporates, for example, an electric hand and elbow together with a body-powered shoulder joint, can be quite significant and increases as the level of limb absence rises and additional components are required. The lack of comfortable and functional devices likely plays a dominant role in the high rates of prosthesis rejection associated with high-level limb absence (i.e., above-elbow) (Biddiss et al. 2007).

Activity-Specific Prostheses

Children's social bonding, neuromuscular development and psychosocial development depend largely on participation in sports and recreational activities (Webster et al. 2001). As such, specialised recreational devices are an extremely important consideration in childhood prostheses. As reported in Biddiss et al. (2007), highly desirable activities frequently reported as particularly challenging with a prosthesis included cycling, swinging sports (e.g., golf, baseball, tennis), climbing and monkey bar activities, swimming, ball sports and playing musical instruments. Multiple and specialised prostheses are often required to meet the full range of activities that mark a healthy child's active lifestyle. In some cases, these needs may be met with commercial products either off-the-shelf or custom ordered. Hosmer Dorrance, for example, offers specialised prosthetic attachments for baseball, fishing, driving, bowling and skiing. In other cases, it may be necessary to design a specific attachment to meet the recreational needs of the child. The design of sports prostheses can be particularly challenging due to the potentially repetitive and high biomechanical forces and vibrations that must be transmitted. Generally, in the design of recreational prostheses, the functional requirements of the device tend to supersede cosmetic considerations.

No Prosthesis

The decision to reject prosthesis use altogether is also an important and common prosthetic option for children with upper limb differences and their families. Prosthesis acceptance and rejection is largely an individual choice. For some, the prosthesis is an enabler and is essential for daily activities and participation; it fulfils an established set of needs. For others, it is an impediment. In a study of 96 children with upper limb differences, 25% had never worn a prosthesis, 15% no longer wore a prosthesis, and 60% reported using a prosthesis (Biddiss et al. 2007). Overwhelmingly, the most common reason for rejecting a prosthesis was lack of functional benefit (Biddiss et al. 2007). There are certainly factors that are associated with a heightened risk for prosthesis abandonment (i.e., high- or low-level limb absence, bilateral limb absence, delayed time of fitting, age and lack of involvement in the selection of a prosthesis) (Biddiss and Chau 2008a). However, prosthesis acceptance or rejection is extremely difficult to anticipate. In fact, the journeys and choices preceding prosthesis acceptance or rejection may be of greater value to the individual's psychosocial well-being and overall quality of life than the ultimate decision. In general, paediatric prosthesis wearers and non-wearers both reported very high levels of quality of life and adjustment to their limb differences (James et al. 2006).

Each of the prosthesis options described in this section has a distinct set of advantages and disadvantages that affect its suitability for different activities and functions. When considering prosthetic options, it is unlikely that a single prosthesis will excel over the range of activities that characterise a busy childhood. Instead, a set of prostheses is more apt to provide the versatility required to meet the diversity of needs.

PROSTHETIC FITTING AND TRAINING

It is the primary goal of prosthetic rehabilitation to appropriate or improve functionality; namely, mobility in the case of lower limb rehabilitation and fine motor skills in the case of upper limb rehabilitation (Vannah et al. 1999; Sener et al. 1999). The effectiveness of function and mobility is dependent on the physiological quality of the residual limb (which is affected by surgery), the physical quality of the prosthesis (which is influenced by the availability of functional prosthetic technologies), and the interaction of these biological and mechanical systems (which may be influenced during prosthetic fitting, training or physical therapy). As such, prosthetic fitting and physical therapy are the means by which the biological and artificial systems are functionally consolidated. The effectiveness of a prosthetic intervention depends not only on the performance of individual prosthetic components, but also on the prosthesis as a whole and its interaction with the human body. Numerous factors such as the child's physical and psychological state, the child's functional and mobility goals and the social support available to the child can also influence the overall efficacy of the various rehabilitation initiatives. Effective surgical, prosthetic and therapeutic rehabilitation at the early stages of life, while the child is developing physically, intellectually and emotionally, provides the important foundation to help the child mature into a well integrated and productive member of society.

The earliest phase of a successful paediatric program for children with limb differences hinges on providing parents with healthy coping strategies and nurturing a strong bond between parent and child (Jain 1996). At these early stages and throughout the lifetime of the child, providing accurate and accessible information is vital. In particular, information on prosthetic and non-prosthetic options, avenues for funding and opportunities for peer support are essential. Parents and children should be provided with realistic expectations with respect to prosthetic options and should be involved as much as possible in the selection of a prosthesis or set of prostheses to best meet the child's goals. Personal goal attainment is a fundamental metric used throughout childhood, adolescence and adult life, to guide rehabilitation strategies and to assess the efficacy of interventions (Wright 2006). Paediatric prosthetic programs require on-going vigilance to monitor and anticipate the developmental progress and needs of the child. Particularly during adolescence, youth may require additional support and revisit the use of a prosthesis and how it fits in with their personal identity and goals. Furthermore, throughout childhood and adolescence, frequent maintenance of the prosthesis is required to accommodate for growth and the everyday wear and tear encountered in child activity. Preschoolers may require a new upper limb prosthesis on a yearly basis, while in adolescence, devices may last for 18 to 24 months (Edelstein 2000). A new lower limb prosthesis is typically required annually up to the age of 5 years, bi-annually from 5 years through puberty, and once every 3 to 4 years thereafter due to wear and tear and physical changes due to growth (Nelson et al. 2006; Lambert 1972). In consequence, provision of a useable prosthetic system often requires much customization and interaction between the client, prosthetist and therapist.

FITTING AND TRAINING STRATEGIES SPECIFIC TO LOWER LIMB ABSENCES

For children requiring lower limb prostheses, prosthetic fitting can start as early as 9 to 16 months of age as the child begins to pull him or herself up. Children with acquired amputations can be fitted with a prosthesis as soon as physically possible. Because individual cases greatly vary, a team approach should be implemented to assess and determine when a child is physically, intellectually and emotionally ready for particular prosthetic interventions. Generally accepted guidelines outlining specific developmental milestones for the prescription and fitting of various prosthetic technologies have been established (Boonstra et al. 2000; Jain 1996).

Typically bench, static and dynamic alignments are performed by prosthetists to determine and provide the 'optimal' prosthesis setup. A technology to assist the prosthetist with the alignment of the prosthesis includes the Laser Assisted Static Alignment Reference (L.A.S.A.R) Posture (Blumentritt 1997). With L.A.S.A.R Posture, a force plate measures the GRFV when an individual stands on it with his or her prosthesis, and a laser projects the GRFV onto the prosthesis. In this way, the prosthetist can determine whether the prosthesis is aligned appropriately based on the manufacturer's specific criteria as well as other factors.

The greater challenge of lower limb prosthesis fitting has been to quantify and evaluate alignment dynamically, during gait. Typically, dynamic alignment alterations are based on a heuristic process that includes observational gait analysis, patient feedback, and the consideration of functional characteristics of different prosthetic components, patient abilities, patient biomechanics and even mobility goals. The application of quantitative gait analysis (i.e., in a gait lab) on a per-client basis is not common practice, due to the associated cost, time and resource commitments and, most importantly, the expertise needed to collect and interpret the data. To address these issues, researchers have recently developed a computer load measurement system that can easily be incorporated into prostheses (Henry 2010). This system measures forces and moments during dynamic tasks, such as walking, and using specially designed algorithms provides information to the prosthetist about the adequacy of the alignment.

Once fitted with the prosthesis, functional exercises are administered by the physical therapist at the medical facility and by the family at home. These exercises, for example, weight shifting from side to side, are meant to encourage the child to better utilise the prosthetic limb and develop a trust in the support it affords. With therapy, the child will typically increase weight-bearing on the prosthetic limb resulting in a more symmetrical loading of the intact and prosthetic limbs (in the case of unilateral amputees) during standing and gait, thus improving gait and lessening potential long-term complications such as back pain and joint degeneration (Stam et al. 2004; Royer and Koenig 2005). The often tedious and repetitive nature of these exercises can hinder compliance, so other modalities are being investigated. One such alternative involves the use of affordable commercial gaming systems that employ a force platform on which the child stands (Steinnagel 2010). By shifting his or her weight over the platform, the child controls the avatars in the game. On-going work is examining the biomechanics that are elicited through the game-playing movements and the therapeutic effect of game-playing on balance and gait performance, in order to evaluate the potential benefits to rehabilitation.

FITTING AND TRAINING STRATEGIES SPECIFIC TO UPPER LIMB ABSENCE

The timing of prosthetic fittings will depend on the child, but generally a first passive prosthesis is provided between the ages of 3 and 6 months when the child begins to have the requisite trunk stability and balance for sitting (Hubbard et al. 2004b). The precise age at which transition to an active device is desirable is controversial and depends largely on the child's and parents' emotional readiness (Hubbard et al. 2004b). For parents, the decision to fit or not to fit a child with an upper limb can be difficult. Parents struggle between wanting to give their child the opportunity to develop prosthetic skills at an early age, while not wanting to impair their child's body image or impart the message that the child is not complete without the prosthesis. For these reasons, some parents choose to delay prosthetic fitting until the child can participate in the discussion. Conversely, evidence indicates that prosthetic fitting before 2 years of age or within 6 months of amputation may be optimal for increasing prosthesis acceptance (Biddiss and Chau 2008a). Either way, it is imperative that the child develops a healthy body image and is comfortable with, or without, the prosthesis.

With regard to training strategies, a few important considerations pertaining to motor learning and motor control are reviewed herein. First, movement is generally goal-directed. Second, there are many ways to accomplish any given task. Last, individuals develop preferences to movements that minimise effort and discomfort (Bowers and Lusardi 2006). The caveat to the latter is that our preferential movement patterns often make us prone to repetitive motion injuries. Inefficient or unhealthy movements can cause secondary musculoskeletal complications such as inflammation or tissue remodelling. It is essential that individuals with upper limb absence be trained in techniques to avoid secondary complications irrespective of prosthesis use or non-use. For a child with a prosthesis, this three-stage model of motor learning involves first a discovery stage wherein the child becomes aware of the prosthesis and his or her ability to control it through simple trial and error. The second stage involves further skill acquisition and development, while in the third, the child learns to apply his or her skills and adapt them to his or her environment and activities of daily living. Vital to skill development is practice and repetition. For this reason, parents are instructed to encourage their child to consistently wear his or her prosthesis and practice bimanual hand use. Targeted functional use training to refine skills may also be conducted within the clinic where occupational therapists teach prosthesis use through individualised and age-appropriate play and activities of daily living (Hubbard et al. 1985). The importance of this occupational training, particularly for myoelectric prostheses, is well documented in the literature (Egermann et al. 2009; Hubbard et al. 1985; Hermansson et al. 1991; Sorbye 1980). Family involvement throughout the process is also critical for successful training (Egermann et al. 2009).

EVALUATION OF PROSTHETIC INTERVENTION OUTCOMES

Developing and implementing new prosthetic treatments requires an intimate understanding of existing limitations. It also requires a means to evaluate these treatments once they have been developed. Both of these tasks require the use of outcome measures, many of which have already been developed and deployed in prosthetic rehabilitation.

Outcome evaluation measures are designed to detect 'clinically important' changes following an intervention (e.g., provision of a prosthesis, fitting adjustments, training provided). In 2001, the World Health Organization's International Classification of Functioning, Disability, and Health formalised the shift in clinical focus from body functions and structures to levels of activity and participation (World Health Organization 2001). This was paralleled by the development of outcome measures that increasingly focus on meeting goals, carrying out tasks and assessing involvement in life situations. Use of standardised outcome measures is important in paediatric prosthetic rehabilitation for the following reasons:

- To provide information about human and prosthetic performance, patients' well-being, and various facets of their functioning (Condie et al. 2006);
- To monitor each individual child's progress toward goals (Hill et al. 2009);
- To evaluate the efficacy of prosthetic rehabilitation programs and strategies (Hill et al. 2009);
- To provide evidence to substantiate funding decisions given the often high costs of prosthesis fitting, training and maintenance (Hill et al. 2009); and
- To enable multi-centre comparisons and databases populated by standardised assessments which, given the small numbers of children with upper limb absence, will allow for the formulation of results with greater statistical significance (Wright 2006).

The psychometric properties of an outcome measure must be rigorously quantified in order for it to be considered scientifically valid and useful. Widespread acceptance of outcome measures is often challenged by the difficulty of applying a single standardised measure for treatment of many individuals. Often, it is the case that some items may not apply and others may not fully capture an individual's unique circumstances, goals and activities. The validity of an outcome measure (i.e., its responsiveness, test-retest reliability, inter-rater reliability and construct validity) is compromised by changes and additions to, or deletion of, its items (Wright 2006). Likewise, the outcome measure must be used only for the specific population for whom it was validated with.

The acceptability of an outcome measure can be improved by providing electronic versions with automated scoring, ensuring ease of interpretation and limiting the resources needed for its administration (Wright 2006). It is also important to consider validating functional sections of an outcome measure such that they may stand alone for more targeted and abbreviated use. Future work on context-aware, quantitative measurements of prosthesis use and function, outside of clinical environments, may provide an additional tool to support the evaluation of outcomes. For example, one approach could be to log frequency of activation of the prosthesis in daily living using the microcontroller inherent in electric prostheses.

Outcomes Evaluation Measures for Lower Limb Rehabilitation

Based on the results of systematic reviews that were performed in this area, prosthetic outcome measures are categorised into 'general aspects of rehabilitation,' 'mobility,' 'functional outcomes,' 'quality of life,' 'predictive factors,' 'phantom pain' and 'skin problems'(Condie et al. 2006; Geertzen et al. 2001). Outcome measures used in the evaluation of prosthetic components on the functioning of lower limb amputees specifically include, in order of prevalence, spatiotemporal and kinematic parameters, oxygen uptake, heart rate and the Borg scale to measure aspects of physical exertion (Linde et al. 2004). The above reviews are not children specific, but studies focusing on children with limb loss also implement biomechanical, functional and health-related quality-of-life measures (Vannah et al. 1999; Boonstra et al. 2000; Colborne et al. 1992; Pruitt et al. 1997, 1999; Engsberg et al. 1993).

Reliable and validated measures (biomechanical, functional and quality of life), spanning the breadth of human health and well-being, are an essential part of research and clinical evidence-based practice. However, at the inceptive stages of device development and evaluation, biomechanical and certain functional measures afford the greatest utility and applicability in particular, as they more directly map to the physical features of the device, allowing the designer or developer to ascertain the potential advantages, drawbacks and necessary improvements of their design. Biomechanical, and to a lesser degree, functional measures are typically obtained using specialised and often technically complex instruments, techniques or procedures, as discussed later. The development, evaluation and application of these represent an important facet of rehabilitation engineering work.

The primary goal of lower limb prosthetic rehabilitation is to enable mobility and physical activity in a comfortable, efficient and cosmetic fashion (Wenz et al. 1998).

In this regard, establishing or re-establishing walking function is of primary importance, and as such, the study of prosthetic gait has become the focus of many research and development initiatives in prosthetics (Lindie et al. 2004). The assessment of gait can simply involve observation techniques (requiring essentially no instrumentation) or conversely the use of complex instrumentation capable of accurately measuring the kinematics and kinetics of body segments in three-dimensional space. A brief overview of the most common gait and mobility assessment techniques is presented here.

Gait and Mobility Analysis

Analysis of human gait involves the study of (1) specific features that constitute gait, such as body movements, weight-bearing load patterns and muscle activity patterns; and (2) the effects of these features on gait mechanics, including stride characteristics and energy expenditure. Body segment movements are expressed in terms of kinematic and spatiotemporal parameters. Loading patterns, in conjunction with movement patterns, are used to calculate kinetic parameters, as well as energy and power at the respective lower limb joints. Within modern instrumented gait laboratories, all of these gait parameters can be readily and accurately measured and analyzed.

A typical modern gait laboratory is comprised of a camera-based motion analysis system for three-dimensional tracking of the movements of markers that are strategically placed on the subject. The trajectories of the markers are computationally determined, and applied to a link-segment model that represents the anatomical structure of the subject. In this way, kinematic parameters, such as the angular changes between the shank and thigh segments, can be accurately measured. Spatial measures, such as stride length, stride width or toe in/out, can also be determined from marker position data. Kinetic parameters are more difficult to obtain, but with additional information such as the segmental moments of inertia and the external loads affecting a given anatomical segment, they can be determined using inverse-dynamics methods (Whittle 2002). During weight-bearing, the major component of external loads is ground reaction forces, which are typically presented as GRFVs and are measured using force plates. Energies and powers at the joints (inter-segmental) can subsequently be derived from kinematic and kinetic data (Whittle 2002). In prostheses, these biomechanical measures are important because they can be directly related to prosthesis or patient function, making it possible for researchers, designers or prosthetists to establish cause-and-effect relationships between features of the intervention and the characteristics of the gait. As a simple example, excessive swing phase heel rise at the prosthetic knee joint (measured as higher than normal peak knee flexion angles) may be due to inadequate prosthetic swing phase control (Hicks et al. 1985). The ability to relate specific gait parameters to the performance of the prosthetic or human systems makes quantitative gait analysis a valuable tool in prosthetics.

Energy expenditure associated with walking is an important indicator of overall mobility function in prosthetics. However, while it can help assess which prosthetic intervention is more effective in providing more efficient ambulation, unlike gait analysis, it does not directly disclose information about the specific mechanism to which the difference may be attributed. Energy expenditure can be estimated by measuring an individual's oxygen consumption or by monitoring heart rate (Whittle

2002). On a related topic, joint moments and powers, which can be measured at different joints as mentioned previously, can provide important information about the amount of work required at a particular joint to perform a task (Umberger and Martin 2007; Seroussi et al. 1996).

Ecologically relevant gait studies are being seen as an important next step in the assessment of mobility. A wide range of instruments can be used outside of the laboratory in quasi-controlled experiments. For example, subjects may go about their daily lives while some aspect of their mobility is being monitored. Least obtrusive instruments for monitoring include pedometers, activity monitors, global positioning systems (GPS), as well as self-reports, which all provide a general picture of the individual's activity and mobility habits (Stepien et al. 2007; Harris et al. 2010; Dudek et al. 2008). It is possible to apply other sensors assuming they do not adversely affect the subject's normal physical function. For example, footswitches, electrogoniometers and accelerometers can provide temporal and kinematic measures. With respect to children with amputations, the opportunity to incorporate load transducers into prostheses makes it possible to measure kinetics of prosthetic limbs (Nietert et al. 1998; Frossard et al. 2000, 2003). Novel technologies, such as the MVN (inertial motion capture) system by Xsens Technologies (used to capture full body kinematics) are continually evolving, and paving the way for a more informative and ecologically relevant evaluation of mobility.

The following basic considerations should be made when designing studies to evaluate the efficacy or effectiveness of prosthetic interventions. In trying to measure the effects of an intervention, for example, comparing two types of foot components, sample heterogeneity can often play an undesirable role. This is especially true when dealing with children, where mobility performance may be confounded by factors relating to physical and mental maturity. For children with congenital deficiencies, additional confounding factors may also include biomechanical deviations stemming from, for example, inadequate proximal joint musculature, the dependence on other assistive devices, or the presence of multiple deficiencies. It is therefore preferable in many cases to apply repeated measures or crossover study designs to reduce the influence of these confounding covariates and effectively have subjects act as their own controls in the study. These studies are also statistically efficient and therefore do not require large sample sizes, which is a major benefit in paediatric prosthetic studies (Normann and Steiner 2000). Other design considerations include randomization, which helps to reduce 'order effects,' and blinding, to reduce placebo effect or observer/rater bias, or both. However, single and double blind trials are typically difficult to administer due to concealment issues, since prosthesis wearers tend to be well informed and acquainted with their prosthetic components. As such, blinding is not commonly used in prosthetic studies. Acclimation is also a very important factor, since it takes about 3 weeks for an individual's gait parameters to stabilise after being fitted with a new prosthesis (English et al. 1995). Lastly, working with children poses an extra set of challenges, especially when the child is very young. For one, their small bodies are more likely to be affected by obtrusive instruments and sensors, which may result in unnatural gait changes during data collection. Additionally, children have shorter attention spans than do adults, and therefore long and highly repetitive data collections are usually not feasible. In summary, careful planning at the inception of the study is pivotal in helping to generate data that are accurate, reliable and clinically relevant.

OUTCOME EVALUATION MEASURES FOR UPPER LIMB REHABILITATION

It is unlikely that one measure can be used to capture the many elements (i.e., technical function, activity and participation) that are needed to fully evaluate prostheses, how they are used, and how they are integrated into daily life (Hill et al. 2009). To accomplish this, a set of validated tests to measure function, activity and participation are needed (Wright 2006). Likely, this set will be composed of a mixture of child or parent reports, observational measures and timed measures that include a combination of pre-prescribed, semi-naturalistic and child-selected activities (Wright 2006; Hill et al. 2009). In order to be internationally acceptable, the tools included in this set must transcend cultural and language differences (Hill et al. 2009). Table 7.1 presents a summary of a number of outcome measures relevant to upper limb prosthesis use and function in paediatrics. Particularly for paediatric outcome measures, it is important to consider age-appropriate development and activities. For this purpose, outcome measures such as the Child Amputee Prosthetics Project-Functional Status Inventory (CAPP-FSI) and the Prosthetic Upper extremity Functional Index (PUFI) offer multiple versions designed for specific age groups. For more information on clinical measures for assessment of upper limb function and activity, the interested reader is referred to an excellent review on the subject by Wright (2009).

TABLE 7.1
Summary of Paediatric Upper Limb Prosthetic Outcome Measures

Outcome Measure	Structure	Focus
Assessment for capacity of myoelectric control (ACMC)	Observational	Ability to control a myoelectric hand during tasks of everyday living.
Paediatric outcomes data collection instrument (PODCI)	Parent or child/ adolescent report	Measure of overall health (physical, mental, attitudinal), pain and ability to participate in normal to vigorous activities. Also measures treatment expectations.
Unilateral below elbow test (UBET)	Timed measure	Time to complete task.
University of New Brunswick test (UNB)	Observational	Ease and method of performance with and without prosthesis.
Child amputee prosthetics project — functional status instruments (CAPP-FSI)	Parent or child report	Frequency of performance and use of prosthesis.
Prosthetic upper extremity functional status index (PUFI)	Parent or child report	Method of performance, ability to perform bimanual tasks and use of prosthesis.

FUTURE DIRECTIONS IN PAEDIATRIC
PROSTHETICS AND REHABILITATION

Very little recent research has focused specifically on paediatric prosthetics development with the exception of a handful of programs (e.g., the Wilmer Group at Delft
Institute for Prosthetics and Orthotics, Bloorview Kids Rehab, Rancho Los Amigos
National Rehabilitation Center, and Open Prosthetics Project), of which some have
led to tangible advances and marketable products (Cummings 2006). New products
and strategies (as will be detailed in subsequent sections) are generally first developed
to meet the needs of adult populations before translation to paediatrics (Cummings
2006). Design challenges such as size, weight and durability are generally magnified in paediatric populations, rendering practical advancements in this area elusive
(Cummings 2006). The following describes a number of on-going innovations in
biomedical and rehabilitation engineering, robotics, informatics and medicine that
are accelerating the development of smarter and more functional prostheses.

ADVANCING HUMAN-MACHINE INTERFACES

CAPTURING AND PROCESSING THE INFORMATION IN BIOLOGICAL SIGNALS

The ability to extract more information from residual muscle activity is an important
area requiring development in order to enable more functional prosthesis control.
Weir and colleagues (2009) developed and demonstrated the potential of implantable, wireless myoelectric electrodes, inserted with a syringe directly in the muscle,
to increase the signal-to-noise ratio and reduce muscle cross-talk (Weir 2009). These
sensors have been used to detect individual finger movements in monkeys and a
fully functional 32-channel system has undergone testing in cats (Baker et al. 2008).
Latest reports indicate no adverse infection and continued operation following 12
months of implantation (Schorsch et al. 2008).

Mechanomyography (MMG) is another approach under exploration (Alves and
Chau 1997; Silva et al. 2005) that uses low-frequency muscle vibrations (i.e., the
sound that occurs when the muscle contracts) as the control input. Using MMG,
different information can be drawn from the muscle activity than through EMG. In
particular, changes in motor recruitment strategies (i.e., the beginning of fast-twitch
fibre recruitment and increased firing rate once full motor recruitment is obtained)
may be more discernable through changes in the MMG signal RMS and frequency
than through EMG (Akataki et al. 2004).

Lastly, the development of soft electrodes, fabricated from textiles or polymers,
may also have implications for collecting physiological signals while enhancing user
comfort (Finni et al. 2007; Pylatiuk et al. 2009). In a comparison of a number of electrode materials, Pylatiuk concluded that dry electrodes, fabricated from polysiloxane
loaded with particles (e.g., carbon) to achieve electrical conductivity, performed well
in comparison with standard Ag/AgCl electrodes (Pylatiuk et al. 2009). Textile electrodes, fabricated from galvanically modified silvered threads made of polyamide,
also performed well if saturated with an electrolyte dilution, but were not as yet
comparable to the standard Ag/AgCl electrodes when dry. Motion artefacts and high

skin-electrode impedance remain as challenges in the design and implementation of textile electrodes to capture biological signals for more comfortable prosthesis control.

Communication Pathways

Establishing a connection to the biological system is important not only from a mechanical or structural perspective, but also from a communication perspective, as this connection can serve as a means for sending signals between the human and prosthetic systems. Neuroprosthetics are designed to operate at the cortical level, bypassing the peripheral nervous system. Electrode arrays are implanted in the motor cortex of the brain to measure the cortical activity within the part of the brain associated with the desired movements. These signals or intents are then interpreted by microcomputers and used to control the movements of the prosthesis. This concept has been demonstrated in human trials with an implantable silicone electrode array called the Braingate, wherein it was established that (1) the areas of the motor cortex mapped to limb function remain viable even in the absence of the actual limb and (2) the tissue-electrode interface remains stable and functional for over 3 years (Hochberg et al. 2006). More recently, Song (2009) demonstrated in primates the second-generation wireless version of the Braingate for implantable, microelectronic transmission of transcutaneous cortical signals. This development is a clear step toward the realization of feasible, thought-controlled prostheses.

Targeted reinnervation, under investigation at the Neural Engineering Center for Artificial Limbs (NECAL) at the Rehabilitation Institute of Chicago, also taps directly into the nervous system in order to attain more natural and intuitive prosthesis control (Kuiken et al. 2009) and sensory feedback (Sensinger et al. 2009; Marasco et al. 2009). In this approach, the residual nerves of the affected limb are surgically redirected and attached to a deinnervated and sectioned muscle, the use of which is not functionally critical (e.g., the pectoral muscle for control of the upper limb). Neuromuscular motor commands originating in the brain are transmitted to this target muscle. In response to these signals, the target muscle is activated and contracts. The activity of the target muscle is detected by an array of electromyography (EMG) sensors on the surface of the muscle and the pattern of EMG signals detected is used to activate the prosthetic components. As such, the target muscle functions as a biological amplifier. By mapping the natural motor commands to their respective prosthesis functions (e.g., elbow extension, wrist rotation and grip), this technique provides a medium for neural control of the prosthesis without the need for brain implants or a specially designed prosthesis. To date, this technique has been demonstrated successfully with a handful of adults with high-level traumatic amputations of the upper limb, with future efforts targeted at improving response times (Kuiken et al. 2009) and online classification accuracy (Simon et al. 2009). Given that this is a surgical technique, there are associated risks of infection, neurotoma and paralysis of the target muscle. Although eventually rectified, one case study reports the return of phantom limb pain following surgery (Kuiken et al. 2009).

It is unknown to what extent these techniques may be applicable to the paediatric population. For children with congenital limb absence, neuromuscular mappings associated with the missing limb will not be established. One might hypothesise that, at an early age, given an interface for direct neural communication with a prosthetic device, a child will learn to control the prosthesis in a similar manner as he or she might learn to use a natural limb. However, these strategies may still be challenged by the need for invasive surgeries. Before undertaking these elective procedures, it is likely that parents may deem it appropriate to wait until their child can actively participate in the discussion and decision processes. Nevertheless, targeted reinnervation and neuroprosthetics are exciting areas of development with particular relevance, at present, to adults with acquired, high-level limb absence for whom conventional control strategies are difficult or non-effective.

Sensory Feedback

Much of the dexterity and motor control of the limbs hinges on proprioceptive and tactile feedback. For instance, reflex control, sensing the position of the limb in space, and assessing the level of force needed to securely grip an object are all largely unconscious processes that rely on the integration of vast quantities of information derived from nocio-, thermo- and mechano-receptors on the hand, together with stretch receptors within the muscles and joints. Without tactile feedback, grip forces applied via prosthesis tend to be considerably higher than requisite for activities of daily living (Inmann et al. 2004), which is wasteful of user effort and battery life. For prosthesis wearers, visual attention is the primary mode of sensory feedback, augmented by subtle cues such as motor noise in the case of electric devices, or harness movements and resistance in the case of body-powered devices (Scott et al. 1980; Silcox et al. 1993). Sensory feedback is particularly important during early childhood exploration and learning to the point that children may at first ignore their limb when the prosthesis is first applied, owing to the decrease in sensory feedback (Jain 1996). For both children and adults, provision of sensory feedback in a natural and cognitively undemanding way promises great improvements in overall function and control of movements.

At present, prosthetic hands are typically limited to a single force sensor on the thumb and a strain sensor incorporated into the transmission system to regulate grasp and to protect the drive mechanism from damage (Carozza et al. 2003). Several research initiatives (Carpaneto et al. 2003; Cotton et al. 2007; Riso et al. 1999; Zecca et al. 2004; Edin et al. 2008; Wettels et al. 2009) are engaged in the development of sensory mechanisms for upper limb prostheses with a primary focus on sensor design for slip and force detection, as reviewed in Biddiss and Chau (2006). These designs often incorporate a combination of technologies that include potentiometers, accelerometers, Hall effect sensors, strain gauges, piezoelectric vibration sensors and force or contact sensors (often arranged in a matrix) that are integrated into the design of the terminal device [e.g., the Cyberhand (Carrozza et al. 2003)]. Recently, microfabrication techniques and the use of novel, electroactive materials have been applied to produce small-scale sensors comparable in size to the finger tip. For example, Cotton (2007) presented experimental results for a thick-film, piezoelectric sensor intended for slip detection, while Beccai (2005) demonstrated a microfabricated three-axial force sensor.

Advancements in sensor designs and sensory systems have not made the transition from the research laboratory to clinical use. The majority of sensor systems developed thus far may be considered most appropriate for closed-loop control, wherein the prosthesis automatically processes and responds to sensor stimuli (e.g., adjusting grip to prevent slip) (Beccai et al. 2005). While the high plasticity of the young brain and its capacity for nerve repair may mitigate some of the challenges associated with presenting sensory information to the user (Rosen et al. 1994), steep learning curves are still expected to be associated with sensory substitution and processing of sensory information presented through alternative feedback mechanisms (e.g., tactile, auditory, neural interfaces) (Beccai et al. 2005). Targeted reinnervation, as described previously, in the future may provide a medium for multi-channel communication of sensory feedback. In an accidental discovery, it was found that pressing on the skin associated with the reinnervated target muscle caused sensory sensations to occur in the phantom limb (Kuiken et al. 2009). This implies that sensors on the prosthesis could be coupled to actuators on the target muscle to provide a medium for communicating sensory messages directly to the brain. Sensinger (2009) demonstrated that subjects could descry force gradations through this mechanism. Perception of temperature, pain and sharp/dull discrimination also proved intact. Development in this area is in the exploratory stages.

Osseointegration

While various socket technologies can help to enhance prosthetic fit and function, the soft tissue of the residual limb was never meant to be encased in a socket and subjected to repetitive compressive and shear loads. An alternative technique, still in development, is to attach the prosthesis directly to osseous tissue of the residuum. Osseointegration, whereby the prosthesis is directly anchored to the living bone of the residual limb, has been shown to be an excellent alternative for adult amputees experiencing complications or limitations in using conventional prosthetic socket technologies. Direct attachment to the bone increases control of the limb, eliminates pain and perspiration issues associated with sockets, decreases perception of weight, and improves osseoperception (Fairley 2006). Although still perceived as investigational, osseointegrated prostheses are associated with positive clinical outcomes such as increased prosthesis use, mobility and quality of life for adults (Hagberg et al. 2008; Staubach and Grundei 2001). A disadvantage of this technology includes the risk of deep infections, although the incidence of this adverse event is decreasing with the improvement of treatment procedures (Fairley 2006). Furthermore, the surgical procedures required entail lengthy recovery times between surgeries and before the prosthesis can be attached. This technique is also not intended for the elderly or persons with vascular disease, diabetes, excess weight or for those prone to infection (Fairley 2006; Hagberg 2008).

Thus far, osseointegration has not been applied to children for the purposes of limb prostheses, although it has been used successfully for bone-anchored hearing aids and craniomaxillofacial implants (Soo et al. 2003). Special considerations are needed given the softness and thinness of young children's bones and their dynamic growth patterns. The medullary canal also widens as young people age, which may be a risk factor for implant loosening (Pitkin 2009). However, osseointegration is certainly an emerging option that in the future may be appropriate for selected active individuals, particularly those who experience severe complications at the skin-prosthesis interface and who require the prosthesis to function in everyday life.

Hand Transplantation

A final future direction worthy of note with regard to biological interfacing is composite tissue allotransplantation. As of the beginning of 2009, 44 hand transplants had been conducted worldwide (Kaufman et al. 2009). Kaufman et al. (2009) describe successful results with five patients, one of whom was monitored for over 10 years. At present, this procedure is under clinical review and is deemed appropriate only for selected individuals, generally adults with traumatic limb amputations at the transradial level with few secondary health concerns, who are likely to psychologically embrace the transplanted hand and to follow the regimen of immunosuppressive drugs prescribed.

INTELLIGENT PROSTHESES

Lower Limb Prostheses That Adapt to User Needs

The use of computers has brought new levels of performance, adaptability and autonomy to both upper and lower limb prostheses. Microprocessor-based prosthetic ankles, such as the Proprio Foot™ by Össur, sense the terrain of the surface and respond by altering the plantar/dorsiflexion angles to enhance foot compliance with the terrain (Agrawal et al. 2007). Future designs can aim to extend this function by increasing the degrees of freedom of the foot, and by allowing the stiffness attributes to adapt as needed. One such idea uses an innovative frame design and pneumatic rubber bellow air muscles (Zahedi ND). Microprocessor-based prosthetic knee joints sense a variety of gait conditions and autonomously respond to provide optimal braking or damping levels for the prevailing gait conditions. For example, these knees can detect and respond to the onset of instability, which could cause a person to fall, and can compensate accordingly to increase resistance at the knee (Kahle et al. 2008). The knee also monitors gait conditions to adapt to changes, such as walking speed, thus decreasing gait deviations. Suction socket technologies for adults, such as the LimbLogic™ VS from Ohio Willow Wood, are now augmented with pumps that automatically adjust the vacuum levels in the socket ensuring that optimal socket suspension is achieved. The use of computer control also has the potential to deal with volumetric changes in residual limbs, as had originally been developed for smart variable geometry socket technology (Greenwalk et al. 2003). This system works by adding and removing liquid from the intra-socket environment, regulated dynamically by intra-socket pressures. The performance of all these aforementioned systems is dependent on the number and types of sensors used to collect data about the status of the prosthesis, user and environment, and the sophistication of the algorithms used to interpret the data and output appropriate control signals.

It is necessary to move beyond conventional passive prosthetic systems to attain greater control and overall functionality. Activities such as fast walking, stair or hill climbing, sitting up and running all necessitate mechanical power generation and therefore prosthetic joint actuation. To address this need, a prototype power ankle has recently been developed that provides active plantar flexion in terminal stance to more closely match the function of the human leg, potentially improving fluidity and efficiency of walking (Au et al. 2007, 2008). For above-knee amputees, the first actuated prosthetic knee, the Power knee™ from Össur, has recently been introduced on the market. Using a powerful actuator, the knee is capable of mimicking concentric muscle activity at the knee joint (Gailey 2007; Cutti et al. 2007). One of the disadvantages of this, and all electronic-based systems, is the need for onboard energy sources which increases the size, weight and maintenance, and is thus currently restricting application of these technologies primarily to adult populations.

Upper Limb Prostheses That Provide Multifunctional Control

The need for more effective signal detection stems from the desire for enhanced life-like movement and multifunctional control. The extraction of additional and reliable information from residual muscle activity can be translated into control strategies for a great range of movements for both lower and upper limb prostheses. Such multifunctional control strategies must be customised to the individual's distinct physiology and neuromuscular characteristics. As such, in lieu of intensive user training, intelligent system design, wherein the controller learns and adapts to the abilities and physiology of the user, is a desirable approach. A number of research groups are utilizing novel signal processing and pattern classification techniques to extract information from greater numbers of EMG and MMG sites (Cipriani et al. 2008; Kurzunski and Wolczowski 2009; Chan et al. 2003; Nishikawa et al. 2000; Ajiboye et al. 2005; Khadivi et al. 2005; Sebelius et al. 2005). For most, the goal is not individual finger control, but control of common grasp configurations (e.g., spherical or pinch) as used in activities of daily living. The same approach to controlling common mobility tasks is suggested for lower limb prosthetics (Huang et al. 2009).

Evidently, the development of multifunctional control software must be paralleled by advances in hardware. To this end, several research groups, including most recently the Deka Research and Development Corporation, have developed multi-articulated prosthetic hands capable of life-like movement (Zollo et al. 2007; Kyberd et al. 2001, 2007; Gow et al. 2001; Yang et al. 2004). Prosthetic hands based on micromotors (Kyberd et al. 2001), pneumatics or hydraulics (Gaiser et al. 2009; Kargov et al. 2008; Caldwell et al. 2002), and shape memory alloys (Price et al. 2006; De Laurentis et al. 2002; dos Santos et al. 2003) have all been conceived and are at varying stages of development. Commercially, the iLimb, an electric upper limb prosthesis driven by micromotors and provided by Touch Bionics, is the only commercially available prosthetic hand with the potential for multifunction control. More recently, the potential of electroactive polymers has been reviewed (Biddiss and Chau 2008b). Electroactive polymers are an emerging class of materials that offer response characteristics reminiscent of the behaviour of natural muscles. Specifically, some electroactive polymers (e.g., dielectric elastomers, polyaniline) respond mechanically to an electrical input (and, vice versa, respond electrically to a mechanical input) and, in certain configurations (e.g., when rolled or layered), have been suggested for use as 'artificial muscles.' These materials could be used to realise linear actuators which may lead to more biomimetic prosthetic actuation. Electroactive polymers are still in the very early stages of refinement and, as yet, do not have the combined force and strain characteristics needed to match their biological counterparts in strength, density and energy efficiency (Biddiss and Chau 2008b).

VIRTUAL REALITY THERAPY AND TRAINING

For children and adults alike, training and skill development are required for the efficient use of myoelectric prostheses in particular, as well as for balance in lower limb rehabilitation. As the complexity of control systems grows to enable more sensory feedback and multifunctional or complex control, the training required may also increase despite efforts focused on the design of intelligent and adaptive learning algorithms. Virtual reality tools and games are emerging as fun alternatives to traditional therapy regimes (Steinnagel 2010). Virtual reality rehabilitation is well aligned with market trends toward active video gaming as exemplified by the Nintendo Wii, the Sony Eyetoy and Microsoft's Project Natal. This area of research is particularly suited to children.

TRENDS IN DESIGN AND MANUFACTURING

Modular Component Design

The iLimb (Touch Bionics), as described by Bogue (2009), is an excellent example of another trend in prosthetics development — modular design (Bogue 2009). Modularity in design is an approach wherein a system is subdivided into a number of smaller components that can be interchanged independently to offer greater multifunctionality and to facilitate maintenance and repairs. In prosthetics, this may include the design of easily interchangeable terminal devices that may offer more activity-specific functionality or it may enable quick and economical replacement of components prone to failure or outgrowth. The iLimb embraces modularity with replaceable fingers and interchangeable wrist, elbow and shoulder joints that facilitate cost- and time-effective maintenance and replacement of components. This is particularly important for paediatric prosthetics where growth and play activities place stringent demands on prosthetic components. Gow and Kybert (2001, 2007) discuss modular designs for commercial and research platforms in upper limb prosthetics.

The need for greater attention to joint design (e.g., knee and shoulder components) is also evident in the literature (Cummings 1997) and is particularly relevant to individuals with high-level limb absence. For example, recent advancements in two degrees of freedom electric shoulder joints may augment the functional potential of upper limb prostheses for individuals with high-level humeral or interscapulothoracic amputees (Troncossi et al. 2009). At present, no powered shoulder joints are commercially available, with previous efforts thwarted by limitations in size, weight, cost, cosmesis and control (Troncossi et al. 2009).

Computer Aided Design-Computer Aided Manufacturing

Despite the availability of Computer Aided Design-Computer Aided Manufacturing (CAD-CAM) systems, the fabrication of sockets is still performed at many facilities using conventional hand casting and forming techniques. In this process, plaster casting is often used to capture the size and shape of the residual limb. The socket is then formed from this positive model. CAD-CAM has the potential to facilitate the fabrication and fitting process in a number of ways. First, CAD-CAM systems allow for more efficient fabrication and higher quality control and duplicability of sockets.

The geometry of the limb can be conveniently captured and digitised using a variety of techniques based on optics (e.g., laser scanning and reconstruction from camera images) or contact scanning techniques that use electromagnetic fields (McGarry and McHugh 2005; Smith and Burgess 2001). This may be particularly relevant to children for whom the plaster casting process can be undesirably lengthy. Electronic representations of the residuum can be manipulated within the CAD program in the same way that a prosthetist might refine the plaster cast to improve the fit. Additionally, these files can be sent electronically to a centralised fabrication facility and filed as part of the client's digitised medical records. Furthermore, digital images of the residual limb can be used in biomechanical assessments to better understand the prosthesis-body interface and optimise load transfer. Scientific studies of surface pressure, socket shear, friction and slippage, using a variety of techniques and instruments combined with computational modelling including linear and non-linear finite element analyses, are providing a firmer foundation for the biomechanical principles relating to socket fabrication and fitting techniques presently used in clinical practice (Mak et al. 2001). For example, scientific studies are affirming the benefits of suction socket technologies and soft socket interfaces (Mak et al. 2001). In a recent study by Dumbleton (2009), pressure mapping techniques indicated that the interface pressures were higher for sockets constructed using CAD-CAM techniques compared to the hand-crafted alternative. Interestingly, the pressure distribution and user satisfaction were comparable. In terms of fabrication techniques, the hope is that one day empirically and computationally derived information may be used to develop more intelligent CAD-CAM systems capable of automatically determining and adjusting inner socket topographies to optimise pressure distributions and ensure optimal socket fit. At present, this is a manual process requiring the knowledge, expertise and judgment of the prosthetist.

Several prosthetics companies offer commercial CAD-CAM systems to manufacture prosthetic components. Traditionally, these systems are used for rapid prototyping of the positive model from which the socket or alternative component is made. As the technology improves, it is likely that this intermediate step will be eliminated entirely and CAD-CAM, in conjunction with rapid prototyping techniques such as laser sintering or fused deposition modelling, will be used directly to create the final product. This will likely increase widespread acceptance of the technique and improve time and cost efficiency.

Drawbacks to CAD-CAM include substantial monetary, resource and time investments upfront, to acquire the system and properly train the technicians and clinicians who will be using it. Moreover, clinical expertise is still needed to design and alter the shape of the socket, a task that may be more intuitively performed on the physical part (i.e., via conventional fabrication techniques) than within three-dimensional computer models (i.e., via CAD-CAM). CAD-CAM also tends to be less effective in dealing with complex residual limb deformities, such as those of many children with congenital limb deficiencies. Lastly, high-strength materials amenable to the processes of rapid prototyping are also essential to the acceptance of these methods of prosthetic fabrication. Examples of prosthetic designs incorporating high-strength plastics are evident in both upper limb (e.g., Touch Bionics' iLimb) and lower limb (e.g., LCKnee described in Andrysek et al. 2010) prostheses.

Low-Cost Prosthetic Components for Developing Nations

A lack of appropriate medical and prosthetic equipment, inexperienced personnel and information provision, unsuitable amputation practices, monetary limitations, geographic barriers and absence of government support are just a few factors inhibiting effective health care and prosthesis provision in developing nations (Cummings 1996). Recycled limbs obtained from developed countries are often mismatched in size and colour and do not address the functional needs of these populations. The cost of maintaining a prosthesis alone can be prohibitive, as reported in studies conducted in countries such as India (Bhaskaranand et al. 2002), Vietnam (Fernandez-Palazzi et al. 1991) and Haiti (Bigelow et al. 2004). A number of technologies and initiatives have been proposed to assist in the design and provision of low-cost prostheses. First, use of videoconferencing services (e.g., as provided by Biodesigns Inc.) may allow specialised expertise to be provided to remote geographic and rural areas. Second, through CAD-CAM, the economic advantages of a centralised manufacturing centre may be realised. Last, design expertise may be amalgamated and advanced through initiatives such as the Open Prosthetics Project, which provides a framework for free collaborations between users, designers and funders (http://openprosthetics.org).

In terms of prosthetic components specifically, challenges include the development of more durable foot components, sockets fabrication techniques that require less training to implement, less time to apply, and result in better socket fit and simple but functional prosthetic knee joints that eliminate the need to walk with a stiff-legged gait, as is the case with manually locking knees that are commonly deployed in developing countries (Anon 2006; Day 1996; Cummings 1996). A number of innovative projects are being undertaken to develop more functional and durable prosthetic foot components (Meier et al. 2004; Pearlman et al. 2008), technologically appropriate socket casting methods to provide a more uniform and comfortable socket fit in less time (Wu et al. 2003, 2009) and functional knee joint mechanisms that provide a safely locked knee in stance phase and controlled knee flexion during swing phase (Anon 2006; Andrysek et al. 2010; LeTourneau University Web site). In contrast, research and development activities relating to upper limb prostheses for developing nations are considerably less extensive when compared to lower limb prostheses and, consequently, the clinical usage of these devices is also less (Anon 2006). Hence, experts agree that more research is needed in both upper and lower limb prostheses for developing countries (Anon 2006).

Strategies for Energy Harvesting

To decrease the reliance on large and heavy onboard energy sources, a number of alternative approaches are being investigated. In place of motors, exploration of potentially more efficient electroactive polymer materials with attributes matching those of biological muscles has potential in prosthetic applications (Biddis and Chau 2006) as do other innovations such as pneumatic artificial muscles (Hannaford et al. 1995). High-density energy storage, such as lithium ion batteries, is also helping to make the utilization of electronics and actuators in prosthetics a reality.

Moreover, energy re-absorption techniques are helping to increase the utility of prostheses with electronics, microprocessors and actuators (Andrysek and Chau

2007; Andrysek et al. 2009). In essence, these systems work in synergy with the human body to provide more efficient transfers and conversions of segmental energies. With conventional prosthetic systems, energy is dissipated during numerous passive gait events using brakes, dampers or cushions. Energy re-absorption is being investigated in prosthetic knee joints for converting mechanical power (which would otherwise be dissipated primarily in the form of heat) into electrical energy to power on-board prosthetic control systems (Andrysek and Chau 2007; Andrysek et al. 2009). In sockets, harnessing of human power is being used to operate pumps that assist in managing residual limb volume changes either by decreasing intra-socket pressures (e.g., the Harmony® System from Otto Bock) or by modifying socket fit through the expansion of bladders at relevant locations in the socket (Greenwald et al. 2003). In both cases, the cyclic nature of changing loads in the prosthesis during walking is used to provide the pumping action. The effectiveness of such systems is directly related to the volume of air or fluid being moved. For small limbs or limbs with space limitations such as paediatric prostheses, the usefulness of these systems may be more limited.

Bridging the Gap between Adult and Paediatric Prosthetics

Existing paediatric prosthetic components incorporate many of the same underlying technologies as those used in adult prostheses, although some of the more sophisticated adult systems have yet to translate to paediatrics. For example, since the 1950s, hydraulics have been widely adopted to provide swing and stance phase control in adult prosthetic knee joints. To date, there are no prosthetic knee joints with hydraulic stance phase control available for children (Cummings 2006). Hydraulic mechanisms provide a greater range of stability during stance (resistance to flexion even with a flexed knee joint) and allow yielding to facilitate stair and slope descents. They also provide better swing phase control during walking. However, while enhancing performance, these more sophisticated systems are more costly to implement, repair, maintain and use, making them presently impractical for use in certain situations and with some populations, including small children. In the future, advancements in materials science, mechanical and electrical engineering and medical sciences should help to bridge the gap between adult and paediatric prosthetic technologies. Stronger materials can help to miniaturise mechanical components and the development of simpler kinematic mechanisms can enhance function without added weight or size. In addition, miniaturization and increased durability of electronic components may make it feasible to develop more intelligent, computer-based systems.

CONCLUDING REMARKS

Children require prosthetic technologies that consider their unique physiological, biomechanical and cognitive attributes as well as their functional demands. When developing new prosthetic technologies for children, these factors should be carefully considered. Historically, major technological progress has predominantly focused on adult rather than on paediatric prostheses. Arguably, one reason for this is that there exists a larger market in adult prostheses, making it easier for a company to recover its research and development investments once a product has been released to market

(Cummings 2006). Furthermore, from a technical perspective, it is easier to develop more sophisticated technologies for the adult population given the looser technical constraints (i.e., size and weight). Since children with amputations are typically very active, they place significant structural demands on their prostheses. Therefore, in order to maintain strength and ensure durability of their devices, less sophisticated and therefore less functional mechanisms typically need to be incorporated to achieve compact designs.

Moreover, possibly as a result of funding reasons and to serve the widest possible customer base, manufacturing companies develop prosthetic components that cover a broad range of ages. Some components are therefore designed to be light and small enough for a 5-year-old child, but strong enough for the added weight and activity of a 12-year-old child. Consequently, compromises occur on both ends of the age spectrum. For the 5-year-old child, a prosthetic component will be structurally over-designed, while for the 12-year-old child, it will be functionally under-designed.

The human limbs serve an incredible variety of functions. Replacing all of these functions with a prosthetic device presents a considerable challenge that, at times, seems insurmountable. While we are making gains, at present, even the most advanced prosthetic interventions have substantial limitations that become more evident with higher levels of impairment. Technological advancements are making it possible for individuals with amputations to achieve basic mobility and functionality more naturally and efficiently than in the past but, as depicted in Figure 7.7, there is still a long road ahead. The primary focus of lower limb prosthetics has been to restore one's ability to stand, sit and walk due to the high importance of these three functions. In upper limb prosthetics, the focus has been on prehension grasp in the form of a pinch grip. Unfortunately, these actions represent only a fraction of the functions and activities that are possible with a human leg or hand. Dedicated prostheses, for example, a limb designed for swimming in water, are helping to extend the functionality envelope. In fact, dedicated sprinting transtibial prostheses have

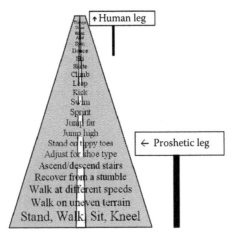

FIGURE 7.7 Despite significant technological advancements in the development of artificial limbs, we still have a ways to go to develop devices that are as functional as a human limb.

recently made it possible for amputee sprinters to compete against world-class able-bodied athletes (Longman 2007). However, it is important to remember that, to date, prostheses do not possess the multifunctionality of their natural counterparts and that a prosthesis designed for a specific activity (e.g., sprinting) will generally not perform well during other activities (e.g., walking). As a result, an individual with an amputation may possess several prostheses to serve various functions. In this way, prostheses of today continue to be used and viewed as 'tools' or 'assistive devices' rather than replacements of the biological system.

Fortunately, on-going and future advancements in medicine, biology, engineering and other related fields hold promise for prostheses. One day, these devices may be as effective as their biological counterparts in restoring function and allowing individuals to participate in activities without major restrictions. An overview of some of this work was provided earlier in this chapter, while research in other disciplines, such as regenerative medicine and tissue engineering, may make it possible, one day, for limbs to be re-grown (Viola et al. ND). For children with amputations, however, there are many more immediate aspects of the rehabilitation process that can be improved. To this end, further research is needed toward the development of better prosthetic components and fitting procedures, physical therapies that are both effective and engaging, and surgical procedures that maximise function of the remaining anatomy. Rehabilitation engineering is, and will continue to be, an integral part of this advancement.

REFERENCES

Agrawal, V.R. et al. 2007. Plantar pressure comparisons: Bionic foot & ankle system versus conventional foot designs. Paper presented at *12th World Congress — International Society for Prosthetics and Orthotics*, Vancouver, British Columbia.

Ajiboye, A.B., and R.F. Weir. 2005. A heuristic fuzzy logic approach to EMG pattern recognition for multifunctional prosthesis control. *IEEE Trans Neural Syst Rehab Eng* 13(3):280–291.

Akataki, K., K. Mita, and M. Watakabe. 2004. Electromyographic and mechanomyographic estimation of motor unit activation strategy in voluntary force production. *Electromyogr Clin Neurophysiol* 44(8):489–496.

Aksnes, L.H. et al. 2008. Limb-sparing surgery preserves more function than amputation: A Scandinavian sarcoma group study of 118 patients. *J Bone Joint Surg Br* 90(6):786–794.

Alves, N., and T. Chau. 1997. Stationarity distributions of mechanomyogram signals from isometric contractions of extrinsic hand muscles during functional grasping. *J Electromyogr Kinesiol* 8(3):509–515.

Andrysek, J. et al. 2010. A new stance-phase controlled prosthetic knee joint for low-income countries. Paper presented at *13th ISPO World Congress*, Leipzig, Germany.

Andrysek, J., T. Liang, and B. Steinnagel. 2009. Evaluation of a prosthetic swing-phase controller with electrical power generation. *IEEE Trans Neural Syst Rehabil Eng* 17(4):390–396.

Andrysek, J., and G. Chau. (2007). An electromechanical swing-phase-controlled prosthetic knee joint for conversion of physiological energy to electrical energy: Feasibility study. *IEEE Trans Biomed Eng* 54(12):2276–2283.

Andrysek, J., S. Redekop, and S. Naumann. 2007. Preliminary evaluation of an automatically stance-phase controlled pediatric prosthetic knee joint using quantitative gait analysis. *Arch Phys Med Rehabil* 88(4):464–470.

Andrysek, J., S. Naumann, and W.L. Cleghorn. 2005. Design and quantitative evaluation of a stance-phase controlled prosthetic knee joint for children. *IEEE Trans Neural Syst Rehabil Eng* 13(4):437–443.

Andrysek, J., S. Naumann, and W. Cleghorn. 2004. Design characteristics of pediatric prosthetic knees. *IEEE Trans Neural Syst Rehabil Eng* 12(4):369–378.

Anon. 2006. State-of-the-science on appropriate technology for developing countries – roundtable session. Paper presented at *State-of-the-Science on Appropriate Technology for Developing Countries*, Chicago, IL.

Atkins, D., D. Heard, and W. Donovan. 1996. Epidemiologic overview of individuals with upper-limb loss and their reported research priorities. *J Prosthet Orthot* 9(1):2–11.

Au, S., M. Berniker, and H. Herr. 2008. Powered ankle-foot prosthesis to assist level-ground and stair-descent gaits. *Neural Net* 21(4):654–666.

Au, S.K. et al. 2007. Powered ankle-foot prosthesis for the improvement of amputee ambulation. *Conf Proc IEEE Eng Med Biol Soc* 3020–3026.

Baker, J.J., D. Yatsenko, J.F. Schorsch, G.A. DeMichele, P.R. Troyk, D.T. Hutchinson, R.F. Weir, G. Clark, and B. Greger. 2008. Decoding individuated finger flexions with implantable myoelectric sensors. *Conf Proc Eng Med Biol Soc* 193–196.

Beccai, L., S. Rocella, F. Arena, P. Valvo, A. Menciassi, M.C. Carrozza, and P. Dario. 2005. Design and fabrication of a hybrid silicon three-axial force sensor for biomechanical applications. *Sens Actuators A* 120:370–382.

Beccai, L., S. Roccella, A. Arena, F. Valvo, P. Valdastri, A. Menciassi, M.C. Carrozza, and P. Dario. 1985. Design and fabrication of a hybrid silicon three-axial below-elbow absence. *Prosthet Orthot Int* 9(3):137–140.

Bhaskaranand, K., A.K. Bhat, and K.N. Acharya. 2003. Prosthetic rehabilitation in traumatic upper limb amputees (an Indian perspective). *Arch Orthop Trauma Surg* 123(7):363–366.

Biddiss, E., and T. Chau. 2008a. Dielectric elastomers as actuators for upper limb prosthetics: Challenges and opportunities. *Med Eng Phys* 30(4):403–418.

Biddiss, E., and T. Chau. 2008b. Multivariate modeling for prediction of prosthesis use or rejection. *Disabil Rehabil: Assit Technol* 3(4):181–192.

Biddiss, E., and T. Chau. 2007. Upper extremity prosthesis use and abandonment: A survey of the last 25 years. *Prosthet Orthot Int* 31(3): 236–257.

Biddiss, E., and T. Chau. 2007b. The roles of predisposing characteristics, need, and enabling resources on upper extremity prosthesis use and abandonment. *Disabil Rehabil* 2(2):71–84.

Biddiss, E., D. Beaton, and T. Chau. 2007. Consumer design priorities for upper limb prosthetics. *Disabil Rehabil: Assit Technol* 2(6):346–357.

Biddiss, E., and T. Chau. 2006. Electroactive polymeric sensors in hand prostheses: Bending response of an ionic polymer metal composite. *Med Eng Phys* 28(6):568–578.

Bigelow, J., M. Korth, J. Jacobs, N. Anger, M. Riddle, and J. Gofford. 2004. A picture of amputees and the prosthetic situation in Haiti. *Disabil Rehabil* 26(4):246–252.

Blumentritt, S. 1997. A new biomechanical method for determination of static prosthetic alignment. *Prosthet Orthot Int* 21(2):107–113.

Bogue, R. 2009. Exoskeletons and robotic prosthetics: A review of recent developments. *Industrial Robot* 36(5):421–427.

Boonstra, A.M. et al. 2000. Children with congenital deficiencies or acquired amputations of the lower limbs: Functional aspects. *Prosthet Orthot Int.* 24(1):19–27.

Bossert, J.L. 1991. *Quality function deployment.* Milwaukee, WI: ASQC.

Bowers, D.M., and M.M. Lusardi. 2006. Motor learning and motor control in orthotic and prosthetic rehabilitation. In *Orthotics and prosthetics in rehabilitation*, M.M. Lusardi, C.C. Nielsen, and M.J. Emery, Eds. Philadelphia: W.B. Saunders Company, 93–108.

Buckley, J.G., W.D. Spence, and S.E. Solomonidis. 1997. Energy cost of walking: Comparison of "intelligent prosthesis" with conventional mechanism. *Arch Phys Med Rehabil* 78(3):330–333.

Caldwell, D.G., and N. Tsagarakis. 2002. Biomimetic actuators in prosthetic and rehabilitation applications. *Technol Health Care* 10(2):107–120.

Caldwell, R.R., and D.F. Lovely. 2004. Commercial hardware for the implementation of myoelectric control. In *Powered upper limb prostheses: Control, implementation, and clinical application*, Ashok Muzumdar, Ed. Berlin: Springer Press, 55–72.

Carpaneto, J., S. Micera, F. Zaccone, F. Vecchi, and P. Dario. 2003. A sensorized thumb for force closed-loop control of hand neuroprostheses. *IEEE Trans Neural Syst Rehabil Eng* 11:346–353.

Carroll, K., and J.E. Edelstein. 2006. *Prosthetics and patient management: A comprehensive clinical approach.* Nottingham: Slack Incorporated.

Carrozza, M.C., P. Dario, F. Vecchi, S. Roccella, M. Zecca, and F. Sebastiani. 2003. The CyberHand: On the design of a cybernetic prosthetic hand intended to be interfaced to the peripheral nervous system. *IEEE/RSJ Int Conf Intelligent Robots Systems* 3:2642–2647.

Carrozza, M.C., B. Massa, S. Micera, R. Lazzarini, M. Zecca, and P. Dario. 2002. The development of a novel prosthetic hand—ongoing research and preliminary results. *IEEE/ASME Trans Mechatronics* 7:108–114.

Chan, A.D.C., and K.B. Englehart. 2003. Continuous classification of myoelectric signals for powered prostheses using Gaussian mixture models. In *Proc 25th Annu Int Conf IEEE Eng Med Biol Soc* 2(4):275–294.

Cipriani, C., F. Zaccone, S. Micera, and M. Chiara Carrozza. 2008. On the shared control of an EMG-controlled prosthetic hand: Analysis of user–prosthesis interaction. *IEEE Trans Robotics* 24(1):170–184.

Colborne, G.R. et al. 1992. Analysis of mechanical and metabolic factors in the gait of congenital below knee amputees. A comparison of the SACH and Seattle Feet. *Am J Phys Med Rehabil* 71(5):272–278.

Condie, M.E., H. Scott, and S. Treweek. 2006. Lower limb prosthetic outcome measures: A review of the literature 1995 to 2005. *J Prosthet Orthot* 18(1S):13–45.

Cotton, D.P.J., P.H. Chappell, A. Cranny, N.M. White, and S.P. Beeby. 2007. A novel thick-film piezoelectric slip sensor for a prosthetic hand. *IEEE Sensors J* 7(5):752–761.

Crandall, R.C., and W. Tomhave. 2005. Pediatric unilateral below-elbow amputees: Force sensor for biomechanical applications. *Sens. Actuators A* 120:370–382.

Crandall, R.C., and W. Tomhave. 2002. Pediatric unilateral below-elbow amputees: Retrospective analysis of 34 patients given multiple prosthetic options. *J Pediatr Orthop* 22(3):380–383.

Cummings, D.R. 2006. Pediatric prosthetics: An update. *Phys Med Rehabil Clin N Am* 17(1):15–21.

Cummings, D.R. 2004. General prosthetic considerations. In *Atlas of limb prosthetics: Surgical, prosthetic, and rehabilitation principles*, D.G. Smith, J.W. Michael, and H.K. Bowker, Eds. Rosemont, IL: American Academy of Orthopedic Surgeons, 789–799.

Cummings, D.R. 1997. The missing link in pediatric prosthetic knees. *Biomechanics* 4(2):163–168.

Cummings, D. R. 1996. Prosthetics in the developing world: A review of the literature. *Prosthet Orthot Int* 20(1):51–60.

Cutti, A.G. et al. A motion analysis protocol for comparing active and reactive prosthetic knees. Paper presented at *12th World Congress — International Society for Prosthetics and Orthotics*, Vancouver, British Columbia, July 29–August 3, 2007.

Datta, D., B. Heller, and J. Howitt. 2005. A comparative evaluation of oxygen consumption and gait pattern in amputees using intelligent prostheses and conventionally damped knee swing-phase control. *Clin Rehabil* 19(4):398–403.

Day, H.J. 1996. A review of the consensus conference on appropriate prosthetic technology in developing countries. *Prosthet Orthot Int* 20(1):15–23.

De Laurentis, K., and C. Mavroidis. 2002. Mechanical design of a shape memory alloy actuated prosthetic hand. *Technol Health Care* 10:91–106.

Dechev, N., W.L. Cleghorn, and S. Naumann. 2001. Multiple finger, passive adaptive grasp prosthetic hand. *Mechanism Machine Theory* 36(10):1157–1173.

Dillingham, T.R., L.E. Pezzin, and E.J. Mackenzie. 2002. Limb amputation and limb deficiency: Epidemiology and recent trends in the United States. *South Med J* 95(8):875–883.

Dormans, J.P., B. Erol, and C.B. Nelson. 2004. Acquired amputations in children. In *Atlas of limb prosthetics: Surgical, prosthetic, and rehabilitation principles,* D.G. Smith, J.W. Michael, and H.K. Bowker, Eds. Rosemont, IL: American Academy of Orthopedic Surgeons, 841–852.

Dos Santos C.M.L., F.L. da Cunha, and V.I. Dynnikov. 2003. The application of shape memory actuators in anthropomorphic upper limb prostheses. *Artificial Organs* 27(5):473–477.

Dudek, N.L. et al. 2008. Ambulation monitoring of transtibial amputation subjects with patient activity monitor versus pedometer. *J Rehabil Res Dev* 45(4):577–585.

Dumbleton, T.A., W.P .Buis, A. McFadyen, B.F. McHugh, G. McKay, K.D. Murray, and S. Sexton. 2009. Dynamic interface pressure distributions of two transtibial prosthetic socket concepts. *J Rehabil Res Dev* 46(3):405–415.

Edelstein, J. 2000. Rehabilitation for children with limb deficiencies. In *Orthotics and Prosthetics in Rehabilitation,* M.M. Lusardi and C.C. Nielsen, Eds. Boston: Butterworth-Heinemann, 553–568.

Edin, B.B., L. Ascari, L. Beccai, S. Roccella, J.J. Cabibihan, and M.C. Carrozza. 2008. Bio-inspired sensorization of a biomechatronic robot hand for the grasp-and-lift task. *Brain Res Bull* 75(6):785–795.

Egermann, M., P. Kasten, and M. Thomsen. 2009. Myoelectric hand prostheses in very young children. *J Int Orthop* 33(4):1101–1105.

English, R.D., W.A. Hubbard, and G.K. McElroy. 1995. Establishment of consistent gait after fitting of new components. *J Rehabil Res Dev* 32(1):32–35.

Engsberg, J.R. et al. 1993. Normative ground reaction force data for able-bodied and below-knee-amputee children during walking. *J Pediatr Orthop* 13(2):169–173.

Fairley, M. 2006. Osseointegration: In the wave of the future? *O&P Edge*. http://www.oandp.com/articles/2006-09_03.asp (accessed January 12, 2010).

Fernandez-Palazzi, F., D.P. de Gutierrez, and R. Paladino. 1991. The care of the limb deficient child in Venezuela. *Prosthet Orthot Int* 15(2):156–159.

Finni, T., M. Hu, P. Kettunen, T. Vilavuo, and S. Cheng. 2007. Measurement of EMG activity with textile electrodes embedded into clothing. *Physiol Meas* 28:1405–1419.

Fishman, S., J.E. Edelstein, and D.E. Krebs. 1987. Icelandic-Swedish-New York above-knee prosthetic sockets: Pediatric experience. *J Pediatr Orthop* 7(5):557–562.

Fisk, J.R., and D.G. Smith. 2004. The limb-deficient child. In *Atlas of amputations and limb deficiencies*, D.G Smith, J.W. Michael, and H.K. Bowker, Eds. Rosemont, IL: American Academy of Orthopedic Surgeons, 3:773–778.

Frossard, L. et al. 2003. Development and preliminary testing of a device for the direct measurement of forces and moments in the prosthetic limb of transfemoral amputees during activities of daily living. *J Prosthet Orthot* 15(4):135–142.

Frossard, L. et al. 2000. Forces acting on the residuum of above-knee amputees during activities of daily living. *Proc Joint Local Symp Physical Sciences and Engineering in Medicine: The Local Scene in Queensland XI*, Brisbane, Australia.

Froster, U.G. and P.A. Baird. 1993. Congenital defects of lower limbs and associated malformations: A population based study. *Am J Med Genet* 45(1):60–64.

Gailey, R. 2007. Gait and functional training for bionic prosthetic feet and foot/ankle components. Paper presented at *12th World Congress — International Society for Prosthetics and Orthotics*, Vancouver, British Columbia.

Gaiser, I.N., C. Pylatiuk, S. Schulz, A. Kargov, O. Reinhold, and T. Werner. 2009. The FLUIDHAND III: A multifunctional prosthetic hand. *J Prosthet Ortho* 21:91–96.

Galiano, L., E. Montaner, and A. Flecha. 2007. Research, design & development project myoelectric prosthesis of upper limb. *J Phys: Conf Ser* 90:7.

Gard, S.A., and D.S. Childress. 1999. The influence of stance-phase knee flexion on the vertical displacement of the trunk during normal walking. *Arch. Phys Med Rehabil* 80(1):26–32.

Geertzen, J.H., J.D. Martina, and H.S. Rietman. 2001. Lower limb amputation. Part 2: Rehabilitation—a 10-year literature review. *Prosthet Orthot Int* 25(1):14–20.

Gow, D.J., W. Douglas, C. Geggie, E. Monteith, and D. Stewart. 2001. The development of the Edinburgh modular arm system. *Proc Instit Mechanical Engineers* 215(3):291–298.

Graham, L.E. et al. 2007. A comparative study of conventional and energy-storing prosthetic feet in high-functioning transfemoral amputees. *Arch Phys Med Rehabil* 88(6):801–806.

Granstroem, G. 2000. Osseointegrated implants in children. *Acta Otolaryngol* 543:118–121.

Greenwald, R.M., R.C. Dean, and J.B. Wayne. 2003. Volume management: Smart variable geometry socket (svgs) technology for lower-limb prostheses. *J Prosthet Orthot* 15(3):107–112.

Hagberg, K. et al. 2008. Osseointegrated trans-femoral amputation prostheses: Prospective results of general and condition-specific quality of life in 18 patients at 2-year follow-up. *Prosthet Orthot Int* 32(1):29–41.

Hannaford, B. et al. 1995. The anthroform biorobotic arm: A system for the study of spinal circuits. *Ann Biomed Eng* 23(4):399–408.

Harris, F. et al. 2010. The participation and activity measurement system: An example application among people who use wheeled mobility devices. *Disabil Rehabil Assist Technol* 5(1):48–57.

Heller, B.W., D. Datta, and J. Howitt. 2000. A pilot study comparing the cognitive demand of walking for transfemoral amputees using the intelligent prosthesis with that using conventionally damped knees. *Clin Rehabil* 14(5):518–522.

Henry, K. 2009. Alignment systems step forward, *O&P Edge*. http://www.oandp.com/articles/2009-10_03.asp (accessed January 12, 2010).

Hermansson, L., A.C. Eliasson, and I. Engstrom. Psychosocial adjustment in swedish children with upper-limb reduction deficiency and a myoelectric prosthetic hand. *Acta Paediatr* 94 (2005): 479–488.

Hermansson, L.M. 1991. Structured training of children fitted with myoelectric prostheses. *Prosthet Orthot Int* 15:88–92.

Hicks, R. et al. 1985. Swing phase control with knee friction in juvenile amputees. *J Orthop Res* 3(2):198–201.

Hilhorst, M. 2005. Prosthetic fit: On personal identity and the value of bodily difference. *J Med, Health Care Philosophy* 7(3):303–310.

Hill, W., P. Kyberd, L. Norling Hermansson, S. Hubbard, Ø. Stavdahl, and S. Swanson. 2009. Upper limb prosthetic outcome measures (ULPOM): A working group and their findings. *J Prosthet Ortho* 21(9):P69–P82.

Hochberg, L.R., M.D. Serruya, G.M. Friehs, J.A. Mukand, M. Saleh, A.H. Caplan, A. Branner, D. Chen, R.D. Penn, and J.P. Donoghue. 2006. Neuronal ensemble control of prosthetic devices by a human with tetraplegia. *Nature* 442:164–171.

Hofstad, C. et al. 2004. Prescription of prosthetic ankle-foot mechanisms after lower limb amputation. *Cochrane Database Syst Rev.* 1:CD003978.

Huang, H., T.A. Kuiken, and R.D. Lipschutz. 2009. A strategy for identifying locomotion modes using surface electromyography. *IEEE Trans Biomed Eng* 56(1):65–73.

Hubbard, S., W. Heim, S. Naumann, S. Glasford, G. Montgomery, and S. Randall. 2004a. Powered upper limb prosthetic practice in paediatrics. In *Powered upper limb prostheses: Control, implementation, and clinical application,* A. Muzumdar, Ed. Berlin: Springer Press, 85–116.

Hubbard, S., D. Stocker, and H. Heger. 2004b. Training. In *Powered upper limb prostheses: Control, implementation, and clinical application,* A. Muzumdar, Ed. Berlin: Springer Press, 147–174.

Hubbard, S., W. Heim, and B. Giavedoni, B. 1997. Paediatric prosthetic management. *Curr Orthop* 11(2):114–121.

Hubbard, S., H.R. Galway, and M. Milner. 1985. Myoelectric training methods for the preschool child with congenital below-elbow amputation. A comparison of two training programmes. *J Bone Joint Surg Br* 67:273–277.

Inmann, A., and M. Haugland. 2004. Functional evaluation of natural sensory feedback incorporated in a hand grasp neuroprosthesis. *Med Eng Phys* 26:439–447.

International Organization for Standardization. 1996. International Standard (ISO 10328) — Prosthetics — Structural Testing of Lower-limb Prostheses. Geneva, Switzerland: International Organization for Standardization Press.

Jain, S. 1996. Rehabilitation in limb deficiency: The pediatric amputee. *Arch Phys Med Rehabil* 77(3):S9–S13.

James, M.A., A.M. Bagley, K. Brasington, C. Lutz, S. McConnell, and F. Molitor. 2006. Impact of prostheses on function and quality of life for children with unilateral congenital below-the-elbow deficiency. *J Bone Joint Surg (Am)* 88:2356–2365.

Kahle, J.T., M.J. Highsmith, and S.L. Hubbard. 2008. Comparison of nonmicroprocessor knee mechanism versus c-leg on prosthesis evaluation questionnaire, stumbles, falls, walking tests, stair descent, and knee preference. *J Rehabil Res Dev* 45(1):1–14.

Kallen, B., T.M. Rahmani, and J. Winberg. 1984. Infants with congenital limb reduction registered in the Swedish register of congenital malformations. *Teratology* 29(1):73–85.

Kapp, S.L. 2000. Transfemoral socket design and suspension options. *Phys Med Rehabil Clin N Am* 11(3):569–83.

Kapp, S.L. 1999. Suspension systems for prostheses. *Clin Orthop Relat Res* 361:55–62.

Kargov, A., T. Werner, C. Pylatiuk, and S. Schulz. 2008. Development of a miniaturized hydraulic actuation system for artificial hands. *Sensors and Actuators: A. Physical* 141(2):548–557.

Kaufman, C.L., B. Blair, E. Murphy, and W.B. Breidenbach. 2009. A new option for amputees: Transplantation of the hand. *J Rehabil Res Dev* 46(3):395–404.

Kestner, S. 2006. Defining the relationship between prosthetic wrist function and its use in performing work tasks and activities of daily living. *J Prosthet Ortho* 18(3):80–86.

Khadivi A. K. Nazarpou, and H.S. Zadeh. 2005. SEMG classification for upper-limb prosthesis control using higher order statistics. In *IEEE Int Conf Acoustics, Speech and Signal Processing (ICASSP)* V385-V388. New York: IEEE.

Krajbich, J.I. 1998. Lower-limb deficiencies and amputations in children. *J Am Acad Orthop Surg* 6(6):358–367.

Krebs, D.E., J.E. Edelstein, and M.A. Thornby. 1991. Prosthetic management of children with limb deficiencies. *Phys Ther* 71(12):920–934.

Kruger, L.M., and S. Fishman. 1993. Myoelectric and body-powered prostheses. *J Pediatr Orthop* 13(1):68–75.

Kruit, J., and J.C. Cool. 1989. Body-powered hand prosthesis with low operating power for children. *J Med Eng Technol* 13(1–2):129–133.

Kuiken, T. 2006. Targeted reinnervation for improved prosthetic function. *Phys Med Rehabil Clin N Am* 17(1):1–13.

Kuiken, T.A., G. Li, B.A. Lock, R.D. Lipschutz, L.A. Miller, K.A. Stubblefield, and K.B. Englehart. 2009. Targeted muscle reinnervation for real-time myoelectric control of multifunction artificial arms. *J Am Chem Soc* 301(6):619–628.

Kurzinsky, M., and A. Wolczoski. 2009. Control of dexterous bio-prosthetic hand via sequential recognition of EMG signals using fuzzy relations. In *Medical informatics in a united and healthy Europe*, K.-P. Adlassnig, B. Blobel, J. Mantas, and I. Masic, Eds. Amsterdam: IOS Press, 799–803.

Kyberd, P.J., A.S. Poulton, L. Sandsjo, S. Jonsson, B. Jones, and D. Gow. 2007. The ToMPAW modular prosthesis: A platform for research in upper-limb prosthetics. *Journal of Prosthetics and Orthotics* 19(1):15–21.

Kyberd, P.J., D. Gow, and P.H. Chappell. 2004. Research and the future of myoelectric prosthetics. In *Powered upper limb prostheses: Control, implementation, and clinical application*, A. Muzumdar, Ed. Berlin: Springer Press, 175–190.

Kyberd, P.J., C. Light, P.H. Chappell, J.M. Nightingale, D. Whatley, and M. Evans. 2001. The design of anthropomorphic prosthetic hands: A study of the Southampton Hand. *Robotica* 19:593–600.

Lambert, C.N. 1972. Amputation surgery in the child. *Orthop Clin North Am* 3(2):473–482.

Landsberger, S., J. Shaperman, A. Lin, V. Vargas, R. Fite, Y. Setoguchi, and D. McNeal. 1998. Child's hand with self-energizing grasp. *Am Soc Mech Eng, Bioeng Div* 39:309–310.

LeTourneau University. LEGS Program — Uncrippling the World. http://www.legsforall.com/index.php?lang-english. (accessed January 12, 2010).

(van der) Linde, H. et al. 2004. A systematic literature review of the effect of different prosthetic components on human functioning with a lower-limb prosthesis. *J Rehabil Res Dev* 41(4):555–570.

Loder, R.T., and J.A. Herring, 1987. Disarticulation of the knee in children. A functional assessment. *J Bone Joint Surg Am* 69(8):1155–1160.

Longman, J. 2007. An amputee sprinter: Is he disabled or too-abled? *New York Times*, May 15.

Lovely, D.F. 2004. Signals and signal processing for myoelectric control. In *Powered upper limb prostheses: Control, implementation, and clinical application*, A. Muzumdar, Ed. Berlin: Springer Press, 35–54.

Lusardi, M.M., and C.C. Nielsen. 2000. *Orthotics and prosthetics in rehabilitation*. Boston: Butterworth-Heinemann.

Madigan R.R., and K.D. Fillauer. 1991. 3-S Prosthesis: A preliminary report. *J Pediatr Orthop* 11(1):112–117.

Mak, A.F., M. Zhang, and D.A. Boone. 2001. State-of-the-art research in lower-limb prosthetic biomechanics-socket interface: A review. *J Rehabil Res Dev* 38(2):161–174.

Marasco, P.D, A.E. Schultz, and T.A. Kuiken. 2009. Sensory capacity of reinnervated skin after redirection of amputated upper limb nerves to the chest. *Brain* 132(6):1441–1448.

McGarry, T., and B. McHugh. 2005. Evaluation of a contemporary CAD/CAM system. *Prosthe Ortho* 29(3):221–229.

McGuirk, C.K., M.N. Westgate, and L.B. Holmes. 2001. Limb deficiencies in newborn infants. *Pediatrics* 108(4):E64.

Meier, M.R. et al. 2004. The 'Shape&Roll' prosthetic foot, II. Field testing in El Salvador. *Medicine, Conflict & Survival* 20(4):307–325.

Mendez, M.A. 1985. Evaluation of a myoelectric hand prosthesis for children with a below-elbow absence. *Prosthet Orthot Int* 9(3):137–140.

Mensch, G., and P. Ellis. 1986. *Physical therapy management of lower extremity amputations*: Rockville, MD: Aspen Publishers, Inc.

Metcalf, C., J. Adams, J. Burridge, V. Yule, and P. Chappell. 2008. A review of clinical upper limb assessments within the framework of the WHO ICF. *Musculoskel Care* 5(3):160–173.

Michael, J.W. 2004. Prosthetic suspension and components. In *Atlas of limb prosthetics: Surgical, prosthetic, and rehabilitation principles*, D.G. Smith, J.W. Michael, and H.K. Bowker, Eds. Rosemont, IL: American Academy of Orthopedic Surgeons, 2:409–427.

Michael, J.W. 1999. Modern prosthetic knee mechanisms. *Clin Orthop Relat Res* 361:39–47.

Nagarajan, R.et al. 2002. Limb salvage and amputation in survivors of pediatric lower-extremity bone tumors: What are the long-term implications? *J Clin Oncol* 20(22): 4493–4501.

Nelson, V.S. et al. 2006. Limb deficiency and prosthetic management. 1. Decision making in prosthetic prescription and management. *Arch Phys Med Rehabil* 87(1):S3–S9.

Nelson, V.S., K.M. Flood, P.R. Bryant, M.E. Huang, P.F. Pasquina, and T.L. Roberts. 2006. Limb deficiency and prosthetic management. 1. Decision making in prosthetic prescription and management. *Arch Phys Med Rehabil* 87(1):S3–S8.

Nielsen, C.C. 2007. Etiology of amputation. In *Orthotics and prosthetics in rehabilitation*, M. M. Lusardi, and C. C. Nielsen, Eds. Philadelphia, PA: Elsevier, 2:519–532.

Nietert, M. et al.1998. Loads in hip disarticulation prostheses during normal daily use. *Prosthet Orthot Int* 22(3):199–215.

Nishikawa, D., W. Yu, M. Maruishi, I. Watanabe, H. Yokoi, Y. Mano et al. 2000. On-line learning based electromyogram to forearm motion classifier with motor skill evaluation. *JSME Int J Ser* 43(4):906–915.

Nolan, L. et al. 2003. Adjustments in gait symmetry with walking speed in trans-femoral and trans-tibial amputees. *Gait Posture* 17(2):142–151.

Norman, G.R., and D.L. Streiner. 2000. Two repeated observations — the paired t-test and alternatives. In *Biostatistics — the bare essentials* 2:93-98, Hamilton, Ontario, Canada: BC Decker Inc.

Norman, D. 1988. *The design of everyday things*. New York: Doubleday.

Pearlman, J. et al. 2008. Lower-limb prostheses and wheelchairs in low-income countries. [Review] *IEEE Eng Med Biol Mag* 27(2):12–22.

Pitkin, M. 2009. On the way to total integration of prosthetic pylon with residuum. *Journal of Rehabilitation Research & Development* 46(3):345–360.

Pitkin, M.R. 1997. Effects of design variants in lower-limb prostheses on gait synergy. *Journal of Prosthetics and Orthotics* 9(3):113–122.

Plettenburg, D.H. 2006. The WILMER appealing prehensor. *J Prosthe Ortho*18(2):43–45.

Plettenburg, D. 2009. The WILMER passive hand prosthesis for toddlers. *J Prosthet Ortho* 21(2):97–99.

Postema, K., V. van der Donk, J. van Limbeek, R.A. Rijken, and M.J. Poelma. 1999. Prosthesis rejection in children with a unilateral congenital arm defect. *Clin Rehabil* 13(3):243–249.

Price, A., A. Jnifene, and H.E. Naguib. 2006. Biologically inspired anthropomorphic arm and dextrous robot hand actuated by smart-material-based artificial muscles. *Proc SPIE* 6173:272–283.

Pruitt, S.D. et al.1997. Prosthesis satisfaction outcome measurement in pediatric limb deficiency. *Arch Phys Med Rehabil* 78(7):750–754.

Pruitt, S.D. et al. 1999. Toddlers with limb deficiency: Conceptual basis and initial application of a functional status outcome measure. *Arch Phys Med Rehabil* 80(7):819–824.

Pylatiuk, C., M. Muller-Riederer, A. Kargov, S. Schulz, O. Schill, M. Reischl, and G. Bretthauer. 2009. Comparison of surface EMG monitoring electrodes for long-term use in rehabilitation device control. *Rehabil Robotics* 300–304.

Reid, D., and A. Fay.1987. Survey of juvenile hand amputees. *J Assoc Child Prosthet Orthot Clin* 22(3):51–55.

Revelle, J.B., J.W. Moran, and C.A. Cox. 1998. *The QFD handbook.* New York: John Wiley & Sons.

Riso, R.R. 1999. Strategies for providing upper extremity amputees with tactile and hand position feedback-moving closer to the bionic arm. *Technol Health Care* 7:401–409.

Rosen, B., G. Lundborg, L.B.. Dahlin, J. Holmberg, and B. Karlson. 1994. Nerve repair: Correlation of restitution of functional sensibility with specific cognitive capacities. *J Hand Surg* 19:452–458.

Royer, T., and M. Koenig. 2005. Joint loading and bone mineral density in persons with unilateral, trans-tibial amputation. *Clin Biomech (Bristol, Avon)* 20(10):1119–1125.

Sauter, W.F., S. Naumann, and M. Milner. 1986. A three-quarter type below-elbow socket for myoelectric prostheses. *Prosthet Orthot Int* 10(2):79–82.

Sawamura, C., F.J. Hornicek, and M.C. Gebhardt. 2008. Complications and risk factors for failure of rotationplasty: Review of 25 patients. *Clin Orthop Relat Res* 466(6):1302–1308.

Schneider, K. et al. 1993. Dynamics of below-knee child amputee gait: SACH foot versus flex foot. *J Biomech* 26(10):1191–1204.

Schorsch, J.F., and R.F. Weir. 2008. Reliability of implantable myoelectric sensors (IMES). *Virtual Rehabilitation* 25(27):75.

Scotland, T.R., and H.R. Galway. 1983. A long-term review of children with congenital and acquired upper limb deficiency. *J Bone Joint Surg Br* 65(3):346–349.

Scott, R.N., R.H. Brittain, R.R. Caldwell, and A.B. Cameron. 1980. Sensory-feedback system compatible with myoelectric control. *Med Biol Eng Comput* 18(1):65–69.

Sebelius, F., L. Eriksson, H. Holmberg, A. Levinsson, G. Lundborg, N. Danielsen, et al. 2005. Classification of motor commands using a modified self-organising feature map. *Med Eng Physi* 27(5):403–413.

Segal, A.D. et al. 2006. Kinematic and kinetic comparisons of transfemoral amputee gait using c-leg and mauch sns prosthetic knees. *J Rehabil Res Dev* 43(7):857–870.

Sener, G. et al. 1999. Effectiveness of prosthetic rehabilitation of children with limb deficiencies present at birth. *Prosthet Orthot Int* 23(2):130–134.

Sensinger, J.W., A.E. Schultz, and T.A. Kuiken. 2009. Examination of force discrimination in human upper limb amputees with reinnervated limb sensation following peripheral nerve transfer. *IEEE Trans Neural Syst Rehabil Eng* 17(5):438–444.

Seroussi, R.E. et al. 1996. Mechanical work adaptations of above-knee amputee ambulation. *Arch Phys Med Rehabil* 77(11):1209–1214.

Sewell, M.D. et al. 2009. Total femoral endoprosthetic replacement following excision of bone tumours. *J Bone Joint Surg Br* 91(11):1513–1520.

Silcox, D.H., M.D. Rooks, R.R. Vogel, and L.L. Fleming. 1993. Myoelectric prostheses: Long-term follow-up and a study of the use of alternate prostheses. *J Bone Joint Surg* 75:1781–1789.

Silva, J., Wi. Heim, and T. Chau. 2005. A self-contained mechanomyography-driven externally powered prosthesis. *Arch Phys Med Rehabil* 86(10):2066–2070.

Simon, A.M., L.J. Hargrove, B.A. Lock, and T.A. Kuiken. 2009. A strategy for minimizing the effect of misclassifications during real time pattern recognition myoelectric control. *Conf Proc IEEE Eng Med Biol Soc* 1:1327–1330.

Smith, D.G., and E.M. Burgess. 2001. The use of CAD/CAM technology in prosthetics and orthotics — current clinical models and a view to the future. *J Rehabil Res Dev* 38(3):327–334.

Song, Y.K., D.A. Borton, S. Park, W.R. Patterson, C.W. Bull, F. Laiwalla, J. Mislow, J.D. Simeral, J.P. Donoghue, and A.V. Nurmikko. 2009. Active microelectronic neurosensor arrays for implantable brain communication interfaces. *IEEE Trans Neural Syst Rehabil* 17(4):339–345.

Soo, G., M.C.F. Tong, J. Mak, V.J. Abdullah, and C.A. Van Hasselt. 2003. Extraoral osseointegration in children. *Hong Kong J Paediatr* 8:290–298.

Sorbye, R. 1980. Myoelectric prosthetic fitting in young children. *Clin Orthop* 34–40.

Stam, H.J., A.M. Dommisse, and H.J. Bussmann. 2004. Prevalence of low back pain after transfemoral amputation related to physical activity and other prosthesis-related parameters. *Disabil Rehabil* 26(13):794–797.

Staubach, K.H., and H. Grundei. 2001. The first osseointegrated percutaneous prosthesis anchor for above-knee amputees. *Biomed.Tech. (Berl)* 46(12):355–361.

Steinnagel, B. et al. 2010. Balance and confidence following Wii Fit video game training among children with unilateral lower limb amputation. Paper presented at *13th ISPO World Congress*, Leipzig, Germany.

Stepien, J.M. et al. 2007. Activity levels among lower-limb amputees: Self-report versus step activity monitor. *Arch Phys Med Rehabil* 88(7):896–900.

Suh, P.N. 1990. *The principles of design.* New York: Oxford University Press.

The Open Prosthetics Project: An Initiative of the Shared Design Alliance. The project. http://openprosthetics.org/ (accessed June 1, 2008).

Troncossi, M., E. Gruppioni, M. Chiossi, A. Giovanni Cutti, A. Davalli, and V. Parenti-Castelli. 2009. A novel electromechanical shoulder articulation for upper-limb prostheses: From the design to the first clinical application. *J Prosthet Orthot* 21(2):79–90.

Tyc, V.L. 1992. Psychosocial adaptation of children and adolescents with limb deficiencies: A review. *Clin Psychol Rev* 12:275–291.

Umberger, B.R., and P.E. Martin. 2007. Mechanical power and efficiency of level walking with different stride rates. *J Exp Biol.* 210(18):3255–3265.

Vannah, W.M. et al. 1999. A survey of function in children with lower limb deficiencies. *Prosthet Orthot Int* 23(3):239–244.

Varni, J.W., and Y. Setoguchi. 1991. Correlates of perceived physical appearance in children with congenital/acquired limb deficiencies. *J Dev Behav Pediatr* 12(3):171–176.

Varni, J.W., and Y. Setoguchi. 1993. Effects of parental adjustment on the adaptation of children with congenital or acquired limb deficiencies. *J Dev Behav Pediatr* 14(1)3:13–20.

Varni, J.W., Y. Setoguchi, L.R. Rappaport, and D. Talbot. 1992. Psychological adjustment and perceived social support in children with congenital/acquired limb deficiencies. *J Behav Med* 15(1):31–44.

Varni, J.W., Y. Setoguchi, L.R. Rappaport, and D. Talbot. 1991. Effects of stress, social support, and self-esteem on depression in children with limb deficiencies. *Arch Phys Med Rehabil* 72(13):1053–1058.

Viola, J., L. Bhavya, and G. Oran. 2003. The emergence of tissue engineering as a research field. The National Science Foundation. http://www.nsf.gov/pubs/2004/nsf0450/start.htm. (accessed January 12, 2010).

Walker, J.L. et al. 2009. Adult outcomes following amputation or lengthening for fibular deficiency. *J Bone Joint Surg Am* 91(4):797–804.

Waters, R.L., and S. Mulroy. 1999. The energy expenditure of normal and pathologic gait. *Gait Posture* 9(3):207–231.

Webster, J.B., C.E. Levy, P.R. Bryant, and P.E. Prusakowski. 2001. Sports and recreation for persons with limb deficiency. *Arch Phys Med Rehabil* 82(3):S38–S44.

Weir, R.F., P.R. Troyk, G.A. DeMichele, D.A. Kerns, J.F. Schorsch, and H. Maas. 2009. Implantable myoelectric sensors (IMESs) for intramuscular electromyogram recording. *IEEE Trans Biomed Eng* 56(1):159–171.

Wenz, W., D. Wenz, and L. Doderlein. 1998. Rehabilitation program for children and adolescents with limb defects or amputations of the lower extremity. *Rehabilitation (Stuttg)* 37(3):134–139.

Wettels, N., A.R. Parnandi, J.H. Moon, G.E. Loeb, and G.S. Sukhatme. 2009. Grip control using biomimetic tactile sensing systems. *IEEE-ASME Transactions on Mechanotronics* 14(6):718–723.

Whittle, M.W. 2002. Basic science. In *Gait analysis: An introduction*. Oxford: Butterworth-Heinemann, 3:1-41.

Whittle, M.W. 2002. Normal gait. In *Gait analysis: An introduction*. Oxford: Butterworth-Heinemann, 3:42–86.

Whittle, M.W. 2002. Methods of gait analysis. In *Gait analysis: An introduction*. Oxford: Butterworth-Heinemann, 3:127–160.

Wilk, B., L. Karol, S. Halliday, D. Cummings, N. Haideri, and J. Stepheson. 1999. Transition to an articulating knee prosthesis in pediatric amputees. *J Prosthet Orthot* 11(3):69–74.

Wilson, D.R. 1980. An exploratory study of complexity in axiomatic design, PhD thesis, MIT.

World Health Organization. 2001. *International Classification of Functioning, Disability and Health*. Washington D.C.: World Health Organization Press. http://www.who.int/classifications/icf/en/ (accessed January 12, 2010).

Wright, V. 2009. Prosthetic outcome measures for use with upper limb amputees: A systematic review of the peer-reviewed literature, 1970 to 2009. *J Prosthet Orthot* 21(9):P3–P63.

Wright, V. 2006. Measurement of functional outcome with individuals who use upper extremity prosthetic devices: Current and future directions. *J Prosthet Orthot* 18(2):46–56.

Wu, Y. et al. 2009. CIR casting system for making transtibial sockets, *Prosthet Orthot Int* 33(1):1–9.

Wu, Y. et al. 2003. CIR sand casting system for trans-tibial socket. *Prosthet Orthot Int* 27(2):146–152.

Yang, J., E. Pena Pitarch, K. Abdel-Malek, A. Patrick, and L. Lindkvist. 2004. A multi-fingered hand prosthesis. *Mech Machine Theory* 39:555–581

Zahedi, S. Lower limb prosthetic research in the 21st century. ATLAS of Prosthetics. http://www.endolite.com/pdfs/research/lower_limb.pdf/ (accessed January 12, 2010).

Zecca, M., G. Cappiello, F. Sebastiani, S. Roccella, F. Vecchi, M.C. Carrozza et al. 2004. Experimental analysis of the proprioceptive and exteroceptive sensors of an underactuated prosthetic hand. *Lect Notes Control Inform Sci* 306:233–242.

Ziegler-Graham, K., E. MacKenzie, P. Ephraim, T. Travison, and R. Brookmeyer. 2008. Estimating the prevalence of limb loss in the United States: 2005 to 2050. *Arch Phys Med Rehabil* 89(3):442–429.

Zollo, L., S. Roccella, E. Guglielmelli, M.C. Carrozza, and P. Dario. 2007. Biomechatronic design and control of an anthropomorphic artificial hand for prosthetic and robotic applications. *IEEE/ASME Trans Mechatronics* 12(4):418–429.

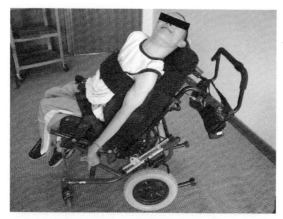

FIGURE 3.2 Client's typical posture in his wheelchair.

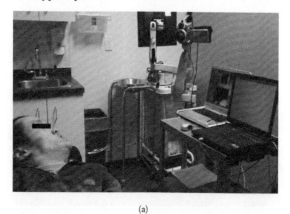

(a)

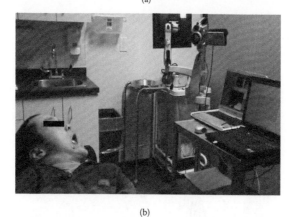

(b)

FIGURE 3.5 Client responding to audiovisual cues generated by Compass Assessment software (Koester Performance Research 2007): (a) client in rest state, (b) client making a switch press by opening his mouth.

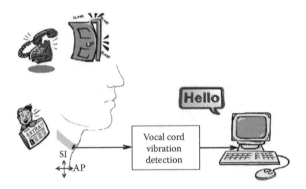

FIGURE 3.8 (a) Block diagram of the vocal cord vibration detection system. Insensitivity to environment noise and user-generated artefacts such as coughs are two major advantages of the system over existing speech-based solutions.

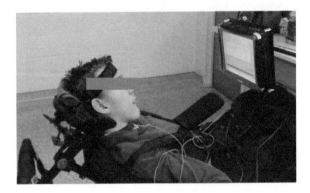

FIGURE 3.10 (b) An adolescent participant with cerebral palsy using the system to access a virtual on-screen keyboard.

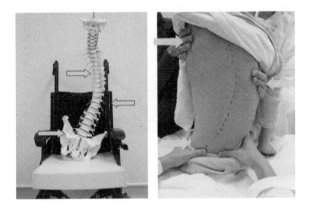

FIGURE 6.4 The three-point force system for the correction of S-curve scoliosis.

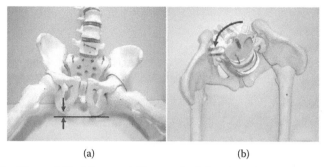

(a)   (b)

FIGURE 6.5   Views of (a) oblique and (b) rotated pelvic orientations.

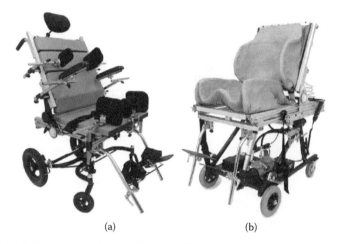

(a)   (b)

FIGURE 6.6   (a) A planar seating simulator and (b) a contoured seating simulator. (Courtesy of Prairie Seating Corporation.)

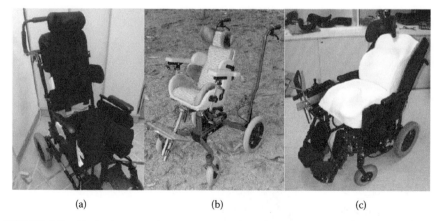

(a)   (b)   (c)

FIGURE 6.7   (a) A planar seating system with flat postural support surfaces (courtesy of Adaptive Engineering Lab, Inc.), (b) a modular seating system and (c) a custom contoured seating system.

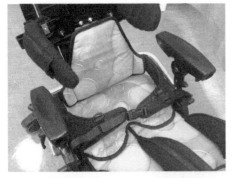

FIGURE 6.12 The Mygo pelvic stabilisation system (Leckey, UK), including a pelvic positioning harness and flexible sacral support. (Courtesy of Leckey, UK.)

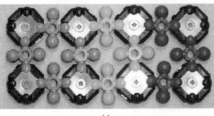

(a)

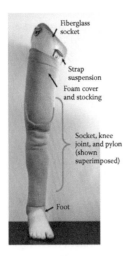

(b)

FIGURE 6.13 (a) An array of interlocking plastic modules that comprise the Matrix seating system and (b) the Matrix seating system mounted on a mobility base. (Courtesy of Southwest Seating & Rehab Ltd., UK.)

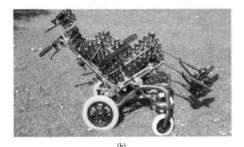

Fiberglass socket

Strap suspension

Foam cover and stocking

Socket, knee joint, and pylon (shown superimposed)

Foot

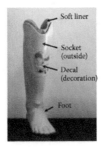

Soft liner

Socket (outside)

Decal (decoration)

Foot

FIGURE 7.3a Paediatric lower-limb prostheses: modular above-knee prosthesis (left); and below-knee prosthesis (right). (Continued)

(a)

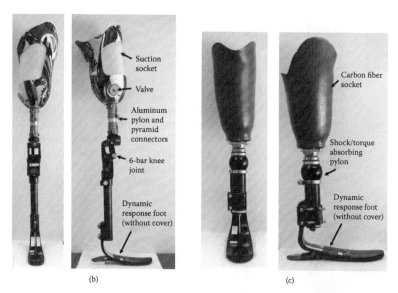

(b)　　　　　　　　　(c)

FIGURE 7.3b,c (Continued) (b) Modern modular above-knee prosthesis for adults showing suction socket, polycentric knee joint and dynamic response foot. A cosmetic foot cover would typically be used. A foam cosmetic cover may also be provided over the rest of the structure. (c) Modern modular below-knee prosthesis for adults showing a shock/torque absorbing pylon and dynamic response foot. Cosmetic finishes are not shown.

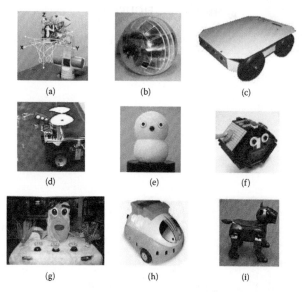

FIGURE 8.5 (a) A robotic basketball hoop used at Vanderbilt University (Conn et al. 2008b). (b) Roball used by Michaud and Theberge-Turme (2002). (c) Labo-1 used by Werry et al. (2001). (d) Mobile base with bubble blower used by Feil-Seifer and Mataric, (2008a). (e) Keepon used by Kozima (2006). (f) Lego robot used by Robins et al. (2008). (©2008 IEEE.) (g) Fishie developed at the Universit´e de Sherbrooke (Michaud and Clavet 2001). (h) Pekee used by Salter (2006). (With permission.) (i) AIBO used by Stanton et al. (2008).

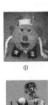
(j)

(k)

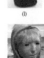
(l)

(m)

(n)

(o)

(p)

FIGURE 8.6 (j) Funny Face developed at the Université de Sherbrooke (Michaud and Clavet 2001). (k) ESRA robot used by Scassellati (2005a). (l) Tito used by Duquette et al. (2006). (m) Infanoid used by Kozima et al. (2004). (©2004 IEEE.) (n) Robota used by Robins et al. (2004a). (With kind permission of Springer Science+Business Media.) (o) Kaspar used by Robins et al. (2008). (p) FACE used by Pioggia et al. (2007). (©2007 IEEE.)

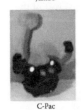
Jumbo

Roball

C-Pac

Bobus

Diskcat

Meastro

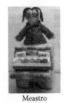

FIGURE 8.7 Examples of the robots used at the École du Touret and S.P.E.C. Tintamarre. (Michaud et al. 2003.)

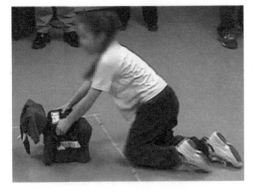

FIGURE 8.9 A child diagnosed with ASD interacts with Jumbo. (Michaud, F. and C. Theberge-Turmel. 2002. Mobile robotic toys and autism. In *Socially intelligent agents — creating relationships with computers and robots*, K. Dautenhahn, A. Bond, L. Cañamero, and B. Edmonds, Eds. 125–132. Kluwer Academic Publishers.)

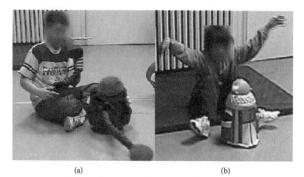

(a)   (b)

FIGURE 8.11   Children diagnosed with ASD interact with robots used at École du Touret and S.P.E.C Tintamarre. (a) C-Pac: we see a child playing with the removable parts. (b) Bobus: we see a female child excited at the interaction with the robot. (Michaud, F. and C. Theberge-Turmel. 2002. Mobile robotic toys and autism. In *Socially intelligent agents — creating relationships with computers and robots*, K. Dautenhahn, A. Bond, L. Cañamero, and B. Edmonds, Eds. 125–132. Kluwer Academic Publishers.)

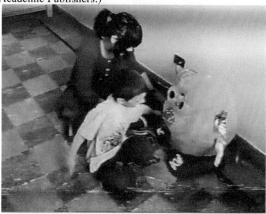

FIGURE 8.12   A child diagnosed with ASD and a care worker interact with Funny Face.

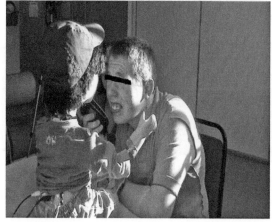

FIGURE 8.18   A participant closely exploring the facial features of KASPAR. (Robins et al. 2009.)

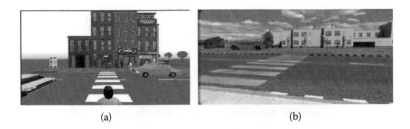

(a)   (b)

FIGURE 9.2 A comparison between the graphics quality of a street crossing virtual environment (VE) available (a) 10 years ago (Katz et al. 2005) and (b) at present (www.dmw.ca). Figure 9.2b shows that much more realistic scenarios can now be displayed even using simple desktop display technology.

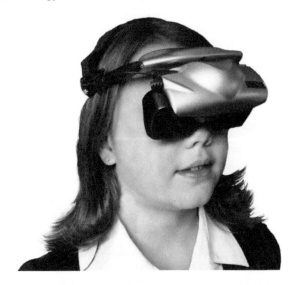

FIGURE 9.3 A head-mounted display (HMD), such as the eMagin unit shown here, is composed of two small screens positioned at eye level within special goggles or a helmet.

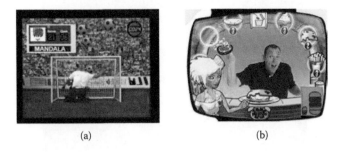

(a)   (b)

FIGURE 9.4 Two examples of video capture VR systems: (a) GestureTek's IREX VR system (http://www.gesturetekhealth.com/) and (b) Sony's PlayStation II EyeToy (http://www.us.playstation.com/PS2/Games/EyeToy_Play). Users see themselves within the simulated environment and are able to interact with virtual objects that are presented.

8 Innovations in Robotic Devices for Autism

Tamie Salter and Francois Michaud

CONTENTS

INTRODUCTION

The idea of using robotic devices in autism therapy began in 1976. The pioneering work of Weir and Emanuel (1976) used a turtle robot with a 7-year-old boy diagnosed with autism. The robot was operated via a set of buttons and was used to catalyse communication. Positive effects were reported from the interaction. Despite this reported success, further research into the effects of robotic devices on children with autism did not begin in earnest until the late 1990s.

Since then, a variety of different robots have been applied within the realm of autism research. These range from robotic balls to toy/cartoon-like robots, to robotic-looking androids, to almost human-looking androids. When developing robots, there are many factors to consider, such as who will be using/interacting with the device, where the device will be used, how long it will be used for, and so on. When developing any device that ultimately interacts with children, there are also considerations of colour, music, lights, safety, etc. Developing a device for those with autism is an even more perplexing task. An understanding of 'autism' is necessary to direct the development of a robotic device for use within this domain. As autism encompasses a spectrum of conditions, and because those with autism often find it difficult to communicate their own likes and dislikes, whether this is through speech or body language, autism is a challenging puzzle to unravel.

In this chapter, we discuss the use of robotic devices, either as a platform for autism research or as a therapeutic or educational device, primarily for children with autism. In the section 'What Is Autism?', we explain the fundamentals of autism from an engineer's perspective. This information has been used to inform the development of robotic devices for children with autism. In the section 'The Potential of Robots', we consider the possibilities that robotic devices may offer those with autism, such as encouraging

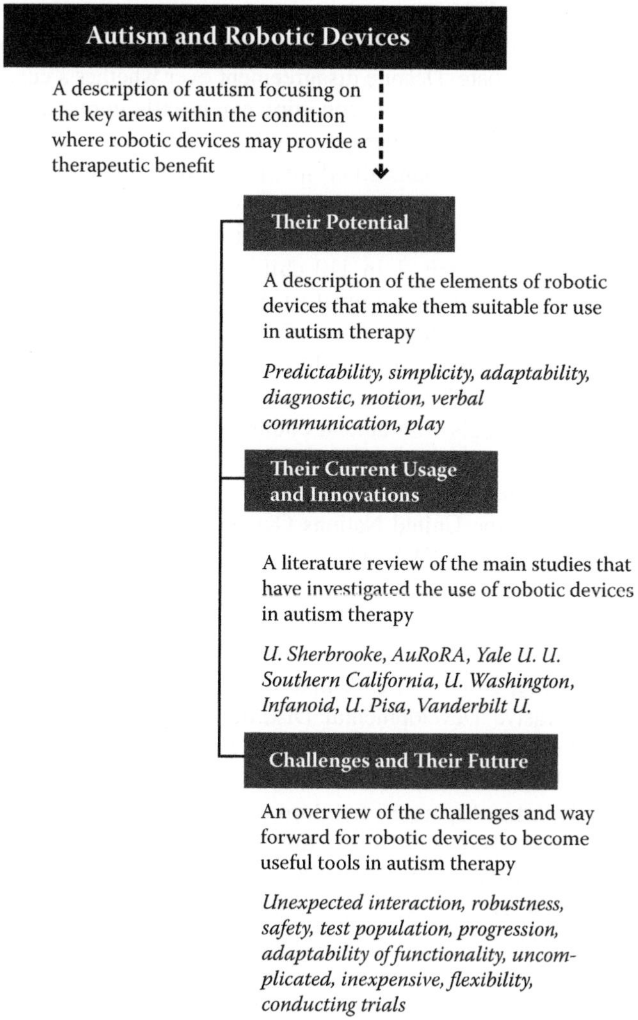

Autism and Robotic Devices

A description of autism focusing on the key areas within the condition where robotic devices may provide a therapeutic benefit

Their Potential

A description of the elements of robotic devices that make them suitable for use in autism therapy

Predictability, simplicity, adaptability, diagnostic, motion, verbal communication, play

Their Current Usage and Innovations

A literature review of the main studies that have investigated the use of robotic devices in autism therapy

U. Sherbrooke, AuRoRA, Yale U. U. Southern California, U. Washington, Infanoid, U. Pisa, Vanderbilt U.

Challenges and Their Future

An overview of the challenges and way forward for robotic devices to become useful tools in autism therapy

Unexpected interaction, robustness, safety, test population, progression, adaptability of functionality, uncomplicated, inexpensive, flexibility, conducting trials

FIGURE 8.1 Conceptual roadmap of chapter content.

verbal communication, enhancing play and breaking repetitive movements. In the next eight sections, we then appraise the contributions of different research groups since the introduction of robots to autism research. Finally, in the section 'Challenges Facing the Use of Robotic Devices', we discuss the outstanding challenges in the development of robotic devices for children with autism. Figure 8.1 provides a conceptual roadmap to help the reader navigate through the content of this chapter.

WHAT IS AUTISM?

Autism can be described as a complex developmental disability that is the result of a neurobiological disorder. It typically appears within the first 3 years of a child's life, and most literature would suggest that autism will last throughout a person's lifetime. However, there are many debates surrounding autism, and the possibility of a cure is just one such debate. Despite disagreement over whether a cure does exist, most experts agree that those with the condition can usually improve their potential through early education, care and therapy.

Autism is a condition that spans all ethnic, racial and social groups. The levels of autism appear to be consistent throughout the world. However, there is one deviation from its path: it is four times more likely to affect boys than girls. Autism is now affecting approximately 1 in 110 children (Centers for Disease Control Prevention 2010a), making it more prevalent than paediatric cancer, diabetes and AIDS combined. The U.S. Department of Education and other governmental agencies have released statistics that indicate that autism is growing at a rapid rate of 10 to 17% per year. The Autism Society of America (2010) estimates that the population of individuals with autism could reach 4 million Americans in the next decade.

Autism has gained recognition globally as a condition affecting children and youth. In fact, in 2007, the United Nations General Assembly declared April 2nd World Autism Awareness Day (WAAD).

How to Categorise Autism

The umbrella term that is used to encompass the group of disorders under which autism falls is Pervasive Developmental Disorders (PDDs), as described in *The Diagnostic and Statistical Manual of Mental Disorders, Fourth Edition, Text Revision edition* (DSM-IV, TR). Conditions that fall under the PDD 'umbrella' include Autistic Disorder, Asperger's Syndrome, Pervasive Developmental Disorder Not Otherwise Specified (PDD-NOS), Rett Syndrome and finally Childhood Disintegrative Disorder. Within the PDD group there is a sub-group called autism spectrum disorders (ASDs). The term *spectrum* is used because people on the ASD spectrum can be affected in many ways. Symptoms of the condition can occur in any combination and can range from very mild to quite severe. Each person with the diagnosis will be affected in unique ways.

The term *autism spectrum disorder* generally refers to the first three disorders of PDD: Autistic Disorder, Asperger's Syndrome and PDD-NOS. There are three core features associated with this spectrum (see Figure 8.2): social impairments, speech deficits and restricted and repetitive behaviours. Out of the PDDs, Asperger's Syndrome is the condition most closely linked with autism. There are many similarities between the two conditions. However, generally people with Asperger's have fewer language problems (see Figure 8.3) and no cognitive deficits. Throughout this text, our discussions surrounding the use of robotic devices with those who have autism include individuals with any of the three conditions under the ASD umbrella.

What Causes Autism?

The actual cause of autism is still being investigated and currently remains unknown. Research indicates no one single factor will ultimately be the cause, and it is likely

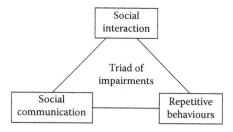

FIGURE 8.2 Graphic depicting the triad of social impairments that those with autism face (as identified by Wing and Gould 1979).

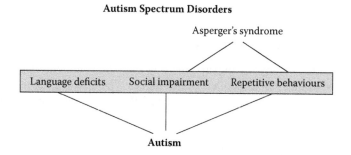

FIGURE 8.3 Graphic depicting the three main threads that affect ASD.

to be a combination of elements that are involved (National Institute of Child Health and Human Development 2010). This may include factors that can occur before, during and after birth, genetic factors, possible environmental influences and certain types of infections. In the past, children with autism were given various labels and were diagnosed as suffering from mental retardation or childhood schizophrenia. Over the years, there have been various theories as to the cause of autism ranging from environmental effects, bad parenting, cognitive deficits and birth defects to genetics. There is no conclusive evidence to support one single theory — although bad parenting is now ruled out. Evidence suggests that the cause will come from a variety of different physical factors that affect brain development and has nothing to do with parenting or emotional deprivation.

There is an increased frequency of autism within families, and this would seem to support a genetic link to the disorder. Researchers believe the aetiology is likely to be a combination of different genes rather than one single genetic defect (National Autistic Society 2010a). Despite much controversy on the subject at this point, there is no evidence or known link that immunisations, specific diets, toxins or immunologic differences cause autism. Researchers believe that the aetiology will vary between individuals and will likely come from some combination of genetic, environmental and neuropathological factors (Autism Society of America 2010).

DIAGNOSING AUTISM

Currently, there is no medical test available for diagnosis. Diagnosis must be achieved by observing the behaviour of a child and seeing if his or her behaviour fits a set of criteria required to assign the label of 'autistic.' The DSM-IV gives guidelines as to the exact criteria. A diagnosis considers the triad of impairments: social interaction, social communication and repetitive behaviours. Diagnostic tools include the Childhood Autism Rating Scale (CARS) (Van Bourgondien et al. 1992) and the Autism Diagnostic Observation Schedule (ADOS) (Lord et al. 1989; Gotham et al. 2008). These diagnostic tools are all based on observations of the child's behaviour. The section 'The Potential of Robots' discusses the possibility of using robotic devices to complement these observational tools in the diagnosis of autism.

HOW DOES AUTISM AFFECT A PERSON?

Autism affects (and many say impairs) the way a person communicates and relates to others around them. It seems that autism makes typical social human-to-human communication and interaction more complex, difficult to understand, and also difficult to perform for those with the condition. Those diagnosed have difficulty initiating and maintaining social interaction. Typically, they also have an impaired ability to recognise and understand emotions. Also, it has been said that people with autism do not possess a 'theory of mind' (Baron-Cohen 1995), a term that was coined to describe their difficulty with recognising, understanding, processing and appreciating the thoughts and feelings of others. Literally, those with autism do not realise that those around them have different thoughts and feelings from their own. Typically someone with autism struggles with communication in various forms (speech, body language, facial expressions). Communication may vary from individual to individual, as each person's ability will fall on a spectrum. Another often observed effect of autism is repetitive and stereotypic behaviours that can manifest themselves as complex rituals, extreme difficulty or reluctance to accept change and transition, and unusual movements such as hand flapping or whirling. The main effects of autism are elaborated upon in the following subsections.

Impairments with Social Communication

Social communication is a complex skill that typically developing people often can achieve without much thought. Social communication involves picking up on extremely subtle cues involving verbal and non-verbal language. Verbal and non-verbal language is often impaired in individuals with autism, making social communication a very difficult, if not impossible, task for them to achieve. Many may not speak at all, or have a limited amount of speech. Also, their general understanding of language may be different from a typically developing person. They can have difficulty understanding the nuances of speech; for example, if a person says something is 'cool', they will take this literally to mean that the temperature is low. Some with autism may understand what other people say to them, but will not respond in a typical manner; they may prefer to respond with methods such as sign language or visual symbols. Tone of voice is another area of language that can prove perplexing to someone with autism — not only can they find it difficult to pick up on the connotations of tone, but they can find it hard to adopt (Wang et al. 2007). Facial expression is yet another area that proves perplexing. Again, those with autism find both the understanding of facial expressions difficult and also have trouble using their own facial expressions to convey meaning of emotion (Phillips 2004).

Impairments with Social Interaction

Social interaction could be considered an art. The way we interact with people is governed by subtleties involving many different facets. We adjust our behaviour to fit our social setting. People with autism will often have difficulty with recognising or understanding these subtle rules that govern social interaction (The National Autistic Society 2010b). For instance, they discuss inappropriate subject matter or they may stand too close to another person and not realise that this is inappropriate. They often struggle to understand other people's emotions and feelings and have difficulty expressing their own feelings, thoughts and emotions. They may have difficulty understanding the emotions of others and consequently do not react appropriately, and therefore they may be judged as insensitive. People with autism may not even want to spend time with others and may prefer to spend time by themselves, sometimes appearing withdrawn. They can appear to be aloof, distant and uninterested in social interaction. They may not feel the need to seek comfort from other people and may not appear to pay attention to other people. They may have behaviour that is perceived as strange or inappropriate. They can have trouble understanding another person's body language and can have body movements that do not fit with typical forms of expression (Perks 2007).

Restricted and Repetitive Behaviours

Many with autism are most comfortable in a fixed, rigid routine. This desire can cover various aspects of life such as what they eat, how they get dressed, which way they walk to a familiar place or when they do a certain activity (The National Autistic Society 2010c). They can be easily disrupted by unplanned events, for example, a rainy day. There can also be a heightened need to follow rules (The National Autistic Society 2010b). Thus, individuals with autism may find it difficult to change the way they do something; once they have established a particular way of carrying out a task, they may not want to deviate from this routine. Advance preparation for change can help those with autism cope with a new way of doing things or a new situation. Those with autism can also focus on a specific routine or ritual that appears to have no practical function. Those with autism can become obsessed with a certain topic or object. It is not that the interest in the topic itself is abnormal, but rather the degree with which they become obsessed with the topic. The same can be said regarding their focus or attention; a great amount of attention can be directed to a particular object or an intense preoccupation with a part of an object can be observed. Those with autism can also exhibit repetitive actions such as hand flapping, spinning or body movements (The National Autistic Society 2010b).

Impairments with Social Imagination

As typically developing children develop, they acquire the ability to pretend play. They develop the capacity to substitute one object for another in their mind. They can conjure make-believe situations and act them out. This social imagination gives people the ability to imagine various situations, to make sense of what it would be like to be in a given situation. Social imagination gives people the ability to predict and possibly gain some understanding or insight into other people's behaviour. As part of their impairment in social interaction, those with autism have difficulty with social imagination, making it a challenge to gain insight, understand and interpret the thoughts, actions and feelings of others. Those with autism often have impairments in predicting the outcome of events or actions. This can therefore make it difficult for them to understand and cope with new events or situations that are not familiar to them.

THE POTENTIAL OF ROBOTS

Models with clockwork mechanisms that mimic human and animal behaviour were first developed in the 17th century. By the 18th century, Pierre Jacquest-Droz had built three mechanical dolls — one could play music on an organ, one could write and the other could draw a simple picture. 'Robot's were first popularised by Czechoslovakian playwright Karel Capek. In his play 'Rossums' Universal Robots,' humans created humanoid robots that were designed to work for humans. The word 'robota' means worker or slave in Czchoslovakian. The play made the front cover of *The Tatler* in 1923 and brought robots to the attention of the general public.

The challenge of designing robots is to create machines that can perceive the world around them using sensor data, make decisions based on this data and then take appropriate actions using the actuators and mechanisms available to them. Scientists hope to develop robots that can live alongside humans, helping us and making our lives easier. The design and capabilities of robots are influenced by the environments in which they must exist and the tasks they must perform (see Figure 8.4). These constraints may or may not lead to the traditional humanoid appearance that springs to mind when people think of robots.

Currently there are many different kinds of robots. However, they can be split into the following categories: assistive, industrial, service, social, search and rescue, and health care. Robots designed for autism therapy would fall into the assistive category.

What are the possibilities for robotic devices aiding those who have autism? Pioggia et al. (2008) have suggested that the use of robotic devices in autism therapy could 'be of tremendous clinical significance'. Early work conducted by Werry et al. (2001) showed the potential for robotic use by initially investigating whether children with autism would enjoy interacting with a robot. Others have also documented success when using robotic devices to engage children. A team from the University of Alberta (Cook et al. 2002) has adapted a robotic arm to facilitate learning in children. They found that the children 'were highly responsive to the robotic tasks. This was in marked contrast to other interventions using toys and computer games.' This section looks at why robotic devices have been used within the domain of ASD research.

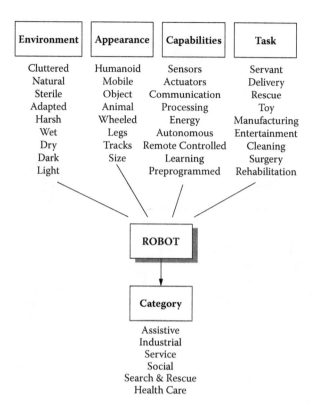

Environment	Appearance	Capabilities	Task
Cluttered	Humanoid	Sensors	Servant
Natural	Mobile	Actuators	Delivery
Sterile	Object	Communication	Rescue
Adapted	Animal	Processing	Toy
Harsh	Wheeled	Energy	Manufacturing
Wet	Legs	Autonomous	Entertainment
Dry	Tracks	Remote Controlled	Cleaning
Dark	Size	Learning	Surgery
Light		Preprogrammed	Rehabilitation

ROBOT

Category

Assistive
Industrial
Service
Social
Search & Rescue
Health Care

FIGURE 8.4 The operational environment, appearance and capabilities of the robot, and the intended tasks determine the categorisation of the robot.

From observations, it would seem that robots possess many appealing qualities when it comes to interaction with children diagnosed with autism. It is known that some people diagnosed with autism incline towards predictability (see section Restricted and Repetitive Behaviors); they seem to have a fascination with mechanical objects and respond well to objects of a simple appearance. Another potential of robotic devices is adaptability. As discussed in section How to Categorise Autism, all children diagnosed with autism are actually on a spectrum and therefore the condition affects each person individually, and each child with autism has varying individual needs. In light of the individuality of the condition, robots offer customisability; every aspect of a robot can be tailored to fit the child. When all this is coupled together, that is, mechanical appeal, adaptability and simplicity, it is clear that robots show great potential. In Figures 8.5 and 8.6, we see a selection of robots that have interacted with children diagnosed with autism. These figures depict the wide variation in the appearance and ultimately the abilities and behaviour of the robots.

Robots may also become a useful tool for autism diagnosis, helping children with autism break repetitive movement, diversifying the range of physical activities, and encouraging verbal communication and play. These possibilities are presented in the following subsections. Note that here we present only the key concepts regarding the

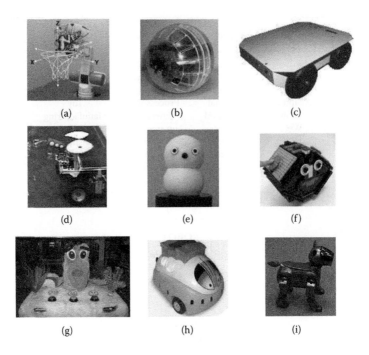

FIGURE 8.5 (See color insert following page 240.) (a) A robotic basketball hoop used at Vanderbilt University (Conn et al. 2008b). (b) Roball used by Michaud and Theberge-Turme (2002). (c) Labo-1 used by Werry et al. (2001). (d) Mobile base with bubble blower used by Feil-Seifer and Mataric, (2008a). (Reprinted with permission from Feil-Seifer, D.J. and M. Mataric. 2008b. Robot assisted therapy for children with autism spectrum disorders. In *Proceedings of the Interaction Design for Children: Children with Special Needs*, Chicago, IL, 49–52.) (e) Keepon used by Kozima (2006). (f) Lego robot used by Robins et al. (2008). (Reprinted with permission from Robins, B., E. Ferrari, and K. Dautenhahn. 2008. Developing scenarios for robot assisted play. In *17th IEEE International Symposium on Robot and Human Interactive Communication* (RO-MAN 2008), University Munchen, Munich, Germany, 180–186. IEEE Press © [2008] IEEE.) (g) Fishie developed at the Universit´e de Sherbrooke (Michaud and Clavet 2001). (h) Pekee used by Salter (2006). (With permission (l) AIBO used by Stanton et al. 2008). (i) AIBO used by Stanton et al. (2008).

previously mentioned areas of potential. Detailed appraisals of research supporting the identified potential areas follow in later sections.

MECHANICAL OBJECTS AND PREDICTABILITY

It is known that children with autism are attracted to mechanical objects such as toy cars, trains and computers (see Shives 2007; Gabriels and Hill 2007; Robins and Dautenhahn 2004; Colby 1973; Moor 2008). In addition, it is known that some people diagnosed with autism incline towards predictability and robots can be predictable. Many believe that it may be possible to exploit this interest in mechanical objects. Scassellati (2009) says, 'Our hope is to exploit this motivation and interest [in mechanical objects], to construct systems that provide social skills training, to

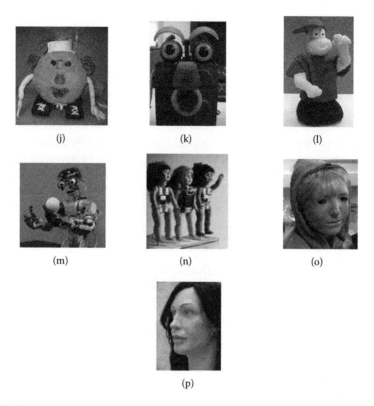

FIGURE 8.6 (See color insert following page 240.) (j) Funny Face developed at the Universit´e de Sherbrooke (Michaud and Clavet 2001). (k) ESRA robot used by Scassellati (2005a). (l) Tito used by Duquette et al. (2006). (m) Infanoid used by Kozima et al. (2004). (© 2004 IEEE.) (With permission from © (2007) IEEE.) (n) Robota used by Robins et al. (2004a). (Reproduced from Robins, B., K. Dautenhahn, R. te Boekhorst, and A. Billard. 2004a. Effects of repeated exposure of a humanoid robot on children with autism. In *Designing a more inclusive world* (Cambridge Workshop on Universal Access and Assistive Technology), ed. S. Keates, J. Clarkson, P. Langdon, and P. Robinson, 225–236. Cambridge: Springer-Verlag (London with kind permission of Springer Science+Business Media.) (o) Kaspar used by Robins et al. (2008). (p) FACE used by Pioggia et al. (2007). (With permission from Pioggia, G., M.L. Sica, M. Ferro, R. Igliozzi, F. Muratori, A. Ahluwalia, and D. De Rossi. 2007. Human-robot interaction in autism: FACE, an android-based social therapy. In *16th IEEE International Conference on Robot & Human Interactive Communication* (RO-MAN 2007), 605–612. IEEE Press © [2007] IEEE.)

supplement the activities therapists and families already engage in.' When talking about children with autism, Colby (1973) says, 'We can try to devise a remedial treatment which takes advantage of the fact that he is often fascinated by machines.' In 2001, the National Autistic Society in the U.K. commissioned a study called 'Making Connections. A Report on the Special Relationship between Children with Autism and Thomas & Friends' (The National Autistic Society, 2009). From the findings in this study, it would appear that robotic devices have the potential to exploit the fascination those with autism have with mechanical objects.

SIMPLISTIC SOCIAL TOYS

In work that investigated how children with autism respond to both social and non-social toys, Ferrara and Hill (1980) found that the children 'approached social objects more readily than non-social objects when both were simple in appearance.' This may suggest that children with autism are attracted to social objects as long as their outward appearance is sufficiently simplistic. Robins et al. (2006) investigated how children with autism responded to a robot that displayed two different appearances: (1) a plain robotic appearance or (2) a typical doll appearance (see Figure 8.16). The results of the trials clearly indicate the children's preference to interact with a plain, featureless robot rather than with a human-like robot. This would again seem to make robots an ideal choice for interaction with children with autism. It is easy to create simple but social robotic devices.

ADAPTABILITY

As those with autism are each so individual (see 'How to Categorize Autism'), it would follow that no one device would be right for all. A shortcoming of conventional toys is that they do not change to aid a specific child. Traditional toys are developed to encompass the largest range of children possible. McConkey and Jeffree (1981) write, 'that it is a matter of finding the right toy for the right child.' Robotic devices may help to simplify this search, as long as they remain adaptable. Otherwise, robots will not succeed in meeting the needs of a large population. Robins writes, 'Autism does not occur to the same degree and in the same form in all cases, so, as robotic systems are developed to aid in the therapy and education of children with autism, it is unlikely that they can be used generically to satisfy all needs and requirements' (Robins et al. 2004b).

A similar view has been expressed by Michaud et al. (2003). 'Since each child is a distinct individual with preferences and capabilities, it might not be possible to design one complete robotic toy that can help capture and retain the interest of every child.'

Scassellati (2005b) investigated a robot with behaviours that could be decomposed arbitrarily, allowing for adaptability. Some of the behaviours could be switched off while others left intact. Section presents a scenario justifying the need for adaptability in robotic devices. Salter has been investigating how to adapt an autonomous robot's behaviour based on sensor readings from on-board sensors on two different robots (Salter 2006; Salter et al. 2005, 2007, 2009). The sensor readings are based on a child's interaction while playing with the robot and, therefore, effectively 'personalising' or 'fitting' the robot to the child. Michaud and Theberge-Turmel (2002) have also discussed similar ideas, advising that, 'since the robot is a device that is programmed, the robot's behaviour can evolve over time, changing the reinforcing loop over time, to make them learn to deal with more sensory inputs and unpredictability.' To adapt mobile robot toys to each child, reconfigurable robots, using different hardware and software components, might be one solution to explore.

Salter et al. (2005, 2007, 2009) have been working on developing an adaptive behaviour for Roball (see Figure 8.5b). The motivation for the new adaptive behaviour is that all children are different. Whether you are looking across age groups or

TABLE 8.1

Coded Video Data. The Coded Behaviours of Smile/Laugh/ Giggle and Asking Questions, for All Children According to the Three Different Interaction Modes

Session	Child (Pseudonymns)	Mode	Smile	Question
1	Edward	B	2	0
1	Evie	A	1	0
1	Gilbert	C	10	0
1	Harold	B	0	0
1	Tyler	A	2	0
2	Edward	C	2	0
2	Evie	B	0	0
2	Gilbert	A	0	0
2	Harold	C	1	0
2	Tyler	B	2	0
3	Edward	B	0	0
3	Evie	C	1	3
3	Gilbert	B	4	0
3	Harold	A	0	0
3	Tyler	C	1	4

A = basic behaviour
B = preprogrmmed behaviour
C = adaptive behaviour

categories (e.g., typically developing, special needs), children all have very different personality traits, for example, shy, boisterous, cautious, outgoing. It is easy to realise that a robot that exhibits only one type of behaviour will not be suitable for all children. This is especially true of children with autism who are on a spectrum and vary greatly in their abilities and personalities. Salter and colleagues based at the Université de Sherbrooke (IntRolab 2010) are developing robotic behaviours that they believe to be encouraging and less daunting for an anxious child. Also, they are developing behaviours that are faster and more exciting for a more confident child.

An adaptation algorithm using touch or contact as a metric was developed, based on the readings coming from sensors on-board Roball. A trial was conducted that investigated which type of behaviour *encouraged* and *sustained* a child's interaction more — adaptive mode or two different pre-programmed modes.

It was found that there was an increase in the amount of smiling/laughing during the adaptive interaction mode. Also, it was observed that only during the adaptive interaction mode did children ask a question to a nearby adult (see results in Table 8.1).

This work showed that a robotic device has the ability to raise the level of communication between typically developing children and the adults around them. The next step was to conduct trials with children who have autism.

Diagnostics

Currently there is no medical test available for the diagnosis of autism (see section Diagnosing Autism). There is a real possibility of using robotic devices as a means to aid the diagnosis of ASD. Robotic devices may introduce an element of objectivity to the diagnostic process. At Yale University, Scassellati (2005a, b) has been looking at how robots can help with the diagnosis of autism. Scassellati hopes to improve the diagnostic standards of autism by using robots to provide quantitative and objective measurements of social response. Using infrared sensor readings, Salter (2006) showed an objective measurable difference in the way a child with autism interacted with a robot when compared to that of typically developing children. Taking a child with autism for clinical observation can be stressful for both the child and parents. Therefore, there would be benefits to collecting data in a place that is familiar to the child, simply by playing with a fun robot. This could reduce the stress on everyone involved. Of course, this is not to say robots would diagnose but that the robot could be a tool for the clinicians to utilise, a tool that could provide the expert with data that may further inform their diagnosis.

Breaking Repetitive Movement

It is known that those with autism show abnormal behaviours including repetitive movements such as spinning and hand flapping (see section Restricted and Repetitive Behaviours). It has been observed that interaction with robotic devices can help decrease the level of repetitive behaviours in children with autism. In work conducted at the Université de Sherbrooke, Duquette conducted a study that paired children with autism with either a robotic mediator or a human mediator (see section Tito). In this work, Duquette et al. (2008) found that the 'children exposed to the robotic mediator showed reduced repetitive play with inanimate objects of interest (their favorite toy), and no repetitive or stereotyped behavior towards the robot.' Others have also found similar results: Stanton et al. (2008) found that children with autism produced less autistic behaviours when playing with a robotic dog (AIBO, equipped with on-board sensors and the ability to respond to a child's interaction) when compared to a mechanical dog; Michaud (see section Diskcat) showed that it is possible for a robot to break a child with autism out of a repetitive routine.

Movement/Motion

There is mounting evidence to suggest that there may be differences in the way children with autism move (Mari et al. 2003; Rinehart et al. 2006). It would follow that due to the triad of social impairments (see section How to Categorise Austism and How Does Austism Affect a Person?), it could prove difficult to instruct and guide them in physical activity. The animated nature and embodiment of robots encourage movement and physical interaction in children: they can follow, jump over, crawl next to, avoid, imitate the robot and so forth. Movement has beneficial qualities both to mental health and in aiding general learning (Barclay et al. 1975). Therefore, it is hoped that the animated interaction that children share with mobile robots could provide additional educational benefits to that of traditional toys. Among other things, learning about interaction would prove more beneficial when experienced in an embodied context rather than attempting to learn through static media such as books. When discussing 'embodied interaction,' Dautenhahn and Werry (2002) tell us that 'bodily interaction itself can be as therapeutically relevant as the content of the interaction.'

Encouraging Verbal Communication

Those with autism can have difficulty in verbal communication (see section Impairments with Social Communication). This can be very limiting; therefore, finding a medium that can encourage children with autism to communicate through language would be very desirable. It has been found that interaction with robots can increase a child's verbal communication in both typically developing children and those with autism. Work by Salter (2009) at the Université de Sherbrooke found that when a robot displayed an adaptive behaviour, it encouraged typically developing children to ask questions to adults in the room. This system will now be tested on children with autism. Werry (2001) found that children with autism were verbally communicative when interacting with a robot: 'children were vocal and talked both about and to the robot throughout the session, in particular about what the robot "should" do' and 'a number of the children asked the teacher present about the robot and it became the focus of attention for child-teacher interaction.' Work by Stanton (2008) has also found an increase in verbal communication when children with autism were with a robotic dog compared to when they were accompanied by a mechanical dog. They hope that 'if (as in the current study) children with autism produce more coherent speech with a robot as compared to other play artefacts, such production would seemingly provide the children with increased capability that they could later utilize in human-human interaction. A second way is that robots might provide autistic children with a pivotal medium for enhanced communication with adults (page 276).'

Play

It may appear that play does not have any apparent reason and all that children are doing is having fun. However, play is an extremely important activity for all children (see Dixon 2009; Power 2000). Play is a necessary part of a child's development, and an activity that children generally perform naturally and with ease. Playtime helps children develop many skills including cognitive learning, symbolic play and learning about social interaction. Play allows children to practice future life scenarios; it enables them to take in information about different situations and to experience different outcomes; and it allows children to understand their environment. Children seem programmed with an innate desire to learn about their own surroundings and use play as the vehicle to make these discoveries (Hyne 2003). Play is a fun, enjoyable experience for most children. It is vital that children partake in this activity.

There are different stages of play according to the age of the child: infant, toddler, preschooler or school age (Children's Hospital of Pittsburgh 2009).

- Infant: During the first year of a typically developing child's life, a series of social and communicative responses will occur between the infant and those around him or her, for example, crying to obtain food or comfort (University of Pittsburgh 2010). Invariably an infant will use eye contact and some form of sound to interact with his or her caregivers (Centers for Disease Control and Prevention 2010b). Infants will begin to find mobility and use their bodies to express emotion, for example, excited arm and leg movements.
- Toddlers: As children grow and develop into toddlers, they enjoy much more physical movement and the accompanying increased freedom (Centers for Disease Control and Prevention 2010c). They begin to explore and understand objects, and how to manipulate and control them. They start to use symbols and begin imaginative play. They become involved in symbolic play. They also begin developing skills for participating with a group, for example, language.
- Preschoolers: At this age we see a heightened level of social skills allowing them to play with others and develop friends. They begin to use symbols in a more complex way. Their language progresses and becomes more complex. They are able to attach language to actions and ideas. They develop a greater understanding of objects and begin exploring their control and manipulation of objects to obtain a desired outcome. Both their fine and gross motor skills begin to refine.
- School age: By school age, children's social interaction skills have developed such that they can play with groups using cooperation and conflict resolution. They can also now follow rules. They have new skills in organising ideas and objects. They are continually developing the ability to use letters and numbers.

But what if a child is not typically developing and does not follow these milestones? 'Some children for various reasons do not have a natural approach to playing, and children with autism, among others, belong to this group' (Gammeltoft and Nordenhof 2007).

It is known that children with autism do not naturally gravitate towards playing (Gammeltoft and Nordenhof 2007). They do not follow typical norms in the way they play. A lot of playing involves social interaction, something that children with autism can actually shy away from and even completely avoid. Typical play involves eye contact, use of language and an understanding of social rules, all areas in which children with autism may have deficits. Therefore, they find this activity difficult to participate in. As described previously, we learn so much through play. Those who do not partake in play greatly compromise their ability to learn the necessary skills for typical interaction with the world in which we live. So how can we attempt to engage a child with autism in play? There are many books written on the subject (Moor 2008; Gammeltoft and Nordenhof 2007; Wolfberg 2009). These involve ideas about games that have clearly defined boundaries and clear instructions to allow a child with autism to play whilst feeling at ease and not confused by what they may perceive as a chaotic experience. We believe that robots may encourage children with autism to play and, therefore, help them to learn some of the skills acquired through play. Researchers have noted that children with autism appear to smile or laugh while with a robot (Dautenhahn and Werry 2004; Duquette et al. 2006; Kozima et al. 2005; Salter 2006; Michaud and Theberge-Turmel 2002; Michaud et al. 2000). As discussed in the section 'Mechanical Objects and Predictability,' children with autism have a natural interest in both mechanical objects and toys that are at a simplistic social level. This makes robots ideal candidates for engaging these children in playful interaction.

UNIVERSITÉ DE SHERBROOKE

We begin our description of robotic devices used in autism by describing the ones from our robot design laboratory at the Université de Sherbrooke because it presents a large variety of robots and shows many of the possibilities for robotic devices being used in autism therapy. While there are investigators from many different disciplines such as education, computer science and psychology involved in our lab, our combined focus is in developing robotic devices that can be used in natural settings. We often use a rapid prototyping method [such as the one suggested by Bartneck and Hu (2004)] to gain information as swiftly as possible, and many of the studies that are conducted are proof-of-concept or exploratory case studies to investigate the effects of different types of robots, with data ranging from narrative observations to qualitative and quantitative information. Iteratively, we develop robots that can eventually be used by a larger population and for longer durations.

Our work with robotic devices for children began in 1999, when the idea of designing custom-made mobile robots to study child development within the paediatric domain that was emerging. This work has continued and now, among other things, we study the use of mobile robotic toys in helping children with autism develop social skills (Michaud et al. 2000, 2003, 2005, 2006; Duquette et al. 2006; Michaud and Theberge-Turmel 2002; Michaud and Clavet 2001). The fundamental goal of this research is to see how mobile robots can help children diagnosed with autism open up to their surroundings, improve their imagination and try to break repetitive patterns, using a combination of autonomous and remote-controlled robots. The following subsections describe trials conducted in different schools and groups with our robots over the last decade.

ÉCOLE DU TOURET

École du Touret (2000) is a school for students with special needs. The school is the regional service centre for students with profound intellectual disabilities, with or without associated impairments and for students with ASD. The school educates children with moderate to severe intellectual disabilities.

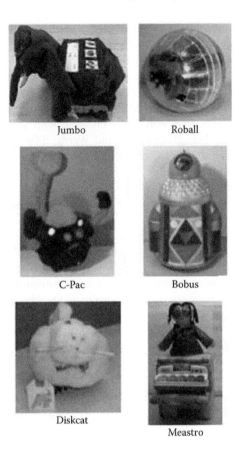

Jumbo

Roball

C-Pac

Bobus

Diskcat

Meastro

FIGURE 8.7   (See color insert following page 240.) Examples of the robots used at the École du Touret and S.P.E.C. Tintamarre. (Michaud et al. 2003.)

We took several robots to see how the children would react to the devices. The trials were conducted on three different occasions in two different rooms: one regular classroom and a $20' \times 20'$ room without tables or chairs. Children were allowed to interact freely with the robots. There was at least one educator present at all times. The role of this person was to introduce the robot to children, or to intervene in case of difficulties of any kind. Each session lasted approximately 1.5 hours. No restriction was imposed on trial length as the goal was to let all the children of the class play with the robots. This allowed 8 to 10 children to play with the robots during one session. None of the children who participated in the trials were capable of fluent speech. However, some were able to understand the short messages generated by the robots. All robots, except one, were developed at the RoboToy Contest (see Michaud and Clavet 2001): Jumbo, C-Pac and Bobus (see Figure 8.7). One robot, Roball, was developed within our laboratory (IntRoLab 2010).

As expected, each child had his or her own way of interacting with the different robots. Some remained seated on the floor, looking at the robot and touching it when it came close to them (if the robot moved away to a certain distance, some children just stopped looking at the robot). Others moved around, approaching and touching the robots and sometimes showing signs of excitement. As we have found in many of our trials, it is very hard to generalize the results of this trial due to the differences between the children and the way they interacted with the different robots. One generalisation that we feel confident in stating is that the robots captured the attention of the children and that in many cases the robots made the children smile, laugh or react vocally. However, we did not notice any increase in eye gaze towards the robots. We give a more detailed description of results from some of the robots used in these trials in the following subsections.

Roball

Apart from the École du Touret trial, Roball (see Michaud and Caron 2002 and Figures 8.4b, 8.6 and 8.7) has been used in numerous interactions with children of all ages, genders and abilities. Roball is 6 in. in diameter and weighs approximately 4 pounds. It consists of a plastic sphere (a hamster exercise ball), which houses the fragile electronics (sensors, actuators, processing elements). Being spherical in shape, Roball encourages a wide range of play situations. Here, we focus on the interaction between Roball and David, a child with autism from École du Touret. We also compare the actions of David against those of the other children involved in the École du Touret trials as well as against those of children who have interacted with Roball in other trials (Michaud and Caron 2000; Salter et al. 2007, 2008).

During the École du Touret trials, Roball exhibited a programmed behaviour that generated a two-phase cycle:

1. Wandering and carrying out obstacle avoidance for approximately 60 sec.
2. Randomly stopping and remaining motionless for a period of time between 30 and 60 sec. While stopped, Roball (using pre-recorded vocal messages) randomly asking for one of three actions:
   - To be spun
   - To be shaken
   - To receive a push to start moving again.If the child responded with the correct action to a request (spinning, shaking or pushing), then Roball thanked the child. If Roball did not perceive any interaction from the child, it indicated that it was getting bored. After a predetermined length of time during which Roball received no interaction, or after the child had given Roball a small push as a response to a pushing request, Roball continued to wander around in the environment.

It seems from our general observations in other trials with Roball (see Salter et al. 2005, 2007, 2009; Michaud et al. 2005; Michaud and Caron 2002) that most children, and certainly most typically developing children, actively try to catch Roball, to grab it or to touch the robot and some will make it spin. David was interested in interacting only with Roball (see Figure 8.8) and none of the other robots present at École du Touret. However, it seemed that David either did not listen to Roball or understand Roball's requests. In other words, he did not respond to the requests in the same manner as did the other children. Also, David did not seem to have typical

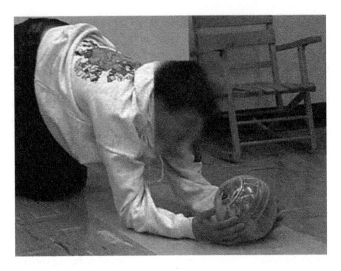

FIGURE 8.8 David, a child diagnosed with ASD, interacts with Roball. (Michaud, F. and C. Theberge-Turmel. 2002. Mobile robotic toys and autism. In *Socially intelligent agents — creating relationships with computers and robots*, K. Dautenhahn, A. Bond, L. Cañamero, and B. Edmonds, Eds. 125–132. Kluwer Academic Publishers.)

play patterns. While Roball was not moving, he played with it by making it roll on the floor between his arms (something not seen with any other children), and he would also bring Roball to his mouth (again not seen with the other children). Also, he did not exhibit as much eye contact towards Roball as the other children. However, this changed when Roball began to move again on its own: David stopped moving, kept looking at Roball, stood up and started to clap his hands and laugh. It would appear that by moving, Roball encouraged and further engaged this child's interest. Overall, it seemed that David enjoyed the interaction with Roball. He did show interest and physically interacted with the robot. He also showed joy by clapping, something that can at times be seen as a breakthrough in those who have autism.

Jumbo

Jumbo is a robot based on an elephant (see Figure 8.7 and Figure 8.9). It has a moving head and trunk, one pyroelectric sensor, an infrared range sensor and three buttons in a line on its back. Above each button is an associated pictogram (these can be easily replaced). Jumbo is programmed to move towards an object (the child) and to stop at a distance of 20 cm. Once close to an object, Jumbo asks for one of the three buttons located on its back to be pressed. The request comes in the form of a verbal prompt to the child. At first, LEDs flash to help the child locate the correct button, but after a preset amount of time, the LEDs are no longer activated to allow the child to determine which button to press on his or her own. If the child is successful in pressing the correct button, Jumbo raises its trunk and plays some music (Baby's Elephant Walk or Asterix the Gaul). If the child does not respond to Jumbo's request, that is to say, no button is pressed, the robot then asks the child to play with it and attempts to reposition itself in front of the child.

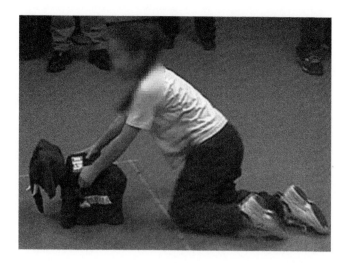

FIGURE 8.9 (See color insert following page 240.) A child diagnosed with ASD interacts with Jumbo. (Michaud, F. and C. Theberge-Turmel. 2002. Mobile robotic toys and
autism. In *Socially intelligent agents — creating relationships with computers and robots,*
K. Dautenhahn, A. Bond, L. Cañamero, and B. Edmonds, Eds. 125–132. Kluwer Academic
Publishers.)

This robot proved to be very robust and even when its pyroelectric lenses got damaged, the robot could still function. The children seemed to enjoy their interaction with
this robot; in particular, they seemed to enjoy the trunk moving and the playing of
music. One child liked to push the robot around when it was not moving (see Figure 8.9).
She would also make the robot stay close to her when it moved away by grabbing it and
pulling it close. Children seemed to enjoy the pictogram game. However, at times the
children would press the pictograms instead of the associated buttons.

Diskcat

One very interesting observation made from the École du Touret trials was with
another robot called Diskcat (see Figure 8.7) and Sarah, a girl 10 years of age. This
robot has a fur exterior and was designed to have the appearance of a cat. The robot
could play games like 'Simon Says' and could dance. In addition, Diskcat could produce visual effects using LEDs, which would light up in the eye area and on the back
of the robot. Resistive bend sensors were used as whiskers.

Sarah's typical behaviour upon entering the recreation room was to immediately
follow the walls, sometimes repeating this action over and over. However, during
the session with Diskcat, she did not follow her normal routine. Figure 8.10 shows
the trajectory Sarah carried out with the robot in the room. Initially, the robot was
near a wall, not moving (location A of Figure 8.10). Sarah started by following the
walls of the room (as was her normal behaviour). As she came across the robot at
location A, she interacted with the robot for a short amount of time when encouraged
by the educator. When the robot moved away from the walls towards location B of
Figure 8.10, Sarah slowly stopped, first at one particular corner of the room (location
1 of Figure 8.10), and then at location 2 (Figure 8.10). Sarah did this to watch the

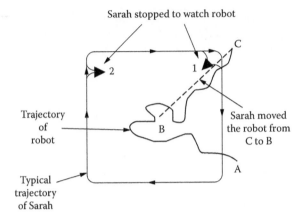

FIGURE 8.10 Overhead view of the trajectory carried out by Sarah with Diskcat in the room.

robot move around. At one point when the robot got to a corner of the room (location C), Sarah was at location 2. Noticing that the robot was not in the centre of the room, she went out of her way to location B and then to location C, to take the robot by its tail and drag it back to the centre of the room. She then went back to her typical trajectory. She even smiled and made eye contact with some of the adults in the room, including those whom she did not know. This was something that she did not normally do. This indicated that having the robot moving in the environment encouraged Sarah to break out of her typical routine and to communicate (by smiling) with others in the room.

C-Pac

C-Pac is a very robust robot that has removable arms and tail (see Figures 8.7 and 8.11). The robot has been designed so that the removable parts use connectors that have different geometrical shapes (i.e., star, triangle and hexagon). The child must align the correct part with the correct connector to connect the two. C-Pac also has a moving mouth, eyes made of LEDs, an infrared range sensor and four pyroelectric sensors that are used to manoeuvre the robot and keep it in close proximity of the child. There are various games that can be played with C-Pac. For example, when successfully assembled (the arms and tail correctly attached), the robot thanks the child and spins. The robot also asks the child to make it dance by pressing its head. When the child presses the head, it becomes illuminated, music (La Bamba) is played and the robot moves to simulate dancing. From these trials, it seems that children really enjoy this dancing function of the robot. The children who interacted with C-Pac quickly learned how to play with it, and even how to assemble the arms and tail. The children found ways to play with the robot that were not expected, such as using the removable parts as toys in their own right. Some children were surprised when they grabbed the robot by its arms or tail, expecting to take hold of the robot but instead removing an appendage from the robot.

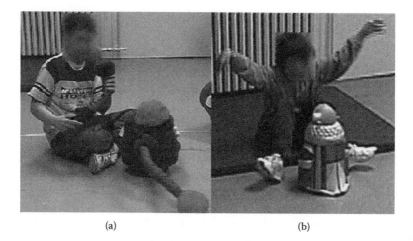

(a)   (b)

FIGURE 8.11   (See color insert following page 240.) Children diagnosed with ASD interact with robots used at École du Touret and S.P.E.C Tintamarre. (a) C-Pac: we see a child
playing with the removable parts. (b) Bobus: we see a female child excited at the interaction with the robot. (Michaud, F. and C. Theberge-Turmel. 2002. Mobile robotic toys and
autism. In *Socially intelligent agents — creating relationships with computers and robots*,
K. Dautenhahn, A. Bond, L. Cañamero, and B. Edmonds, Eds. 125–132. Kluwer Academic
Publishers.)

Bobus

Bobus is an extremely robust robot (see Figures 8.7 and 8.11). It withstood extremely
physical interaction from the children, including one child lying on top of it. This
robot works by detecting the presence of a child using pyroelectric sensors. It then
slowly moves closer to the child, and when close enough, the robot performs simple
movements and plays music. The robot can vocalise simple requests, such as requesting that a button be touched, and if the child responds appropriately, light effects are
generated using the LEDs around the 'neck' of the robot, and the small ventilator on
its head is activated and rotates. Two female participants in particular liked Bobus.
They enjoyed the light effects, the moving head with the ventilator, and the different
textures of the 'body.' One of the participants showed signs of excitement when playing with Bobus. Another participant was very physical in her interaction: she lifted
the robot and made it roll on its side on top of her legs. She then put the robot on the
floor, lay on top of it and made it roll on its side using her legs.

S.P.E.C. Tintamarre Summer Camps

S.P.E.C. Tintamarre is a summer camp specifically aimed at those diagnosed with
some form of pervasive developmental disorders. It offers activities that promote
stimulation, socialisation and integration (S.P.E.C. Tintamarre Summer Camp 2001).
A longitudinal study involving three sets of trials was carried out at this summer
camp over one summer. In general, from these trials we discovered that it is important to let a child become familiar with both the experimental area and the robot.
We also found that having an educator present to encourage the child can positively

impact the child and his or her interaction with robots. In the following subsections, we present the interactions that the children had with two of our robots, namely Jumbo and Diskcat.

Jumbo

In this set of trials, Jumbo (see Figure 8.7) was used 1 day a week over a period of 5 weeks, for 30 to 40 min with four different groups. This trial involved both children and young adults. The participants were grouped according to the severity of their condition, their level of autonomy and their age. Each group contained between 4 and 10 children/young adults, along with 2 or 3 educators, and each group had its own room. The participants were placed in a circle either sitting down on the floor or sitting on small cubes, depending on their physical capabilities. The robot was always on the floor, and each child played with the robot in turn, for example, pressing the buttons. Once each participant had a turn, a new set of pictograms was used.

Many of the children showed interest in Jumbo as soon as it entered the room. This was evident from their looking at the robot, going to touch it, pushing it, grabbing the trunk and pressing on the buttons and pictograms. Again, as we found before (see section École de Touret, Jumbo), the children seemed to enjoy interacting with this robot. They appeared to enjoy the music and some would dance to it. Overall, the amount of interactions varied greatly from one child to another. Some remained seated on the floor and played with the robot when it came close to them. Others would clear the way in front of the robot to make a path so that it could come close to them, while others moved away from its path when it came in their direction. It was communicated by the educators that overall the children seemed to have a higher concentration span when interacting with the robot than they normally did for other activities. One girl who had previously shown a dislike of animals happily petted Jumbo. She would even intervene when other children took too long to respond to a request from Jumbo or did not respond in a correct manner to Jumbo's requests. This action was also seen with another boy, and it was noted that this child was very expressive (by lifting his arms in the air) when he succeeded with the pictograms.

One general observation is that the participants seemed to anthropomorphise Jumbo. They would talk to the robot and show reactions when they believed it was not behaving correctly or when it was not moving towards them. Some of the educators would encourage this behaviour by also exhibiting anthropomorphic tendencies towards Jumbo: they would also talk to Jumbo as if it were a real animal, for example, by calling its name and asking it to come closer. When Jumbo did not respond correctly, that is, moved away when an educator had requested it come closer, the educators would say things like 'Jumbo! You should clean your ears!' or 'Jumbo has big ears but cannot hear a thing!'

One boy showed real progress in his participation, his motivation and his interactions over the 5 weeks. Initially his reaction was to observe the robot from a distance, but he rapidly began to interact with the robot. His overall interest towards the robot seemed greater than that of the other children. He remembered the pictograms and the interactions he had with the robot from 1 week to another. He also understood how to change the pictograms and frequently asked the educators to let him do it.

Another boy also enjoyed cradling Jumbo in his arms like a pet animal and showed improvements in shape and colour recognition.

Diskcat and a Dog

Due to the animal-like appearance of Diskcat (see Figure 8.7 and description in the previous section on Diskcat), we were interested in comparing the level of interaction, attention and interest towards the robot compared to that of a real living animal. In this trial, children entered the experimental room separately. The robot (Diskcat) and a dog were in the room. As mentioned before, it is important for the child to have a familiarisation period with the robot and this seemed equally important for the child to become comfortable with the dog. We found that interest in the dog and the robot varied among the children: some children were more interested in the robot, others in the dog. The children also seemed to be able recognise that the dog was alive and that the robot was not. There are many points of consideration when using animals with children of all abilities: the welfare of the animal must be taken into consideration and this was the case in this trial. The handler of the dog eventually believed that the animal was tired of interacting with children and so it was taken away. Also, the handler would need to intervene if the children did not interact with the dog in a kind or appropriate manner. This, of course, is not usually the case with robots. The only time that the supervisors of our robots needed to intervene was when there was a possibility of damaging the robot, which was something we anticipated and tried to avoid by making our robots as robust as possible. Also, we can replace robots so we do not need to be as attentive to their safety and can allow the interaction to be more free. In contrast, animals can also prove problematic because of allergies and injurious behaviours (e.g., bites or scratches).

Tito

Led by Duquette (2006, 2008), this work began in 2003 and investigated the use of a cartoon-like humanoid robot called Tito (see Figure 8.6l) with children diagnosed with autism. This was a longitudinal study conducted over several weeks by psycho-educators. The objective was to investigate the effects of a mobile robot on the imitation abilities of children diagnosed with autism. The hypothesis presented was that

> an animated object, more predictable and less complex than interacting with humans, can make the child with autism demonstrate reciprocal communication, observed by: 1) the reduction of avoidance mechanisms, namely repetitive and stereotyped play with inanimate objects; 2) an increase in shared focused attention and shared conventions; and 3) the appearance of symbolic mode of communication like verbal language. (Duquette et al. 2006)

The participants were four children who were diagnosed with low-functioning autism. Three of the children were aged 5 and one was aged 4. All the children showed very limited skills in language and symbolic or pretend play. They presented sensory interests similar to 8- to 9-month-old typically developing children.

However, their sensory play patterns showed signs of being more repetitive than typically developing children. The participating children also exhibited deficits in attention (e.g., avoiding eye contact, not responding to smiling), sharing and conventions for communicating common interests (e.g., poor imitation of facial expressions and gestures such as moving the head to say no or raising a hand to say goodbye).

In this work, the participants interacted either with (1) a robotic mobile mediator (Tito) or (2) a human mediator. The participants interacted with only one of the mediators and the sessions were conducted at separate times. During a session, one of the mediators (robot or human) executed a common set of imitation play patterns: (a) facial expressions (joy, sadness, angry), (b) body movements (raise the arms, dance, move forward or backward) and (c) actions with objects (point to the hat and request that it be given back, point at the door, point at the mediators picture) or actions without objects (wave hello or bye-bye, play peek-a-boo).

Each child participated in a total of 22 sessions with his or her paired mediator. This total was made up of three sessions per week over 7 weeks plus one familiarisation trial. There was a limit of two sessions per day, with 15 min of free play between consecutive sessions. Observational data from each of the sessions were analysed. Statistical analysis was organised into four categories, each with a different number of variables: shared focused attention (4 variables), shared conventions (4 variables), absence of sharing (7 variables) and other phenomenon (4 variables). The analysis resulted in the following summary findings: children exposed to the robotic mediator showed reduced repetitive play with inanimate objects of interest (their favourite toy), and no repetitive or stereotyped behaviour towards the robot. They also showed increased shared focused attention (visual contact, physical proximity). Imitation of the facial expression of joy (smiling) appeared more with children exposed to Tito than with children exposed to the human mediator.

ÉCOLE SAINT-MICHEL, QUÉBEC

In a recent study, two robots from the RoboToy Contest at the Université de Sherbrooke (Michaud and Clavet 2001), named Fishie (see Figure 8.5g) and Funny Face (see Figure 8.6j and Figure 8.12), were taken to a school in Québec City that had a large section devoted to autism. This study was in response to a request to bring some robots for interaction with children diagnosed with varying levels of autism. The team did not receive any other information and, as such, this was the first completely unstructured trial in which we had been involved. For example, the team had no control over which room was used, how the room was arranged, the choice of participants, how the trial was conducted or how many children would participate. We simply handed the two robots over to the care workers. It was indeed an interesting trial, as it provided a glimpse of how robots might ultimately be used in a real environment.

In total, six children participated. All were diagnosed with autism, and were non-verbal. The children had been prepared for the trial by previously being shown a picture of Fishie, as a representative robot. When it was their turn, they had to go and get the picture of Fishie and place it on their activity strip to show that it was time to do the 'robot activity.'

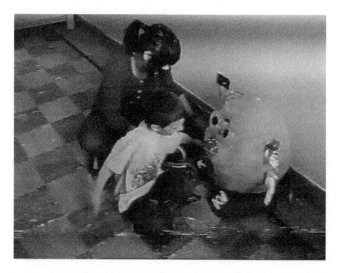

FIGURE 8.12   (See color insert following page 240.) A child diagnosed with ASD and a care worker interact with Funny Face.

One striking observation made by the experimenter in attendance was the need for easily adaptable robots. It is known that those diagnosed with autism can have difficulties with fine motor skills, for example, manipulating small objects. One of the robots (Funny Face) had a game that involved using motor skills (the placing of magnetic objects on the robot). The objects are quite large in size and appear easy to manipulate. The majority of the children found this task to be so difficult that they were unable to accomplish it. However, all of the children did repeatedly attempt to place the magnetic objects and so received practice in gross motor skills. The other robot (Fishie) played lively music when it was initially started. Most of the children did not seem to mind this. However, it seemed to overwhelm one child. The child showed clear signs of not liking the robot. The child seemed distressed and showed that he did not want to participate by continuously signing 'go' to the care worker present and so the trial was ended. Seven days later when it was time for this child's next session with the robots, he did not appear comfortable and so the care worker did not turn either of the robots on. The only robot that could be engaged without being powered on was Funny Face; the child could play by placing the objects on the robot without any power. Therefore, in this particular instance, Funny Face was the best robot for this particular child.

THE AURORA PROJECT

The University of Hertfordshire initiated the AuRoRA Project (AuRoRa Project 2008) in 1997. This program is investigating if and how robots can become a 'toy' that might serve an educational or therapeutic role for children with autism. The group's main aim is to engage children with autism in coordinated and synchronised interactions with the environment. It is hoped that if this can be achieved, it may then enable the children to develop and increase their communication and social interaction skills. This group has used a variety of robots, from mobile to humanoids.

Labo-1

In early work by the AuRoRA project, Werry et al. (2001) used a robot called Labo-1 (see Figure 8.5c) to study 'how mobile robots can be used to teach children with autism basic interaction skills that are important in social interactions among humans.' The robot had eight infrared sensors positioned around its body and one positional heat sensor mounted at the front. It could produce speech and say certain phrases such as 'I can't see you,' triggered by the robot's own state and the way children interacted with it. The primary action of the robot is to avoid obstacles, including people. It also follows heat sources and can generate simple speech and sounds. These behaviours allow the robot to follow children and to be chased by them.

A series of trials conducted by Werry took place in a room at the participants' school (Radlett Lodge School, Hertfordshire, United Kingdom). Six children (all males diagnosed with ASD) participated in the trials, in three pairs (see Figure 8.13). These children had been selected prior to the trial session by the teachers of the school. The children interacted with the robot in a room at the school. The trials lasted until either the teacher or one of the experimenters requested an end, due to the state of the robot or the emotional state of the children. On average, the trials lasted 9 min.

Results from this study are given in a narrative form, and show that, for one pair of children, the robot provided a focus of attention and an opportunity for shared attention. An example of this is given: 'an experimenter showed child "A" how to interact with the robot by demonstrating that it would back away from objects. Later in the session, child "A" then explicitly demonstrated this in order to instruct child "B", showing social interaction, social learning (possibly imitation) and demonstration of a new skill' (Werry et al. 2001). Also reported in this work is the ability of the

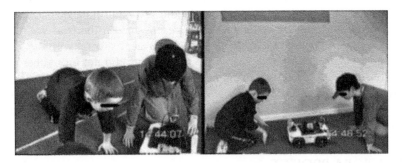

FIGURE 8.13 Children (in pairs) diagnosed with ASD interact with Labo-1 in a school environment. (Werry, I., K. Dautenhahn, W. Ogen, and B. Harwin. 2001b. Can social interaction skills be taught by a social agent? The role of a robotic mediator in autism therapy. In *Cognitive technology: instruments of mind (CT 2001)*, M. Beynon, C.L. Nehaniv, and K. Dautenhahn, 57–75. With kind permission of Springer Science+Business Media; Springer-Verlag Berlin Heidelberg.)

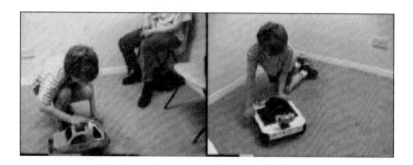

FIGURE 8.14   A child diagnosed with ASD interacts with a toy truck (left) and a robotic platform (right). (Dautenhahn, K. and I. Werry. 2002. A quantitative technique for analysing robot-human interactions. In IROS2002, *IEEE/RSJ International Conference on Intelligent Robots and Systems*, Lausanne, 1132–1138. IEEE Press © 2002 IEEE.)

robot to serve as a means for the children to communicate with the adults present. This observation provides a basis for the findings of Salter et al. (2007).

Another study conducted by Werry involved four children aged 7 to 11 years. All were male and had mid-to high-functioning autism. Again, the trials were conducted in a room at a school. This series of trials studied how children with autism interact with the mobile robot as opposed to a non-robotic toy (see Figure 8.14) (Werry et al. 2001; Dautenhahn and Werry 2002). Trials were split into three sections. Firstly, the child interacted with a toy truck that was similar in size to that of the robotic platform. Secondly, the child interacted with both the toy truck and the robot, although the robot was switched off and therefore passive. Thirdly, the child interacted with the robot in an 'active mode.' Results showed that children with autism are capable of distinguishing between animated and unanimated objects, expressing greater attention, laughter and vocal responses towards a robotised platform than to a toy truck of similar dimensions (Werry et al. 2001).

Videos of the trials were analysed by enumerating the frequency of the following behaviours: eye gaze, eye contact, operate, handling, touch, approach, move away, attention, vocalisation, speech, verbal stereotype, repetition and 'blank' (e.g., when the child is doing nothing).

Robota

In work that was originally separate from the AuRoRA project but later became integrated, Billard (2003) developed a robotic doll 'Robota' (see Figure 8.6n), which was eventually applied in autism therapy. Work with Robota conducted by Dautenhahn and Billard (2002) was based on the assumption that 'bodily interaction in imitative interaction games is normally an important factor in a child's development of social skills and that teaching of such skills (in a playful and exploratory context but nevertheless from an educational point of view focusing explicitly on specific types of interactions) could help children with autism in coping with the normal dynamics of social interactions' (Dautenhahn and Billard 2002 page 3).

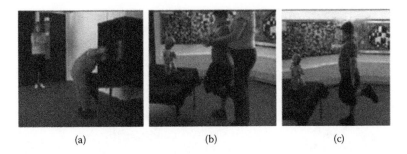

(a)   (b)   (c)

FIGURE 8.15   Pictures from the three different phases, namely, a, b and c, of the longitudi-nal study with Robota. (Robins, B., Dautenhahn, K., te Boekhorst, R., and Billard, A. (2004). Effects of repeated exposure of a humanoid robot on children with autism. In *Designing a More Inclusive World* (Cambridge Workshop on Universal Access and Assistive Technology), ed. S. Keates, J. Clarkson, P. Langdon, and P. Robinson, 225–236. Cambridge: Springer-Verlag, London.)

In work conducted by Robins, Robota has been used to look at 'effects of repeated exposure of a humanoid robot on children with autism' (Robins et al. 2004a). This was a longitudinal study with four children with autism (aged 5 to 10 years). The children were repeatedly exposed to Robota over a period of several months (an average of nine sessions per child). The aim was to encourage imitation and social interaction skills. The average duration of a trial was approximately 3 min. However, some lasted up to 5 min, a few were just less than 3 min, and two ended very shortly after the children left the room (approximately 40 to 60 sec).

The trials were conducted in three phases (see Figure 8.15). Firstly, in phase A, the robot was placed within a black box area. The robot operated in a pre-pro-grammed 'dance' mode. This session was meant to familiarise the child with the robot [similar to the familiarisation stage as suggested by Michaud (2003)]. There was minimal encouragement from the caregiver; the child was left to do as he or she chose. Secondly, in phase B, the box was removed, the robot was placed openly on the table. In this phase, there was active encouragement from the caregiver. The caregiver gave instructions about the robot and about imitating the robot. Here, the robot was used in 'puppet' mode (controlled by the experimenter). Lastly, in phase C, the children did not receive any instruction or encouragement to interact with the robot in 'puppet' mode, and were left to interact and play imitation games on their own initiative if they chose to do so.

Video tapes of the trials were analysed. The following four variables were inves-tigated: eye gaze, touch, imitation and near (i.e., when the child remained in close proximity to the robot). The results showed that interaction with the robot elicited imitative behaviour in children with autism. Also, there were occurrences where the children interacted with the robot and the investigator. It was suggested that the child was using the robot 'as a mediator, an object of shared attention, for their interaction with their teachers' (Robins et al. 2004a).

Another study conducted by Robins et al. (2004b, 2006) investigated whether the appearance of the robots matters to a child with autism. This study looked at how

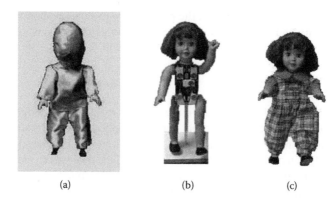

(a) (b) (c)

FIGURE 8.16 Robota shown in different physical manifestations: (a) Robota's appearance as a plain robotic device; (b) Robota shown with the inner robotic workings exposed, and (c) Robota's appearance as a typical doll. (Robins, B., K. Dautenhahn, R. te Boekhorst, and A. Billard. 2004b. Robots as assistive technology — does appearance matter? In *13th IEEE International Workshop on Robot and Human Interactive Communication* (RO-MAN 2004), Kurashiki, Okayama, Japan, 277–282. IEEE Press.)

willing children were to interact with Robota when it was dressed as a typical girl doll, as opposed to Robota being dressed in an outfit that was very plain. In addition, Robota had material placed over its head so that the head appeared featureless (see Figure 8.16).

The participants were four children with autism (aged 5 to 10 years) from the Enhanced Provision unit at a mainstream school. Each child participated in an average of 13 sessions with the robot. The trials lasted 3 min on average. They ended when the child wanted to leave the room. As with the study discussed previously, there were three phases. (1) The familiarisation phase — robot in 'dance' mode, moving its limbs and head to the rhythm of pre-recorded music. This phase was designed mainly for the children to familiarise themselves with the robot, and they were free to do whatever they chose. (2) The learning phase — the teacher showed the child how the robot could imitate his movements. The robot was operating in its 'puppet' mode (being controlled by the experimenter). It is suggested that this was unknown to the child. (3) Free interaction/imitation — the children were free to interact and play imitation games on their own initiative.

Again, video tapes of the trials were analysed and the same four variables were investigated: eye gaze, touch, imitation and near. The results from this study clearly indicated the children's preference for interaction with a plain, featureless robot over interaction with the more complex-featured girl-like robot. This would suggest that when designing robots for children with autism, we should keep features to a minimum.

Finally, another team has also conducted investigations with Robota. In work headed by Nadel et al. (2004) and Billard et al. (2007), Robota has been used in a longitudinal study investigating the use of machines to elicit imitation in children with autism. In this work, children played imitation games with Robota. The first phase consisted of an instructor sitting with a child while demonstrating the imitation game. The second phase consisted of the child positioned in front of Robota but without any instruction. Results from the preliminary evaluation show an 'increase in the interactivity and understanding of the imitation game, demonstrated through spontaneous imitation, in several children' (Billard et al. 2007).

Pekee

In this work, Salter used Pekee (see Figure 8.5h) to investigate whether the use of infrared sensors on-board a mobile robot could be applied beyond the simple task of navigation. Data coming from the infrared sensors were used to detect and record interactions between children and Pekee. The basis of the trial was to see if the robot could detect the type of child playing with it, for example, boisterous or shy, and in later work, to ultimately adapt the robot to this information. Salter conducted a study at a primary school in Hertfordshire, U.K., with nine boys participating in the trial (1 ASD, 8 typically developing). The presence of a child diagnosed with autism also meant that a comparison with typically developing children could be made. In total, five experiments were carried out for each child. They lasted for 5 min each and the robot performed slow obstacle avoidance regardless of the children's activities. Sensor data were recorded for the duration of the trial. It was stored on-board the robot and downloaded after each trial.

Among other statistical techniques, cluster analysis was used to analyse the robot's sensor data. This showed which sensors cluster together based on the activation data, that is, which sensors were activated together. The data showed that the child with autism did not activate the sensors in the same way as the typically developing children did (see Figure 8.17). It is possible to see that the child with autism seemingly would activate sensors 3 and 8 together, and also sensors 5 and 9 together. This shows that in this instance the child with autism did not play with robotic devices in

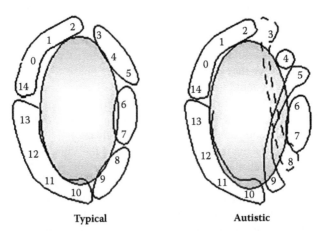

Typical   Autistic

FIGURE 8.17 Results of cluster analysis of sensor activations with only typically developing children (left) and including data from the child with autism (right). Numbers denote sensors around the robot, which is depicted as a shaded ellipse. (Salter, T. 2007. Sensor-based recognition of interaction patterns between children and mobile robots. Ph.D. Thesis, Computer Science Department, University of Hertfordshire, U.K.)

the same way as typically developing children did. Information like this could augment current diagnostic procedures, which only involve observations of the child. Such patterns of sensor activation could provide clinicians with objective, quantitative data, which may inform their decisions.

KASPAR

KASPAR has been used in work by the AuRoRA and IROMEC projects (see 'The AuRoRA Project'). In work conducted for the AuRoRA project, KASPAR was used in a series of trials that investigated whether KASPAR could assume the role of a social mediator — encouraging children with low functioning autism to interact with the robot, and to break their isolation and, importantly, to interact with other people (see Robins et al. 2009 and Figure 8.18). From this trial, Robins et al. (2009) presents a case study of three of the participants, each one at a different location. Two of the participants (two males, one aged 16 and one whose age was not stated) were at different schools in the U.K. These trials were conducted over a period of several months. The third participant in the case study (female, aged 6) was a one-off case held at a medical centre in Germany. It was noted that generally each of the participants showed deficits in interacting with both adults and children. The trials were held in a room familiar to the participants and were designed to allow the children to have unconstrained interaction with the robot, and to build a foundation for further possible interactions with other people using the robot as a mediator. The robot was operated remotely via a wireless remote control (a specially programmed keypad), either by the investigator or by the child (depending on the child's ability). The trials stopped when the child indicated that he or she wanted to leave the room or if he or she became bored. The majority of the interactions involved the participant

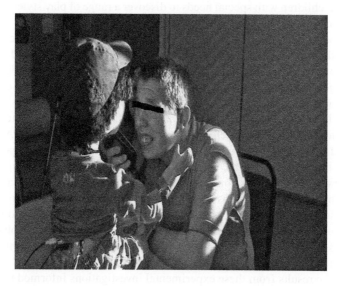

FIGURE 8.18 (See color insert following page 240.) A participant closely exploring the facial features of KASPAR. (Robins et al. 2009.)

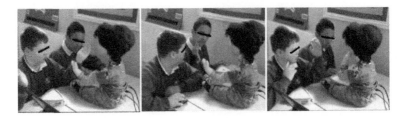

FIGURE 8.19 Two children with ASD interacting with KASPAR. One is imitating and the other is controlling the robot. (Robins, B., K. Dautenhahn, and P. Dickerson. 2009. From isolation to communication: a case study evaluation of robot assisted play for children with autism with a minimally expressive humanoid robot. In *The Second International Conferences on Advances in Computer-Human Interactions, ACHI* 09. 205–211. IEEE Press.)

interacting with the robot while the experimenter and a caregiver were present (also involved in the interaction). However, some of the interactions involved two children interacting with the robot.

Preliminary analysis of the study was conducted by using observational analysis, which applied, in abbreviated form, certain principles from conversation analysis. This preliminary analysis showed positive results for all of the children. Each of the participants appeared to show a level of direct, physical engagement with KASPAR and it also seems that they were able to generalize this behaviour to the adults who were present.

The IROMEC project investigates how robotic toys can become social mediators, encouraging children with special needs to discover a range of play styles, from solitary to collaborative play (with peers, caregivers/teachers, parents, etc.) (IROMEC 2009). Through their work, they aim 'to empower children with special needs to prevent dependency and isolation, helping them develop their potential and learn new skills' (Robins et al. 2008). In this series of trials, both KASPAR (see Figure 8.6o) and the Lego robot (see Figure 8.5f) were used with the primary goal of developing play scenarios (Robins et al. 2008).

In the trials involving KASPAR, two children with autism played a turn-taking and imitation game. The two children were seated in front of KASPAR (which was placed on a table). One child, rather than an adult caregiver/experimenter, controlled the robot, while the other child imitated the robot (see Figure 8.19). The authors tell us that 'this enabled the actors to play together an imitation game (mediated by the robot)' (Robins et al. 2008). In the trials with the Lego robot, the game consisted of turn-taking with a sensory reward. The child played the game with a supportive adult (see Figure 8.20). The authors state that 'the objective of the game is to engage the child in a collaborative turn-taking game with another person, whilst having enjoyment and sensory rewards (lights) as a result' (Robins et al. 2008). The results from these experimental investigations informed the process of developing novel robotic systems that consider specific needs of various target user groups.

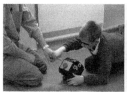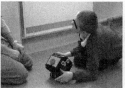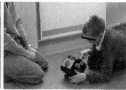

FIGURE 8.20 A child with ASD interacting with Lego robot and the experimenter. (Robins, B., K. Dautenhahn, and P. Dickerson. 2009. From isolation to communication: a case study evaluation of robot assisted play for children with autism with a minimally expressive humanoid robot. In *The Second International Conferences on Advances in Computer-Human Interactions, ACHI* 09. 205–211. IEEE Press.)

YALE UNIVERSITY

At Yale University, Scassellati (2005b,c) has been looking at how robots can help with the diagnosis of autism. In this work, Scassellati hopes to use social robotic devices to improve the diagnostic standards of autism by using robots to provide quantitative and objective measurements of social response.

Similar to the work conducted by Feil-Seifer (see section titled 'University of Southern California'), Scassellati has also looked at the effects of social contingency on children with autism. In this work, Scassellati used a commercially available robot called ESRA (see Figure 8.6k). The robot was able to display both contingent and non-contingent behaviours. In the non-contingent condition, the robot simply performed a short script, which involved a series of actions accompanied by an audio file. The robot did not respond to the actions of the child. In the contingent condition, the robot was used in a 'Wizard of Oz' (puppeteer) mode. The same repertoire of behaviours was used as in the non-contingent condition, but these behaviours were triggered by an experimenter sitting behind a one-way mirror. The experimenter triggered behaviours that seemed to be socially appropriate based on the actions of the child. The robot was able to generate a small set of facial expressions using five servos. The participants were 13 children (mean age 3.4 years, 7 ASD, 6 typically developing). Analysis of the trial revealed that the typically developing children lost interest quickly in the non-contingent condition, while the children with autism did not differ significantly in their interactions between the two experimental conditions. Scassellati found that the children with autism showed positive protosocial behaviours (e.g., touching, vocalising and smiling at the robot), which they did not generally show in a typical day.

In other work, Scassellati is looking at how to diagnose autism, with the conviction that diagnosis may be enhanced 'by the introduction of quantitative, objective measurements of social response' (Scassellati 2005a). This would take on the form of information being gathered from two sources: passive observation of the child and structured interaction with a robot. The passive source would involve recording and interpreting data from cameras, microphones and software, while the subjects are engaged in standard clinical evaluations. Three ways of detecting this passive information have been developed: (1) detecting gaze direction, (2) tracking the position of individuals as they move throughout a room and (3) measuring aspects of prosody from human voices. Scassellati (2005a) states that 'while there is a vast array of information that can be obtained by passive sensing technologies, the use of interactive robots provides unique opportunities for examining social responses in a level of detail that has not previously been available.' The author says that these advantages include (1) being able to selectively probe a social behaviour, (2) providing a robotic system that is a repeatable, standardised stimulus and recording methodology, and (3) data collection outside of the clinic, effectively increasing both the quantity and quality of data that a clinician can obtain without extensive field work. This will provide a system that is free from subjective bias, resulting in a useful tool for evaluating the success of therapeutic programs. The robotic system may also provide a standard for reporting social abilities within the autism literature.

In a reversal of events, autism has even been the inspiration for the design of a robot. In Scassellati (2002), the objective was to give robots a 'theory of mind,' an area in which people with autism are known to have deficits.

UNIVERSITY OF SOUTHERN CALIFORNIA

At the University of Southern California (USC), Feil-Seifer and Mataric (2008a,b, 2009) are developing socially assistive robot (SAR) systems for use as an intervention method with children who have been diagnosed with ASD. They hope that their system will take on the form of a humanoid social partner. The robot is intended to be a catalyst for social interaction, including human-robot interaction and human-human interaction. The latter is intended to aid those with ASD in human-human socialisation. They have added the SAR architecture to two robots: one is a mobile robot that blows bubbles (see Figure 8.5d), and the other is a humanoid robot that has a bubble blower (see Figure 8.21). Their motivation for using bubbles is that 'bubble blowing games are a standard part of ASD diagnosis since bubbles are an effective method of provoking social behaviour such as joint attention and pointing' (Feil-Seifer and Mataric 2008b). Such a feature has also been used in a RoboToy robot (Michaud and Clavet 2001; Michaud et al. 2000).

Initially, Feil-Seifer and Mataric conducted a pilot study with the mobile base robot (see Figure 8.5d). The participants were five children (4 ASD, 1 typically developing) ranging in age from 20 months to 12 years old. The objectives of this initial study were to verify that the robotic architecture worked correctly and to test that the behaviour of the robots actually affected the behaviour of the children. To test the latter, they developed two robotic conditions: contingent and random. The difference between the two conditions was whether the bubble blowing was driven by the child. In the contingent condition, the child must push large buttons mounted on the robot for the bubbles to appear. In the random condition, regardless of whether the buttons are pushed, bubbles automatically appear after a random amount of time.

The trials were analysed by coding the following variables: speech/vocalisations, gestures (pointing, waving, etc.), movement towards/away from/in front of person/ robot, ASD-stereotypical behaviour (hand flapping, etc.), joint attention/eye contact with parent/robot and actions to control robot (button pushes, moving to make the

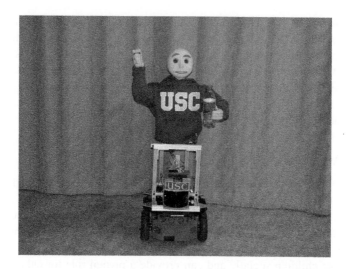

FIGURE 8.21 The robot 'Bandit' being used by Feil-Seifer with children diagnosed with ASD (Reprinted with permission from Feil-Seifer, D.J. and M. Mataric. 2008b. Robot assisted therapy for children with autism spectrum disorders. In *Proceedings of the Interaction Design for Children: Children with Special Needs*, Chicago, IL, USA, 49–52.)

robot move). The analysis revealed that the social interactions of the children were greater when the robot displayed a contingent behaviour, compared to when the robot displayed the random behaviour. Overall, findings showed that the behaviour of the robot does affect the social behaviour of the children (both human-human interaction and human-robot interaction). In particular, going from the random to contingent behaviour condition, the following specific changes were found: total speech increased from 39.4 to 48.4 utterances, speech towards the robot increased from 6.2 to 6.6 utterances, and speech towards parents increased from 17.8 to 33 utterances. Total robot interactions went from 43.42 to 55.31, with button pushes increasing from 14.69 to 21.87 and other robot interactions going from 24.11 to 28. Total directed interactions (interactions that clearly were directed at either the robot or the parent) went up from 62.75 to 89.47. They found that, generally, when the robot was acting contingently, the child was more sociable.

The on-going work of the USC group expands on this set of experiments to use a more sophisticated robot (see Figure 8.21) along with the bubble-blowing functionality (Feil-Seifer et al. 2009).

UNIVERSITY OF WASHINGTON

In work led by Peter Kahn, Stanton et al. (2008) used a robot called AIBO that looks like an animal, that is, a dog (see Figure 8.5i), to investigate possible social development benefits to children with autism. The inspiration behind this approach came from the fact that literature suggests that animals may be effective in increasing social interaction and communication in those who have autism. The participants were 11 children diagnosed with autism (ages 5 to 8 years). All had some verbal ability. The participants interacted with two toy dogs: the robotic AIBO and a simple mechanical (non-robotic) dog called Kasha. AIBO had the ability to respond to actions from the children, but Kasha had no ability to detect or respond. The children spoke more words when they were with AIBO as opposed to Kasha, and more often engaged in verbal, reciprocal and authentic interaction. Also, the authors found that the children interacted more with AIBO and exhibited fewer autistic behaviours. This result echoes the findings of Michaud and Theberge-Turmel (2002).

THE INFANOID PROJECT

Research by Kozima and others in Japan led to a child-like humanoid named 'Infanoid' (see Figure 8.6m), and a small creature-like robot, 'Keepon' (see Figure 8.5e), with which they have investigated human social development, especially 'interpersonal communication.' They have also deployed these robots in autism therapy (Kozima et al. 2004, 2005b, 2006). This work suggests that robotic devices have the potential to engage children socially and can provide a pivotal role for enhancing communication between children and adults. Similar to work done at the Université de Sherbrooke (see 'Université de Sherbrooke'), Kozima often reports his findings in a narrative manner.

In the work with Infanoid and children who have autism, Kozima et al. (2004) observed that contingency games could benefit children in learning communication skills. In what is the longest study investigating the role of robotic devices in the domain of autism, Keepon was used at a day-care centre for children with autism, PDD, Asperger's syndrome, Down's syndrome, and other developmental disorders. This study lasted more than 2 years and contained over 80 sessions (Kozima and Nakagawa 2006). Most of the children at the day-care centre were aged between 2 and 4 years. The children interacted with Keepon in both a relaxed, unconstrained manner and also in organised group activities. Keepon was placed on the floor as just another toy (see Figure 8.22), and its behaviour was controlled by a human.

From this work, Kozima reported that

> the children showed various actions in relation to Keepon. Sometimes they showed vivid facial expressions that even their parents had not seen before. Some of the children extended their dyadic interaction with Keepon into triadic inter-personal interaction, where they tried to share with others the pleasure and surprise they found in Keepon. Each child showed a different style of interaction that changed over time. (Kozima et al. 2005).

UNIVERSITY OF PISA

In recent work, a team based in Pisa, Italy, lead by Pioggia et al. (2007, 2008), have been investigating the use of an anthropomorphic humanoid (named FACE) to 'define and test a therapeutic protocol for autism in order to enhance social and emotive abilities in people with autism' (Pioggia et al. 2007). Due to the flexible artificial muscular architecture, FACE has the ability to express six basic emotions (happiness, sadness, surprise, anger, disgust and fear).

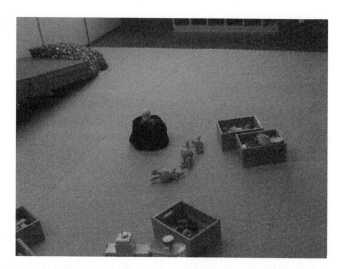

FIGURE 8.22 Keepon placed on the floor next to other toys. (Kozima, H., C. Nakagawa, N. Kawai, D. Kosugi, and Y. Yano. 2004. A humanoid robot in company with children. In *IEEE-RAS/RSJ International Conference on Humanoid Robotics*, Santa Monica, CA., USA. IEEE Press.)

The role of FACE is to engage the participant in simple social interactions (see Figure 8.23). This is achieved by exchanging emotions between the android and the participant. FACE is able to engage in social interaction by modifying its behaviour in response to the participant's behaviour. The participant wears what the team considers an unobtrusive sensitised wearable interface (life-shirt) throughout the

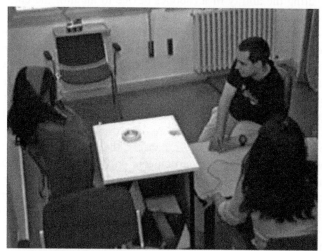

FIGURE 8.23 University of Pisa experiment showing FACE (left), participant (top right) and therapist (lower right). (Reprinted with permission from Pioggia, G., R. Igliozzi, M.L. Sica, M. Ferro, F. Muratori, A. Ahluwalia, and D. De Rossi. 2008. Exploring emotional and imitational android-based interactions in autistic spectrum disorders. *Journal of CyberTherapy & Rehabilitation* 1(1):49–61.)

interaction. This allows for physiological and behavioural information to be acquired in real time. Pioggia et al. have taken the application of robotic devices in autism one step closer to clinical practice; they have introduced a complete framework of what they term the 'FACE-T system' (the T stands for therapy). This complete framework consists of the android FACE, the sensitised life-shirt, a therapeutic protocol between a participant and a trained therapist, and a specially equipped room.

Trials were carried out with four participants diagnosed with ASD (three male and one female) between 7 and 20 years old. The sessions lasted for 20 min. The group looked at the following variables: relating to people, emotional response, imitation, listening response, fear or nervousness, verbal communication, non-verbal communication and activity level. The sessions were scored in terms of these variables using the CARS scale (Childhood Autism Rating Scale). The team conducting the study observed that for two participants, the CARS score decreased or remained the same for all variables after the therapy session. Only one participant (the oldest, with lowest IQ and highest ADOS rating) showed an increase of 0.5 points for listening, fear and verbal communication. Also, the team noted that 'more importantly, all the subjects demonstrated a decrease in the score of emotional response in the CARS scale of between 1 and 0.5 points, and imitation in 3 out of 4 children, so implying a marked improvement in these areas after interacting with FACE' (Pioggia et al. 2007).

VANDERBILT UNIVERSITY

In this work led by Nilanjan Sarkar (Conn et al. 2008b; Liu et al. 2008), a team has been investigating the ability of a robotics device to monitor the emotional state of children who have ASD. They are developing affective models based on physiological data because children with ASD often have communicative impairments (both non-verbal and verbal), particularly regarding expression of affective states (Conn et al. 2008a). They believe that physiological markers will allow the robot to respond automatically to the child's emotional state. Similar to the work by Pioggia (see section titled 'University of Pisa'), the children in this study must have physiological sensors attached to them. In their first set of experiments, they tested six children (aged 13 to 16 years) who were diagnosed with ASD. They developed a two-phase approach to the testing. In Phase 1, they produced affective models. They achieved this by testing the participants on two computer-based cognitive tasks: an anagram-solving task and a Pong-playing task. These tests were designed to evoke varying intensities of the following three affective states: anxiety, engagement and liking. In Phase 2, the participants played a variant of Nerf basketball with the hoop and backboard attached to the end of a robotic arm that moved backward/forward and up/down (see Figure 8.5a). The robotic device used the physiological models developed in Phase 1 to learn about the participants' emotional state and then to select appropriate behaviours. Results showed that the robot could accurately predict the participants' emotional state 80% of the time, and that using this information to alter the robot's behaviour significantly increased the children's degree of engagement.

CHALLENGES FACING THE USE OF ROBOTIC DEVICES

Although the previous sections have presented promising diagnostic and therapeutic applications, robotic devices are still in their infancy and require time to mature. There are many complications when using robotic devices in the real world with any end user, and these can be further complicated when the end user has developmental disorders such as ASD. This section presents the specific challenges encountered in the development and deployment of robotic devices for this unique end user.

UNEXPECTED INTERACTION, ROBUSTNESS, DURATION AND SAFETY

All types of children can be rough in their play styles, and of course those with ASD are no exception. Robots that are meant for interaction with children must be much more robust than robots that are designed to interact with adults. When developing robots, we must plan for the unexpected and we must assume that children will surpass the boundaries of interaction for which the robot was designed. Expecting the unexpected enables designers to plan for interaction that could be destructive or dangerous. Michaud and Theberge-Turmel (2002) tell us about a robot with which they were conducting a study: 'the pyroelectric lenses got damaged by the children, and one even took off the plastic cup covering one eye of the robot and tried to eat it.' Another factor is the duration over which the robot must be able to correctly function. The robot should always be able to function over a period of weeks and always perform in the same way, for example, battery power, general motion. Safety is paramount, particularly when conducting investigations with children. Restrictions must be placed on the design of any hardware to avoid sharp edges and exposed wires.

ACCESS TO AND GENERALISATION FROM A TEST POPULATION

Aside from issues with developing the robot, the next problem researchers typically face is access to the test population. This can be due to many reasons. As described in section Restricted and Repetitive Behaviours, those with autism can find it difficult to accept a change in routine, such as that introduced by playing with a robotic device. Not only is the robot new to the participants, but interacting with it will change the normal routine of the day. There is the possibility for such things to be disturbing to a child with ASD. Also, it can be difficult to find enough participants with ASD to allow for data analysis that will show any sort of statistical significance. Even if a small group of participants can be recruited, the heterogeneity of participant abilities may preclude generalisation of the findings from the study. Therefore, it is common for researchers not to use a control group when studying the interaction between robotic devices and children with ASD. Some researchers will use a control object, such as the work by Werry et al. (2001a,b) comparing a mobile robotic platform with a toy truck of similar dimensions. Work by Stanton et al. (2008) compared a robotic dog with a mechanical dog, and work by Duquette et al. (2006) compared a robotic mediator with a human mediator. 'It is very hard to generalize the results of these tests since each child is so different' (Michaud and Theberge-Turmel 2002). Stanton et al. (2008) also discuss this point:

Given this state of affairs, it is then reasoned that generalizable findings of children with autism interacting with robots should not be expected. Rather, investigations with this population of children should be understood more as case studies. It takes something of the form: "Here, let me show you what worked with at least a few of the children in my study." Then you try it, and maybe you'll find that it will work with some other children with autism. Over time, we'll hope to build up a repertoire of techniques, but we shouldn't be expecting any technique to work for this population as a whole.

TREADING A CAUTIOUS PATH

By developing robots for interaction with those who have autism, we hope to benefit the participants in some way. Potential benefits may include language improvement/development, a better understanding of emotions, opening up to their surroundings, performing imitation, etc. However, in the pursuit of our goals, we must tread a cautious path: we must make sure that our devices do not encourage isolation from the real world. When talking about computers, Moor (2008) says that it can be a

> hugely supportive piece of home technology that can assist us on our journey to find ways for our children to play, learn and engage. Just like the TV it can also be a source of solitary unsociable entertainment that drains the time a child has to learn by engaging, watching and interacting with others — we have to be smart in how we use this technology.

With regard to the use of robotic devices, Robins et al. (2009) also give us a 'cautionary tale':

> This paper exemplifies interaction where social behaviour was directed at the robot which raises awareness of the goal of the research, namely to help the children to increase their social interaction skills with other people and not simply create relationships with a social robot which would isolate the children from other humans even further.

Another factor that should be carefully considered is that some (but not all) of a robot's behaviour can be repetitive. This can be a quality that is both sought after as well as one that ought to be avoided. Some believe that having a repetitive behaviour will provide comfort for the children. For example, Robins et al. (2005) state that, 'We wanted to provide a reassuring environment where the repetitive and predictable behaviour of the robot is a comforting factor.' Yet others believe that we should discourage repetitive behaviours in robots. Dautenhahn et al. (2003) tell us, 'Note, that the robot's behaviours are simple, but not completely predictable. This issue is important since using robots in autism therapy should not perpetuate existing repetitive tendencies.' Michaud and Theberge-Turmel (2002) also talk about the benefit of developing robotic behaviours that begin in a predictable manner and then progress to become unpredictable in gradual steps.

ADAPTABILITY OF FUNCTIONALITY

As with all objects designed for interaction with children, they must be appealing to the child. Often colours, sounds and lights are used to gain the attention of the children. However, when considering interaction with children with autism, it is vitally important that these functions be adaptable, such as having adjustable sound levels and switchable or dimmable lights. The motion of the robot should also be controllable; the speed of a mobile robot or the movement of appendages such as arms ought to be configurable. As children with autism are so individual, the robot must be able to adapt to their preferences in a quick and easy manner.

Uncomplicated, Inexpensive and Flexible

If robots are to be useful for experimentation with children who have autism, they must be able to function correctly in natural human environments (wherever the child is). The robot should not require special markers in the room such as paint on the walls to recognise objects. Also, it must be operable by technically untrained people, for example, caregivers or teachers. The complexity of the robot must be kept to a minimum to enable a range of operators as diverse as possible. Another factor that must be considered is cost. The lower the cost, the more accessible the robot will be.

How to Conduct Trials

There are many different ways to conduct an investigation on the benefits of robotic devices with children who have autism. However, there are some factors that are unique to human-robot interaction.

Should the robot be controlled? A robot can be teleoperated or autonomous, or a combination of the two. If using a teleoperated method, there are two strategies that can be applied: Wizard of Oz or remote-controlled. Wizard of Oz refers to a technique that can be used whereby the participant believes he or she is interacting with an autonomous robot, but in fact the robot is being controlled by an experimenter (the wizard) who is hidden from view. The name comes from the story *The Wonderful Wizard of Oz* whereby a man hides himself behind a curtain and uses technology to talk to people by pretending to be a wizard. In contrast, the remote-controlled strategy involves the robot being controlled by a human clearly visible to the participant. An autonomous robotic device uses sensor technology to sense certain factors and uses this information to control the robot's own behaviour. For example, the robot senses obstacles in the environment and changes its own direction to avoid them. There is also the possibility of combining teleoperated and autonomous modes as necessary for the type of experiment being conducted. Currently, in this field, most researchers use either the Wizard of Oz mode or remote-controlled mode to control the robot (see Robins et al. 2004a, 2006, 2008; Kozima et al. 2004, 2005); Scassellati 2005c; Duquette et al. 2006). However, some researchers have used autonomous robots (see Salter 2006; Werry et al. 2001; Michaud and Theberge-Turmel 2002). There are many reasons for and against the different styles of control. Using a robot in Wizard of Oz or remote-controlled mode means that many risks can be mitigated by the human operator, therefore making the trial run smoother for the participant. Duquette et al. (2006) tell us that 'designing a mobile robot that can implement such scenarios is a challenge, even if teleoperation is used to conduct the navigation and respond to the child's interaction.' Using a robot in an autonomous mode means that you are truly seeing the effects a robotic device can have on children with autism, and often this can bring about unexpected interactions that probably would not have happened had a human controlled the robot (see section Diskcat).

Feedback to the robot. If the robotic system requires feedback to function, how is this to be achieved? Feedback is to be more likely necessary if the robot has some form of autonomy. Scassellati (2005a) tells us that

> For several years, we have used commercial eye-tracking systems which require subjects to wear a baseball cap with an inertial tracking system and camera/eyepiece assembly which allows us to record close-up images of one eye. In addition to this commercial system, we have developed computational systems that give much less accurate recordings but do not require the subject to be instrumented.

In other work by Pioggia et al. (2007), the participants in the study must wear what the group calls an unobtrusive sensorized wearable interface. This allows the real-time acquisition of both physiological and behavioural information. In work conducted by Conn et al. (2008b), participants must wear a commercially available biofeedback sensor system to acquire their physiological data (www.biopac.com). However, it is not always necessary for the participants to have sensors attached to them or to wear some sort of device. If the robot is used in a Wizard of Oz or remote-controlled mode, it is typically the person controlling the robot who gives the necessary feedback. In work conducted by Salter (2006), information about the interaction was obtained from the children touching the robot and the on-board sensors recording the information. In this case, information was obtained while the robot was autonomous and without the need for the participant to remain stationary or have sensors placed on them.

Quantitative versus qualitative evaluations. We recognise and appreciate that there are many benefits when applying both quantitative and qualitative evaluation methods to human-robot interaction studies. However, in our research with robots and children with autism (without discounting quantitative methods), we are increasingly finding it beneficial to use qualitative evaluations of the observed interactions. This is for several reasons, including that we are progressively conducting trials in less controlled conditions and now carry out many of our trials 'in the wild' (i.e., in natural settings) (Salter et al. 2008). Also, the use of autonomous rather than remote-controlled robots can make the trials more unpredictable and therefore harder to precisely replicate. In essence, each trial becomes unique. Another reason for qualitative evaluation is the uniqueness of each child with autism. This uniqueness calls for methods that do not simply enumerate predefined quantifiable cues, but that look at the trial as a whole. Interaction with an embodied, moving robot is a dynamic process. It is important to capture the essence of this interaction and to report observations in a form that is abstract and conveys the most information from the trial.

CONCLUSION

This chapter described the use of robotic devices within the realm of autism research, therapy and education. The research presented herein illustrates the potential of robots in paediatric rehabilitation, from helping those with autism open up to their surroundings, to facilitating the acquisition of social skills, from complementing the current diagnostic tools for autism, to encouraging those with autism to communicate with others around them, and to help children with autism engage in play.

Research in this area is continually growing, with the availability of more robots and new technology, such as sound localisation, tracking and separation (Valin et al. 2007a,b), and torque-controlled actuators that provide safe robot manipulators (Fauteux et al. 2009; Legault et al. 2008). It is hoped that these new technologies will bring about new, natural and interesting ways to interact with robots. We hope that this chapter has provided the reader with insight into an area of robotics research that we believe will eventually evolve into an assistive technology for children and youth in the autism spectrum.

REFERENCES

AuRoRa Project 2009. The AuRoRa Project. A. http://www.aurora-project.com (accessed December 8, 2008).

Autism Society of America 2010. http://www.autism-society.org/ (accessed February 8, 2010).

Barclay, P., R. Barnitt, H. Brand, A. Brown, K. Connolly, N. Finnie, M. Gilberston, A. Harrison, G. Higgon, K. Holt, M. Horton, S. Levitt, M. MacCulloch, J. McGuiness, P. Rosebaum, L. Rosenbloom, D. Shaffer, V. Sherborne, and B. Wyke 1975. *Movement and child development.* London: Spastics International Medical Publications.

Baron-Cohen, S. 1995. *Mindblindness: An essay on autism and theory of mind.* Cambridge, MA: MIT Press.

Baron-Cohen, S., S. Wheelwright, A. Cox, G. Baird, T. Charman, J. Swettenham, A. Drew, and P. Doehring. 2000. The early identification of autism: The checklist for autism in toddlers (chat). *Journal of the Royal Society of Medicine* 93:521–525.

Bartneck, C. and J. Hu. 2004. Rapid prototyping for interactive robots. In *The 8th Conference on Intelligent Autonomous Systems (IAS-8),* Amsterdam, the Netherlands: IOS Press, 136–145.

Billard, A. (2003). Robota: Clever toy and educational tool. *Robotics and Autonomous Systems* 42, 259–269.

Billard, A., B. Robins, K. Dautenhahn, and J. Nadel. 2007. Building Robota, a mini-humanoid robot for the rehabilitation of children with autism. *Assistive Technology Journal* 19(1):37–49.

Black, R. 2009. World Autism Day raises awareness, but what causes the disorder still eludes researchers. http://www.nydailynews.com/lifestyle/health/2009/04/02/2009-04-02_ world_autism_day_raises_awareness_but_wh.html (accessed April 2, 2009).

Centers for Disease Control and Prevention 2010a. Counting Autism. http://www.cdc.gov/ ncbddd/features/counting-autism.html (accessed January 31, 2010).

Centers for Disease Control and Prevention 2010b. Child Development. http://www.cdc.gov/ ncbddd/child/infants.htm (accessed February 9, 2010).

Centers for Disease Control and Prevention 2010c. Child Development. http://www.cdc.gov/ ncbddd/child/toddlers1.htm (accessed February 9, 2010).

Children's Hospital of Pittsburgh 2009. Stages of Play. http://www.chp.edu/CHP/P02266 (accessed 16 June 2009).

Colby, K.M. 1973. The rationale for computer-based treatment of language difficulties in nonspeaking autistic children. *Journal of Autism and Developmental Disorders* 3(3):254–260.

Conn, K., C. Liu, N. Sarkar, W. Stone, and Z. Warren. 2008a. Affect-sensitive assistive intervention technologies for children with autism: An individual-specific approach. In *17th IEEE International Symposium on Robot and Human Interactive Communication (RO-MAN 2008)*, Munich, Germany: IEEE Press, 442–447.

Conn, K., C. Liu, N. Sarkar, W. Stone, and Z. Warren. 2008b. Towards affect-sensitive assistive intervention technologies for children with autism. In *Affective computing: Focus on emotion expression, synthesis and recognition*, J. Or, Ed. Vienna, Austria: ARS/I-Tech Education and Publishing, 365–390.

Cook, A.M., M.Q. Meng, J. Gu, and K. Howery. 2002. Development of a robotic device for facilitating learning by children who have severe disabilities. *IEEE Transactions on Neural Systems and Rehabilitation Engineering* 10(3):178–187.

Dautenhahn, K. and A. Billard. 2002. Games children with autism can play with Robota, a humanoid robotic doll. In *Designing a more inclusive world*, S. Keates, P. Langdon, P.J. Clarkson, and P. Robinson, Eds. Cambridge: Springer-Verlag (London), 179–190.

Dautenhahn, K. and I. Werry. 2002. A quantitative technique for analysing robot-human interactions. In *IROS2002, IEEE/RSJ International Conference on Intelligent Robots and Systems*, Lausanne: IEEE Press, 1132–1138.

Dautenhahn, K. and I. Werry. 2004. Towards interactive robots in autism therapy: Background, motivation and challenges. *Pragmatics and Cognition* 12(1):1–35.

Dautenhahn, K., I. Werry, T. Salter, and T. te Boekhorst. 2003. Towards adaptive autonomous robots in autism therapy: Varieties of interactions. In *IEEE International Symposium on Computational Intelligence in Robotics and Automation*, Kobe, Japan, 577–582. IEEE Press.

École du Touret 2009. http://ecoles-csrs.recit05.qc.ca/fr/page.php?site=st-laurentd (accessed June 16, 2009).

Dixon, E. 2009. Importance of play in child development. http://www.child-development-guide.com/importance-of-play.html (accessed June 16, 2009).

Duquette, A., H. Mercier, and F. Michaud. 2006. Investigating the use of a mobile robotic toy as an imitation agent for children with autism. In *International Conference on Epigenetic Robotics*, Paris, France, 167–168. Morgan Kaufman Publishers.

Duquette, A., F. Michaud, and H. Mercier. 2008. Exploring the use of a mobile robot as an imitation agent with children with low-functioning autism. *Autonomous Robots* 24(2):147–157.

Fauteux, P., M. Lauria, M.A. Legault, B. Heintz, and F. Michaud. 2009. Dual differential rheologic actuator for robotic interaction tasks. In *IEEE International Conference on Advanced Intelligent Mechatronics*. IEEE Press.

Feil-Seifer, D.J., M.P. Black, M.J. Mataric, and S. Narayanan. 2009. Toward designing interactive technologies for supporting research in autism spectrum disorders. Poster presented at the *International Meeting for Autism Research*, Chicago, IL.

Feil-Seifer, D.J. and M. Mataric. 2008a. B³IA: A control architecture for autonomous robot-assisted behavior intervention for children with autism spectrum disorders. In *17th IEEE International Symposium on Robot and Human Interactive Communication*, Ro-Man 2008, University Munchen, Munich, Germany, 701–706. IEEE Press.

Feil-Seifer, D.J. and M. Mataric. 2008b. Robot assisted therapy for children with autism spectrum disorders. In *Proceedings of the Interaction Design for Children: Children with Special Needs*, Chicago, IL, 49–52.

Feil-Seifer, D.J. and M. Mataric. 2009. Towards the integration of socially assistive robots into the lives of children with ASD. Paper presented at Human-Robot Interaction Workshop on Societal Impact: How Socially Accepted Robots Can Be Integrated in our Society, San Diego, CA.

Ferrara, C. and S.D. Hill. 1980. The responsiveness of autistic children to the predictability of social and nonsocial toys. *Journal of Autism and Developmental Disorders* 10(1):51–57.

Gabriels, R.L. and D.E. Hill. 2007. *Growing up with autism.* New York: Guilford Press.

Gammeltoft, L. and M.S. Nordenhof 2007. *Autism, play and social interaction.* London: Jessica Kingsley Publishers.

Gotham, K., S. Risi, G. Dawson, H. Tager-Flusberg, R. Joseph, A. Carter, S. Hepburn, W. McMahon, P. Rodier, S.L. Hyman, M. Sigman, S. Rogers, R. Landa, M.A. Spence, K. Osann, P. Flodman, F. Volkmar, E. Hollander, J. Buxbaum, A. Pickles, and C. Lord. 2008. A replication of the Autism Observation Schedule (ADOS) revised algorithms. *Journal of the American Academy of Child and Adolescence Psychiatry* 47(6):642–651.

Hyne, S. 2003. Play as a vehicle for learning in the foundation stage. Presented at *British Educational Research Association Annual Student Conference*, Edinburgh.

IntRoLab 2009. Intelligent, interactive, integrated interdisciplinary robot lab. http://introlab. gel.usherbrooke.ca/mediawiki-introlab/index.php/Main Page (accessed June 16, 2009).

IROMEC 2009. Interactive robotic social mediators as companions. http://www.iromec.org/ (accessed June 16, 09).

Kozima, H. and C. Nakagawa. 2006. Social robots for children: Practice in communication-care. In *IEEE International Workshop on Advanced Motion Control,* 768–773. IEEE Press.

Kozima, H., C. Nakagawa, N. Kawai, D. Kosugi, and Y. Yano. 2004. A humanoid robot in company with children. In *IEEE-RAS/RSJ International Conference on Humanoid Robotics*, Santa Monica, CA. IEEE Press.

Kozima, H., C. Nakagawa, and Y. Yasuda. 2005. Interactive robots for communication-care: A case-study in autism therapy. In *IEEE Conference on Robot and Human Interactive Communication* (RO-MAN 2005), Nashville, TN, 341–346. IEEE Press.

Kozima, H., C. Nakagawa, and Y. Yasuda. 2006. Wowing together: What facilitates social interactions in children with autistic spectrum disorders. In *International Workshop on Epigenetic Robotics (EpiRob-2006)*, Paris, France, 177.

Legault, M.A., M.A. Lavoie, F. Cabana, P. Jacob-Goudreau, D. Létourneau, F. Michaud, and M. Lauria. 2008. Admittance control of a human centered 3 DOF robotic arm using differential elastic actuators. In *Proceedings of IEEE/RSJ International Conference on Intelligent Robots and Systems,* 4134–4144. IEEE Press.

Liu, C., K. Conn, N. Sarkar, and W. Stone. 2008. Online affect detection and robot behavior adaptation for intervention of children with autism. *IEEE Transactions on Robotics* 24(4):883–896.

Lord, C., M. Rutter, S. Goode, J. Heemsbergen, H. Jordan, L. Mawhood, and E. Schopler. 1989. Autism diagnostic observation schedule: A standardised observation of communicative and social behavior. *Journal of Autism and Developmental Disorders,* 19(2):185–212.

Mari, M., U. Castiello, D. Marks, C. Marraffa, and M. Prior. 2003. The reach-to-grasp movement in children with autism spectrum disorder. *Philosophical Transactions of the Royal Society of London* 358(1430):393–403.

McConkey, R. and M. Jeffree. 1981. *Let's make toys human.* London: Condor Book Souvenir Press (E&A) Ltd.

Michaud, F. and S. Caron. 2000. An autonomous toy-rolling robot. In *PRECARN-IRIS International Symposium on Robotics (ISR)*, Montréal, Québec, 114–119.

Michaud, F. and S. Caron. 2002. Roball, the rolling robot. *Autonomous Robots* 12(2):211–222.

Michaud, F. and A. Clavet. 2001. Robotoy contest — designing mobile robotic toys for autistic children. In *AAAI Spring Symposium on Robotics and Education* Working Notes.

Michaud, F., A. Duquette, and I. Nadeau. 2003. Characteristics of mobile robotic toys for children with pervasive developmental disorders. In *IEEE Conference on Systems, Man, and Cybernetics*, 2938–2943. IEEE Press.

Michaud, F., J.F. Laplante, H. Larouche, A. Duquette, S. Caron, D. Létourneau, and P. Masson. 2005. Autonomous spherical mobile robot for child-development studies. *IEEE Transactions on Systems, Man, and Cybernetics* 35:471–480.

Michaud, F., P. Lepage, J.D. Leroux, M. Clarke, Y. Bélanger, F. Brosseau, and D. Neveu. 2000. Mobile robotic toys for autistic children. In *PRECARN-IRIS International Symposium on Robotics (ISR)*, Montréal, Québec, 180–181.

Michaud, F., T. Salter, A. Duquette, and J.F. Laplante. 2006. Perspectives on mobile robots used as tools for child development and pediatric rehabilitation. *Assistive Technology* 19(1):21–36.

Michaud, F. and C. Theberge-Turmel. 2002. Mobile robotic toys and autism. In *Socially intelligent agents — creating relationships with computers and robots*, K. Dautenhahn, A. Bond, L. Cañamero, and B. Edmonds, Eds. Norwell, MA: Kluwer Academic Publishers, 125–132.

Moor, J. 2008. *Playing, laughing and learning with children on the autism spectrum. A practical re- sources of play ideas for parents and carers.* London: Jessica Kingsley Publishers.

Nadel, J., A. Revel, P. Andry, and P. Gaussier. 2004. Toward communication: First imitations in infants, low-functioning children with autism and robots. *Interaction Studies: Social Behaviour and Communication in Biological and Artificial Systems* 5(1):45–74.

National Autistic Society 2009. http://www.nas.org.uk/content/1/c6/01/40/24/Making%20 Connections.pdf (accessed April 12, 2009).

National Autistic Society 2010a. http://www.autism.org.uk/about_autism/autism_and_ asperger_syndrome_an_introduction/what_is_autism.aspx (accessed September 2, 2010).

National Autistic Society 2010b. http://www.nas.org.uk/nas/jsp/polopoly.jsp?d=1541&a=15189 (accessed February 8, 2010).

National Institute of Child Health and Human Development 2010. http://www.nichd.nih.gov/ autism/presentations/etiology1.cfm (accessed February 9, 2010).

Perks, S. 2007. *Body language and communication: A guide for people on the autism spectrum.* London: The National Autistic Society.

Pioggia, G., R. Igliozzi, M.L. Sica, M. Ferro, F. Muratori, A. Ahluwalia, and D. De Rossi. 2008. Exploring emotional and imitational android-based interactions in autistic spectrum disorders. *Journal of CyberTherapy & Rehabilitation* 1(1):49–61.

Pioggia, G., M.L. Sica, M. Ferro, R. Igliozzi, F. Muratori, A. Ahluwalia, and D. De Rossi. 2007. Human-robot interaction in autism: FACE, an android-based social therapy. In *16th IEEE International Conference on Robot & Human Interactive Communication* (RO-MAN 2007), 605–612. IEEE Press.

Phillips, M.L. 2004. Facial processing deficits and social dysfunction: How are they related? *Brain, Oxford Journals* 127(8):1691–1692.

Power, T. 2000. *Play and exploration in children and animals.* Mahwah, NJ: Lawrence Erlbaum Associates.

Rinehart, N.J., M.A. Bellgrove, B.J. Tonge, A.V. Brereton, D. Howells-Rankin, and J.L. Bradshaw. 2006. An examination of movement kinematics in young people with high-functioning autism and Asperger's disorder: Further evidence for a motor planning deficit. *Journal of Autism and Developmental Disorders* 36(6):757–767.

Robins, B. and K. Dautenhahn. 2004. Interacting with robots: Can we encourage social interaction skills in children with autism? *ACM SIGACCESS Accessibility and Computing* 80:6–10.

Robins, B., K. Dautenhahn, and P. Dickerson. 2009. From isolation to communication: A case study evaluation of robot assisted play for children with autism with a minimally expressive humanoid robot. In *The Second International Conferences on Advances in Computer-Human Interactions, ACHI 09.* 205–211. IEEE Press.

Robins, B., K. Dautenhahn, and J. Dubowski. 2005. Robots as isolators or mediators for children with autism? A cautionary tale. In *AISB'05 Symposium on Robot Companions Hard Problems and Open Challenges in Human-Robot Interaction*, University of Hertfordshire, UK, 82–88. SSAISB.

Robins, B., K. Dautenhahn, and J. Dubowski. 2006. Does appearance matter in the interaction of children with autism with a humanoid robot? *Interaction Studies* 7(3):509–542.

Robins, B., K. Dautenhahn, R. te Boekhorst, and A. Billard. 2004a. Effects of repeated exposure of a humanoid robot on children with autism. In *Designing a more inclusive world* (Cambridge Workshop on Universal Access and Assistive Technology), S. Keates, J. Clarkson, P. Langdon, and P. Robinson, Eds. Cambridge: Springer-Verlag (London), 225–236.

Robins, B., K. Dautenhahn, R. te Boekhorst, and A. Billard. 2004b. Robots as assistive technology — does appearance matter? In *13th IEEE International Workshop on Robot and Human Interactive Communication* (RO-MAN 2004), Kurashiki, Okayama, Japan, 277–282. IEEE Press.

Robins, B., P. Dickerson, and K. Dautenhahn. 2005. Robots as embodied beings — interactionally sensitive body movements in interactions among autistic children and a robot. In *IEEE International Workshop on Robots and Human Interactive Communication* (RO-MAN 2005), Nashville, TN, 54–59. IEEE Press.

Robins, B., E. Ferrari, and K. Dautenhahn. 2008. Developing scenarios for robot assisted play. In *17th IEEE International Symposium on Robot and Human Interactive Communication* (RO-MAN 2008), University Munchen, Munich, Germany, 180–186. IEEE Press.

Salter, T. 2007. Sensor-based recognition of interaction patterns between children and mobile robots. Ph.D. thesis, University of Hertfordshire, U.K.

Salter, T., F. Michaud, K. Dautenhahn, D. Létourneau, and S. Caron. 2005. Recognising interaction from a robot's perspective. In *Proceedings of the 14th IEEE International Workshop on Robot and Human Interactive Communication* (RO-MAN 2005), Nashville, TN, 178–183. IEEE Press.

Salter, T., F. Michaud, and D. Létourneau. 2009. An exploratory investigation into the effects of adaptation in child-robot interaction. In *Proceedings of the International Conference on Social Robotics* (FIRA Congress), Incheon, Korea, 102–109. Berlin: Springer-Verlag.

Salter, T., F. Michaud, D. Létourneau, D. Lee, and I. Werry. 2007. Using proprioceptive sensors for categorizing human-robot interactions. In *Proceedings of the 2nd Human-Robot Interaction* HRI 07, Washington, DC, 105–112. New York: ACM

Salter, T., I. Werry, and F. Michaud. 2008. Going into the wild in child-robot interaction studies — issues in social robotic development. *International Journal of Robotics — Special Issue on Multidisciplinary Collaboration in Socially Assistive Robotics* 1(2):93–108.

Scassellati, B. 2009. http://www.cs.yale.edu/homes/scaz/Research.html (accessed June 2, 2009).

Scassellati, B. 2002. Theory of mind for a humanoid robot. *Autonomous Robots* 12:13–24.

Scassellati, B. 2005a. How social robots will help us to diagnose, treat, and understand autism. In *12th International Symposium of Robotics Research (ISRR)*, San Francisco, CA, 552–563. Berlin: Springer-Verlag.

Scassellati, B. 2005b. Quantitative metrics of social response for autism diagnosis. In *IEEE Workshop on Robots and Human Interactive Communications*, Nashville, TN, 585–590. IEEE Press.

Scassellati, B. 2005c. Using robots to study abnormal social development. In *Fifth International Workshop on Epigenetic Robotics (EpiRob)*, Nara, Japan. L. Berthouze, F. Kaplan, H. Kozima, H. Yano, J. Konczak, G. Metta, G., Sandini, G. Stojanov, and C. Balkenius, Eds. 11–14.

Shives, L.R. 2007. *Basic concepts of psychiatric-mental health nursing*. Philadelphia, PA: Lippincott Williams & Wilkins.

S.P.E.C. Tintamarre Summer Camp 2001. http://www.spectintamarre.qc.ca/index.htm.

Stanton, C., P.H.J. Kahn, R.L. Severson, J.H. Ruckert, and B.T. Gill. (2008). Robotic animals might aid in the social development of children with autism. In *ACM/IEEE International Conference on Human-Robot Interaction (HRI)*, Amsterdam, the Netherlands, 271–278. New York: ACM.

Stone, W.L., E.E. Coonrod, and L.M. Turner. 2004. Psychometric properties of the STAT for early autism screening. *Journal of Autism Developmental Disorders* 34:691–701.

University of Pittsburgh. 2010. Crying and how you can cope. Published at www.pitt.edu/~ocdweb/familyissues/guides

Valin, J.M., F. Michaud, and J. Rouat. 2007a. Robust localization and tracking of simultaneous moving sound sources using beamforming and particle filtering. *Robotics and Autonomous Systems* 55:216–228.

Valin, J.M., S. Yamamoto, J. Rouat, F. Michaud, K. Nakadai, and H.G. Okuno. 2007b. Robust recognition of simultaneous speech by a mobile robot. *IEEE Transactions on Robotics* 23(4):742–752.

Van Bourgondien, M.E., L. Marcus, and E. Schopler. 1992. Comparison of DSM-III-R and childhood autism rating scale diagnoses of autism. *Journal of Autism and Developmental Disorders* 22(4):493–506.

Wang, A.T., S. Lee, M. Sigman, and M. Dapretto. 2007. Reading affect in the face and voice. Neural correlates of interpreting communicative intent in children and adolescents with autism spectrum disorders. *Archives of General Psychiatry* 64(6):698–708.

Weir, S. and R. Emanuel. 1976. Using logo to catalyse communication in an autistic child. Department of Artificial Intelligence, Research Report no. 15, University of Edinburgh.

Werry, I., K. Dautenhahn, and B. Harwin. 2001a. Evaluating the response of children with autism to a robot. In *RESNA 2001, Rehabilitation Engineering and Assistive Technology Society of North America*, Nevada.

Werry, I., K. Dautenhahn, W. Ogen, and B. Harwin. 2001b. Can social interaction skills be taught by a social agent? The role of a robotic mediator in autism therapy. In *Cognitive technology: Instruments of mind (CT 2001)*, M. Beynon, C.L. Nehaniv, and K. Dautenhahn, Eds. Berlin: Springer-Verlag, 57–75.

Wing, L. and J. Gould. 1979. Severe impairments of social interaction and associated abnormalities in children: Epidemiology and classification. *Journal of Autism & Development Disorders* 9:11–29.

Wolfberg, P.J. 2009. *Play and imagination in children with autism,* 2nd ed. New York: Teachers College Press.

9 Virtual Reality Therapy in Paediatric Rehabilitation

Patrice L. (Tamar) Weiss, Naomi Weintraub and Yocheved Laufer

CONTENTS

INTRODUCTION

Virtual reality (VR) has been defined as the use of interactive simulations created with computer hardware and software to present users with opportunities to perform in virtual environments (VEs) that appear, sound and feel similar to real-world objects and events (Sheridan 1992; Weiss and Jessel 1998; Rizzo 2002). Users interact with virtual objects by moving and manipulating in a way that generates a feeling of 'virtual presence' in the simulated world. The therapeutic aim of VR is to provide users with more than just an entertaining experience and thus it differs in scope from conventional computer games as will be described.

Since the mid-1990s, VR has been applied to various rehabilitation populations including those with stroke (Christiansen et al. 1998), autism (Strickland 1996), cerebral palsy (Inman et al. 1997) and phobias (Pugnetti et al. 1998; Wiederhold and

Wiederhold 1998; Rizzo et al. 1997). For the past decade, the number of applications and types of platforms has expanded dramatically, to the point where it has become increasingly difficult to track all new developments and applications.

The use of VR in rehabilitation is based on a number of unique attributes of this technology, including the opportunity for experiential, active learning that is motivating and challenging, yet safe and ecologically valid and that provides the ability to objectively measure behaviour (Rizzo et al. 2002; Schultheis and Rizzo 2001). Importantly, the automated nature of stimulus delivery within VEs enables a therapist to focus on the clients' performance and observe whether they are using effective strategies. These attributes have been reviewed in great detail (e.g., Sveistrup 2004; Rizzo and Kim 2005). Clinicians use VR to achieve a variety of therapeutic objectives by varying task complexity, type and amount of feedback, and extent of independent activity. The ability to provide for these variables depends on the characteristics of the hardware and software, and needs to be taken into consideration.

INSTRUMENTATION

As shown in Figure 9.1, there are a variety of categories of hardware approaches that can be used to implement VEs. These include the use of standard desktop or laptop computer technology, camera-based video capture devices, head-mounted displays (HMDs), haptic and other sensor and/or actuator-based devices [e.g., Novint's Falcon (2010) and Nintendo's Wii (2006)], and large screen immersive systems [e.g., CAVE (2001) or Motek's CAREN (1994)]. Within each category, there is a progression from standard technology to more customised technology, shown schematically as sliders

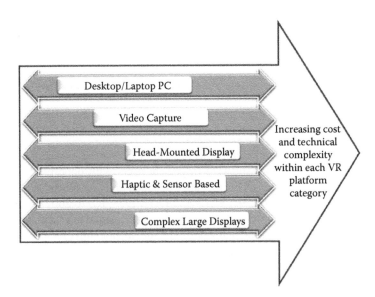

FIGURE 9.1   Different categories of VR platforms. Depending on the quality of the graphics, feedback and other factors, the intensity of the virtual experience can vary within a given platform and across platforms.

on a continuum of technical complexity. This progression is usually accompanied by increases in cost and immersion. Although the assumption is that users' sense of virtual presence tends to increase from one category to the next, and within each category, from the simpler to the more complex systems, there is no clear demonstration that such is the case. Moreover, non-platform related factors such as the meaningfulness of the virtual task (Hoffman et al. 1998) and the fidelity of the feedback (Holden 2005) clearly have an effect on how well the subjective experience within a VE resembles that in a comparable physical setting.

Desktop systems use basic computer hardware with monitors of varying sizes. They have been used extensively in rehabilitation due to their low cost and ready availability (Rizzo and Kim 2005). Despite the low level of immersion generated by such systems, they have been demonstrated to achieve effective intervention and transfer of effects when running a variety of functional environments such as the street crossing simulation shown in Figure 9.2 (Katz et al. 2005). Figure 9.2a shows the VE with the quality of graphics available 10 years ago, whereas Figure 9.2b shows the much more realistic scenarios that can now be displayed even using simple desktop display technology.

HMDs were one of the first instruments used to display virtual environments. An HMD, such as the eMagin unit shown in Figure 9.3, is essentially composed of two small screens positioned, at eye level, within special goggles or a helmet. Users view the VE in three dimensions in high resolution. The more expensive HMDs, for example, Virtual V8 (1998), even provide highly realistic displays of the environment but they tend to be heavier and more encumbering.

Other VR applications use video capture systems whereby the VE is projected onto a large screen located in front of the user. GestureTek's IREX VR system, shown in Figure 9.4a, and Sony's PlayStation II EyeToy, shown in Figure 9.4b, are examples of such systems. Users see themselves within the simulated environment and are able to interact with virtual objects that are presented.

Some expensive projection systems, such as the CAVE, are composed of several large screens surrounding users from all sides such that the VE may be viewed no matter where they gaze. Video capture and CAVE systems do not require the use of devices such as an HMD, which encumber the user and, in some cases, lead to

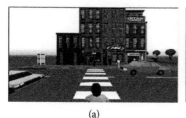 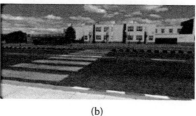

(a)   (b)

FIGURE 9.2 (See color insert following page 240.) A comparison between the graphics quality of a street crossing virtual environment (VE) available (a) 10 years ago (Katz et al. 2005) and (b) at present (www.dmw.ca). Figure 9.2b shows that much more realistic scenarios can now be displayed even using simple desktop display technology.

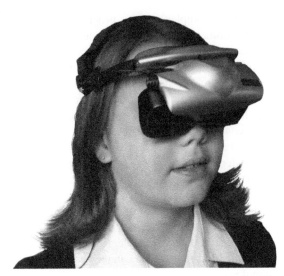

FIGURE 9.3   (See color insert following page 240.) A head-mounted display (HMD), such as the eMagin unit shown here, is composed of two small screens positioned at eye level within special goggles or a helmet.

discomfort, nausea and other side effects; this is particularly a factor to consider when working with children (Reid and Campbell 2006; Mott et al. 2007).

An extremely important component of an effective VR system is the feedback provided to the user. Almost all systems provide visual and auditory feedback as such technologies are standard elements of any computer-based equipment. More recently, the provision of additional sources of feedback is being explored. Haptic feedback enables users to experience the sensation of touch and force, resulting in a much more realistic experience in the virtual world. Haptic information may also be conveyed by simpler means such as a force-feedback joystick (Reinkensmeyer et al. 2003) or a force-feedback steering wheel (Andonian et al. 2003) (Figure 9.5a). Several attempts have been made to use quasi-haptic sensors, such as the small

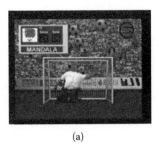
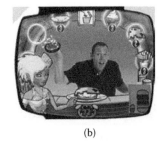

(a)   (b)

FIGURE 9.4   (See color insert following page 240.) Two examples of video capture VR systems: (a) GestureTek's IREX VR system (http://www.gesturetekhealth.com/) and (b) Sony's PlayStation II EyeToy (http://www.us.playstation.com/PS2/Games/EyeToy_Play). Users see themselves within the simulated environment and are able to interact with virtual objects that are presented.

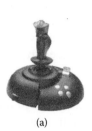
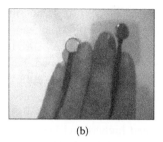

(a)   (b)

FIGURE 9.5   Approaches to providing haptic feedback to users: (a) the simpler Microsoft Sidewinder Precision 2 force-feedback joystick (http://en.wikipedia.org/wiki/Microsoft_ SideWinder#Joystick) and (b) small vibrators to simulate haptic feedback via technologies that are less encumbering and expensive than true haptic devices. (Feintuch et al. 2006.)

vibrators shown in Figure 9.5b, to simulate haptic feedback via technologies that are less encumbering and expensive than true haptic devices (Feintuch et al. 2006).

Vestibular feedback may be provided via moving platforms that are programmed to rotate or translate in tandem or in conflict with the virtual environment (Keshner and Kenyon 2009). These systems tend to be costly and, hence, are not yet in wide clinical use. Still rarer is the provision of olfactory feedback to add odour to a virtual environment. The potential of this feedback channel is now being investigated (Bordnick et al. 2004).

Navigation throughout a VE and manipulation of virtual objects within it are also important elements of any VR system. Each category of VR system tends to have its own particular method for navigation and manipulation. Desktop virtual environments are usually controlled via standard computer input devices such as the keyboard, mouse and joystick. HMDs are instrumented with a tracking device such as Intersense's InterTrax2 (1996), a three-degrees-of-freedom inertial orientation tracker used to track pitch, roll and yaw movements. Video capture systems are controlled via natural movement of the users' limbs, with a camera tracking all actions and responding accordingly.

Presence

Sheridan (1992) has defined presence (also referred to as virtual presence or telepresence) as being '... experienced by a person when sensory information generated only by and within a computer compels a feeling of being present in an environment other than the one the person is actually in' (Sheridan 1992). Presence is thought to be a key element in achieving a strong sense of interaction within a virtual environment (Slater 2003). Slater (1999) suggested that presence includes (1) the sense of 'being there,' (2) domination of the VE over the real world and (3) the user's memory of visiting an actual location rather than a compilation of computer-generated images and sounds. Although numerous studies have attempted to merge the various definitions of presence, it continues to be viewed as a complex concept that may be influenced by numerous interdependent factors (Mantovani and Castelnuovo 2003; Schuemie et al. 2001). Presence is often measured via questionnaires, most notably Wittmer and Singer's (1998) Presence Questionnaire. It has also been assessed via physiological measures such as heart rate or galvanic skin response (Wiederhold et al. 2002). More recently, 'breaks in presence,' wherein the VE is momentarily stopped, have been used to contrast the sense of presence from its absence (Slater et al. 2006).

The intensity of a user's sense of presence is clearly influenced by the extent of immersion achieved by the VR equipment (Slater 2003). High immersion systems such as the CAVE and higher-level HMDs are thought to generate a strong sense of presence (Hoffman et al. 2004). However, immersion is not the only influential factor as demonstrated by the high levels of presence experienced by users of video capture VR systems (Kizony et al. 2003). Diverse additional factors also affect presence. These include the extent to which the user is encumbered with sensors, the way in which the user is represented within the virtual environment (Nash et al. 2000), whether the system supports two- or three-dimensional interactions, and the number and quality of feedback modalities (e.g., Durfee 2001). Another set of factors relates to a given user's characteristics. These include age, gender, immersive tendencies, prior VR experience and disability (e.g., Stanney et al. 1998). With regard to paediatric rehabilitation, it appears that children feel greater presence in VEs than do adults (Sharar et al. 2007). Finally, a third set of factors relates to characteristics of the VE and the task that is being performed within it (Nash et al. 2000). These include the meaningfulness of the task (Hoffman et al. 1998), how realistic it is and the intuitiveness of the interaction (Rand et al. 2005).

The relationship between the sense of presence, immersion and performance within the VEs is still not fully understood (Nash et al. 2001; Mania and Chalmers 2001). Nevertheless, there is considerable evidence indicating that a high sense of presence may lead to deeper emotional response, increased motivation and, in some cases, enhanced performance (Schuemie et al. 2001).

A roadmap depicting the organization of this chapter is shown in Figure 9.6. The introduction has provided an overview of VR including definitions of the key terms and descriptions of the main types of instrumentation used. The important concept of virtual presence was also discussed. In the next sections we present some of the major ways in which VR has been used as a therapeutic and educational tool for children. We present results from various studies on the topics of improving knowledge and achievement, classroom instruction, communication and creativity, disability awareness and functional virtual training. Specifically, we take the task of road crossing to illustrate how VR can implement functional tasks, thereby serving as a medium for the practice of practical skills. Next we explore ways in which VR has been used as a tool for the evaluation and assessment of widely prevalent disabilities including attention-deficit hyperactivity disorder (ADHD), autism spectrum disorder (ASD), intellectual developmental deficits (IDD), cerebral palsy (CP) and for pain relief during burn care. We conclude with thoughts about current VR practice including a consideration of limitations in the literature and recommendations of topics that need to be addressed in order to ensure successful use of VR for paediatric rehabilitation.

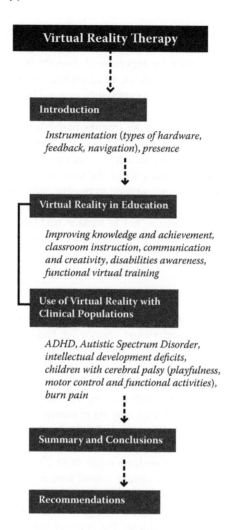

FIGURE 9.6   Conceptual roadmap of chapter content.

USE OF VIRTUAL REALITY IN EDUCATION

IMPROVING KNOWLEDGE AND ACHIEVEMENT

Computer-assisted instruction (CAI) is widely used in the classroom and its advantages have been repeatedly shown in various studies (Vogel et al. 2006). Several attributes of CAI have been identified including reward (feedback), interactivity, self-running simulations, etc. Consequently, CAI is highly motivating for students (Bowman et al. 1999; Kim 2006). In recent years, researchers and educators have realised that VR technologies, which are a type of CAI, may contribute much to the development of curriculum (Kim 2006), learning methods and styles, and consequently to students acquisition of knowledge and achievement (Bowman et al. 1999).

One of the benefits of VR technology is that it provides an authentic (Kim 2006) and life-like experience, which is a major factor in learning (Vogel et al. 2006). For example, some concepts cannot be experienced directly in the world, such as the interactions between subatomic particles. In cases such as this, a VE can assist in understanding this phenomenon. This experience may aid in comprehension of complex ideas, concepts and skills.

An additional assumption is that an inquiry-based learning approach is more effective than traditional instructional methods in the learning process (Kim 2006). VR interactions require that users be active participants, learners and explorers, requiring effort and activity on the part of the user to continuously choose his or her position and actions. Active, as opposed to passive, learning is believed to be an important factor in increasing learning and retention. However, it is also assumed that the purpose of VR programs is not to replace traditional classroom teaching but rather reinforce or supplement the learning process and methods (Bowman et al. 1999; Kim 2006).

CLASSROOM INSTRUCTION

VR has been used as a teaching tool for a variety of classroom subjects. Sun et al. (2008) showed that a Web-based virtual science lab had a positive effect on fifth-grade students' knowledge on a specific topic compared to their peers who learned in a traditional class. Similarly, Kim (2006) found that fifth-grade students who were taught about volcanoes via 3D simulation scored significantly higher on an achievement test than did their peers who studied using traditional 2D visuals.

Based on the assumption that VEs may be effective in conveying spatial information and time chronology, Foreman et al. (2008) developed a simulation to teach sequences of historical events. They examined these programs in three different age groups: university undergraduate students (ages 18 to 22 years), middle-school students (ages 11 to 14 years) and elementary school students (ages 7 to 9 years). They found that the 3D VE technology was more effective than 2D or paper images in conveying the knowledge only among university students. The authors hypothesised that the 3D program may have distracted the younger students, thus affecting their ability to acquire the information conveyed. From the studies reviewed previously, it appears that VE technology does not enhance students' knowledge and achievements in all cases. The effectiveness of VE may depend on the content studied or the simulations used. Additional studies are required prior to drawing conclusions in this area.

COMMUNICATION AND CREATIVITY

One of the common uses of computers today among children is for communicating with their peers and others around the world through chat programs or games. It has been hypothesised that this medium may enhance student's language ability and communication skills. Bailey and Moar (2001) described a shared 3D Internet-based VE simulation whereby the user can enter, navigate in and interact with an avatar, a 3D animated character representing the user. Users can also construct their own environments online, providing opportunities for creativity and active design. Thus, this system enables individuals to share the virtual worlds they developed or to jointly develop worlds. In a pilot study among elementary school students, sole exploration of a virtual world had limited interest for the children. Instead, they focused on searching for other people and were mostly interested in exploring the world with other children. Therefore, it appeared that this system had great potential for developing communication and collaboration skills as well as creativity. These cooperative world systems were also found to be helpful in developing students' narrative abilities. Different 3D text-based VEs (e.g., MOOSE Crossing, Neverwinter Nights) were designed for children to learn to program and to practice reading and creative writing collaboratively. Robertson and Good (2005) showed these programs to be helpful in enhancing students' narrative abilities, most likely because children found them enjoyable, engaging and rewarding.

DISABILITY AWARENESS

Pivik et al. (2002) examined the use of VR in enhancing the awareness of fourth- to sixth-grade students of the needs of individuals with disabilities. The experimental group (n = 30) used the 'Barriers' VR program, where users travel in a 'virtual wheelchair' and explore a virtual school building that includes 24 virtual barriers. As the users navigate within the virtual school, they perform tasks such as opening doors. A message provides feedback when a barrier has been identified. A control group (n = 30) used a second simulation, 'Wheels,' wherein the user navigates within a VE but does not encounter barriers. Although there were no differences between the two groups in terms of their attitudes toward children with disabilities, in comparison to the 'Wheels' simulation, 'Barriers' enhanced the students' knowledge of possible obstacles while driving a wheelchair.

FUNCTIONAL VIRTUAL TRAINING

A number of studies have investigated the use of VR to impart functional skills to children, a common one being road crossing. Road crossing is a task of inherent importance, due to the danger of accidents for children with poor pedestrian behaviours, as well as one of great suitability to VR. Crossing a road safely is a complex cognitive task that requires the integration of well-developed knowledge and skills, including visual and auditory information, and control of attention and executive functions. In addition, there is a need for time and distance estimation of the approaching vehicles as well as combining this knowledge with the individual's awareness of his or her walking pace. Based on this knowledge, the individual needs to develop strategies and make complex judgments and decisions, which enable him or her to decide when to cross, and to adjust his or her crossing pace to the specific situation (Clancy et al. 2006). Therefore, it is not surprising that pedestrian injuries are one of the greatest causes for children's morbidity and mortality (Bart et al. 2008; McComas et al. 2002). Moreover, it is understandable that individuals with cognitive deficits and specifically with ADHD may encounter difficulties with road crossing (Clancy et al. 2006). VR technologies provide a safe and controlled environment to teach children pedestrian skills and behaviours. Moreover, VR enables provision of consistent feedback, practice and repetition in a motivating manner.

Schwebel et al. (2008) examined the validity of an immersive, interactive VR pedestrian environment to understand and prevent children's pedestrian injuries. The study included 102 children between the ages of 7 and 9 years, and 74 undergraduate students between the ages of 17 and 54 years. The participants stood on a simulated curb, and viewed the VE on three monitors arranged in a semicircle in front of them. Noise from the road was transmitted through speakers. Participants also took part in a real road-crossing activity. In the real situation, older participants crossed a real street at a marked crosswalk whereas the children stood at a real crossing, but instead of crossing, they were directed to initiate the crossing by shouting 'now' when they felt it was safe to cross. In both groups of participants, there were low to medium significant correlations between the VR and real environments for the various outcome measures (e.g., start delay time, namely, the time after a car passes and before the participant initiates crossing). In addition, significant differences were found between children and adults (e.g., in start delay time and wait time, namely, the time spent waiting to cross the street). Based on these findings the authors concluded that the VR environment may serve as a valid tool for measuring street-crossing safety.

McComas et al. (2002) investigated whether children can learn pedestrian safety skills via a VE and if these skills transfer to real-world behaviour. The study included 95 fourth- to sixth-grade students who participated in either an intervention or a control group. The simulation ran on a desktop computer with the VE projected onto three synchronised monitors. In addition, a head-tracking device was used to determine head movements (looking to the left and right). There were eight intersections, each designed to teach children about different aspects of pedestrian safety including signage, number of lanes and distractions (e.g., noise, other pedestrians). The children in the training program learned safe street crossing. However, this behaviour transferred to the real-world environment only among the suburban students and not among those from urban homes.

Bart et al. (2008) also evaluated the effectiveness of a VR environment in teaching children how to cross a street safely. The study included 86 typical children between the ages of 7 and 12 years. Children who failed a VR street-crossing safety test were randomly assigned to training (n = 11) and control groups (n = 10). Training took place using Superscape's 3D Webmaster software, which ran on a desktop and was viewed on a 17-in. monitor. Children in the training group had to pass nine stages of increasing difficulty (i.e., greater number of cars travelling at faster speeds). At each stage they had to indicate when it was safe to cross the virtual street. In addition, two independent observers monitored actual street-crossing performance and the children completed a satisfaction and enjoyment questionnaire. Both boys and girls in the training program significantly improved their street crossing in comparison to the control group (who participated in two sessions of computer games). These findings supported McComas et al.'s (2002) results and showed that VR simulation training appears to improve the pedestrian skills of children who live in urban areas and that this improvement can transfer to real street-crossing situations.

ATTENTION-DEFICIT HYPERACTIVITY DISORDER

Attention-deficit hyperactivity disorder (ADHD) is a complex neurodevelopmental condition. The diagnosis of ADHD includes five criteria: (1) a persistent pattern of inattention and/or hyperactivity-impulsivity that is more frequently displayed and more severe than is typically observed in individuals at a comparable level of development; (2) some symptoms that cause impairment must be present before the age of 7 years; (3) some impairment from the symptoms must be present in at least two settings; (4) there must be evidence of interference with developmentally appropriate social, academic or occupational functioning; and (5) disturbance must not occur exclusively during the course of other disorders such as schizophrenia or other psychotic disorders and must not be better accounted for by another disorder (e.g., mood or anxiety disorder) (American Psychiatric Association [APA], 2000).

Individuals with ADHD often encounter multifaceted executive impairment, resulting in the inability to inhibit or delay behavioural responses. Consequently, impulsive behaviour and diminished problem-solving ability and flexibility are observed (Barkley and Murphy, in Clancy et al. 2006). In addition, poor organizational abilities are one of the most common characteristics of children with ADHD (Barkley 1990). Barkley (1997) expressed this deficiency in specific relation to organization of behaviour relative to time.

ADHD is typically diagnosed using clinical interviews, behaviour checklists or rating scales (Barkley 1991). Recently, however, there has been a growing interest in developing alternative diagnostic methods, such as VR, due to the limitations of conventional measures, for example, limited psychometric properties (Rizzo et al. 2004). One major research initiative, investigating the use of VR to assess and rehabilitate attention disorders, was conducted by a group at the University of Southern California led by Rizzo et al. (2004). They developed a virtual classroom, which is a continuous performance task (CPT) embedded within a VR classroom, viewed via an HMD. The system also included a three-position-and-orientation magnetic tracking device that recorded head, arm and leg movements in order to measure activity level. Their premise was that HMDs can provide a controlled-stimulus environment, where attention challenges can be presented in a precise way and with control of the distracting auditory and visual stimuli within the virtual environment. Using these devices allows a high level of experimental control and supports the creation of attention assessment and rehabilitation tasks that resemble the real world (Rizzo et al. 2004, 2006).

Users of the virtual classroom viewed a standard classroom environment containing desks, a female teacher and a blackboard, as shown in Figure 9.7. On one side of the environment, there was a wall with a large window looking out onto a playground and a street with moving vehicles. On the opposite wall there was a pair of doorways through which activity occurred. As the users viewed this scenario, their attention performance was assessed using a Go/No-Go task. The children were tested under two conditions: with common classroom distractions (e.g., noises, activities going on, etc.) and without distractions. The measures for evaluating attention included reaction time performance, number of omission and commission errors on various attention challenges, as well as the extent of head, arm and leg activity.

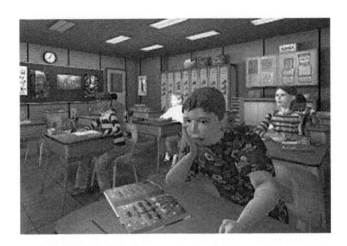

FIGURE 9.7   A virtual classroom. (www.dmw.ca.)

Results of the initial study (Rizzo et al. 2006), which included boys with (n = 8) and without (n = 10) ADHD, aged 6 to 12 years, showed that compared to their non-ADHD peers, the boys with ADHD had significantly slower correct hit reaction time in the distraction condition, and higher reaction time variability and more omission and commission errors under both conditions. In addition, the tracking device indicated that the boys with ADHD had higher activity levels on all metrics compared to their non-ADHD peers across conditions.

A subsequent study (Parsons et al. 2007) included a similar sample size and age group. In this study, a third condition was added that included a more realistic, ecologically valid attention task requiring the integration of audio and visual attention processes [e.g., the stimulus was taken from the Boston Naming Test (Kaplan et al. 1983) and a virtual teacher called out the item's name either correctly or incorrectly]. Similar to the initial study, the authors reported that in both the no-distraction and distraction conditions, boys with ADHD had more commission and omission errors (but they did not differ in hit reaction time). In the more ecologically valid condition, significant differences were seen only in commission errors. In addition, in all three conditions, boys with ADHD showed more overall hyperactivity.

Pollak et al. (2009) expanded the previous studies. Their study included 37 boys, 9 to 17 years, with (n = 20) and without (n = 17) ADHD. In addition, they compared the performance of the children in the two groups using three tasks: (1) VR-CPT (i.e., the system used in the previous studies), (2) No VR-CPT (i.e., the same CPT stimuli as in the first condition but with masking of the virtual classroom, and (3) the TOVA (Test of Variables of Attention), the most commonly used CPT that measures the extent of inattention in this population (Greenberg et al. 1993). The authors reported that significant differences between the groups were noted only in the reaction time in the VR-CPT and in omission errors in both VR-CPT and No VR-CPT. In examining the sensitivity and specificity, the No VR-CPT had the highest sensitivity (84%), and the TOVA and VR-CPT had the highest specificity (94%).

Based on these studies, it appears that the VR classroom (VR-CPT) distinguished between children with and without ADHD on the different measures, yet it did not appear to be more effective or precise in identifying these children. However, in terms of their subjective experience, VR-CPT was perceived as more enjoyable compared to the TOVA (Pollak et al. 2009). Thus, it appears that the virtual classroom has good potential as an efficient, cost-effective and ecologically valid tool for conducting attention performance measurement among elementary-school students (Rizzo et al. 2006).

As indicated previously, assessing and training road-crossing ability is highly suited to VR. For example, Clancy et al. (2006) examined the assumption that individuals with ADHD are more accident-prone in road-crossing situations. The study compared 24 adolescents with ADHD and 24 age and gender matched controls (i.e., children without ADHD), between the ages of 13 and 17 years. The hypothesis was examined by having children attempt to cross a virtual road that was displayed via a V8 HMD and that met the New Zealand Transport Safety Authority regulations. Compared to their peers, both male and female adolescents with ADHD were more prone to accidents based on outcome measures including a margin of safety, walking speed, crossing unsafely and the time that the participant waited before starting to cross divided by the time he or she had before the vehicle arrived.

The studies described previously demonstrate how various VR simulations have great potential in both the diagnosis and the rehabilitation of children with ADHD. Nevertheless, further research relating to this population is required.

AUTISM SPECTRUM DISORDER

Autism spectrum disorder (ASD), or autism, is a complex developmental disability with symptoms that usually emerge during the first years of life. Children with autism often have difficulties in verbal and non-verbal communication, social interactions, and leisure or play activities (Baron-Cohen and Howlin 1998). Those with high functioning autism (HFA) have a close to normal IQ, and some even exhibit exceptional skill or talent in specific areas.

Social interaction is defined as a reciprocal process in which children effectively initiate and respond to social stimuli presented by their peers (Sigman and Ruskin 1999). Social interaction with peers comprises a major component of typically developing children's social competence (Parker et al. 1995). Children who have poor social interactions with peers are considered to be at greater risk for experiencing loneliness and adjustment difficulties (Hay et al. 2004).

The two major capabilities that interchangeably predict competent social interaction with peers during middle childhood include conversational skills (e.g., how to start, maintain and end a conversation; how to switch between topics) and cooperative prosocial skills (e.g., mutual planning, sharing, comforting, providing help, empathy) (Hay et al. 2004). In fact, these two capabilities are recognised as major hallmarks of social deficiency in children with HFA (APA 2000). Children with HFA encounter problems initiating and maintaining an interaction with peers during social activities or games. They also tend to show more parallel play rather than social or coordinated play when interacting with their friends, compared to their typically developing peers (Bauminger 2002). Maintaining interactions, in particular, requires the performance of complex, cooperative, prosocial behaviours that pose difficulty for these children, such as sharing, collaborating and negotiating (Lord et al. 1994). Conversational skills are also very limited for children with HFA who experience difficulties in choosing topics appropriate to the setting and conversational partner as well as difficulties in choosing what is relevant and irrelevant during a conversation. They exhibit problems in initiating and maintaining conversations that are sensitive to the social context and to others' interests and previous knowledge. Taking turns within an on-going conversation or switching between topics to accommodate the conversational partner's perspective also poses difficulty (for extensive information on conversational characteristics of children with HFA; see Landa 2000).

In recent years, technologies, in general, and computer-based activities, specifically, have become increasingly valued as therapeutic and educational tools for children with autism (Grynszpan 2005). Studies have suggested a few reasons for the special interests that children with autism have in computerised learning and have identified several advantages that computers provide with respect to the ASD core deficits. These include, for example, the predictability of software, the safety of a clearly defined task, and the usually specific focus of attention (Murray 1997). Indeed, the inherent structure of computer-based tasks may be used to facilitate simulated social situations. While various advantages for the use of computerised learning have been promoted in recent years, only a few studies have investigated its potential attributes via a systematic intervention with children with autism. Those studies that have conducted systematic interventions suggest that computer-based intervention and VEs appear to offer a useful tool for social skills training in children with ASD (Silver 2001).

The Asperger's syndrome (high-level ASD) interactive study explored the suitability of VR technology to support learning of social communication skills for teenagers with ASD (Cobb et al. 2002). The rationale behind this study was that if social scenarios could realistically be replicated within VEs, the limited personal interaction afforded by the computer interface would be inherently more attractive to children with ASD and would therefore provide a safe and supportive environment for learning (Parsons et al. 2000). Environments were chosen that represented typical social situations that would be familiar to most users, with the objective of supporting social interaction behaviour specific to two tasks: lining up and finding somewhere to sit. This required users to control movement of their avatar through the VE, to respond appropriately to other avatars, and to make decisions about when they should communicate with others in the VE and what they should say. Observations of how teachers used the VE to support teaching of these specific skills in the classroom showed that they used the VE as a visual prompt to promote discussion about what was happening in the social scenario and why characters behaved as they did (Neale et al. 2002). Teachers found that the VE helped students to talk about their anxieties or worries in dealing with these situations. Case studies showed that rehearsing with the VE gave students confidence to do things independently in the real world (Wiederhold and Wiederhold 2004). Experimental studies examined the navigation patterns of participants in the VEs, documenting how much time they spent at specific locations (e.g., near or far from virtual people) and whether their behaviour was appropriate (e.g., did they sit at a free table in the café or one that was already occupied) (Parsons 2001). The results showed that people with ASD know how to interpret VEs in a non-literal manner, imbuing avatars with 'people-like' behaviour. Moreover, the VEs were used and understood appropriately by young people with ASD and were effective in supporting learning about social skills (Parsons et al. 2004, 2005, 2006; Mitchell et al. 2007).

As is the case for typically developed children and for those with ADHD, a number of studies have investigated the use of VR to impart skills to children and youth with ASD. In a pioneering study, Strickland (1996) used a desktop environment to teach two children with ASD, aged 7.5 and 9 years, to cross a street. She found that both participants succeeded in adjusting to the HMD (which was much heavier than those currently used) and in concentrating on the task. They both learned to navigate within the VE and to locate and approach objects that moved. Only one of the two learned to stop when he reached the object, which constituted the goal of this task. Although the initial results were encouraging, the implications of the study are limited due to the small number of participants and concerns related to the use of an HMD with this population (Parsons 2004).

A second street-crossing environment was used by children and youth with ASD to examine whether they were able to learn street-crossing skills with the aid of the simple, desktop environment, and whether the simulation helped them to improve their pedestrian behaviour in a real road street-crossing setting (Josman et al. 2008). The findings demonstrated that the research and control groups differed in their initial ability to succeed in VE, but no significant differences were found between groups in measures related to pedestrian behaviour (e.g., number of times looked to the left and right). This finding is similar to that of Parsons et al. (2004, 2005) who found no differences between youth with ASD and youth with normal development on all measures in their virtual pedestrian and coffee shop simulations.

Cassell (2004) and colleagues (Cassell and Bickmore 2002; Ryokai et al. 2003) have developed the novel 'Virtual Peer,' a life-sized, language-enabled and computer-generated animated character that resembles the children with whom it interacts. Virtual peers appear to give children with autism opportunities to repeatedly rehearse both verbal and non-verbal interaction skills. They also appear to empower children, offering the ability to be manipulated by their users and to encourage the creation and practice of dialogue and sharing behaviours.

An 'enforced cooperation' paradigm has been used, with virtual storytelling environments, implemented via a multi-user touch table (i.e., the Mitsubishi Electronic Laboratory's DiamondTouch) (Deitz 2001). This paradigm aims to support and promote cooperation within small groups by requiring that designated actions and manipulations at the interface be physically performed together by the group of participants (Zancanaro et al. 2007). The nature and distribution of those multi-user actions can be varied to affect the degree of cooperation among the group members. The enforced cooperation paradigm was used to enhance the ability of six boys, aged 8 to 10 years, with high functioning ASD, to interact in social situations while they narrated a shared story (Gal et al. 2009). Pre- and post-intervention tasks included a 'low-technology' version of the storytelling device and a non-storytelling play situation using a free construction game. The outcome measure was a structured observation scale of social interaction. Results demonstrated progress in three areas of social behaviours. First, the level of shared play of the children increased from the pre-test to the post-test and they all increased the level of collaboration following the intervention. Second, the participants were more likely to initiate positive social interaction with peers after the intervention. Third, the children with ASD demonstrated lower frequencies of autistic behaviours while using the StoryTable in comparison to the free construction game activity.

The studies described in this section demonstrate how VR has been used to ameliorate the core ASD symptoms. There has been particular success in using VR simulations to promote positive social behaviours and to provide these children with opportunities to practice functional skills in a safe setting.

Intellectual Developmental Deficits

Intellectual developmental deficit (IDD) is a generalised disorder, characterised by sub-average cognitive functioning and deficits in two or more adaptive behaviours that are observed in childhood (Chakrabarti and Fombonne 2001). IDD includes both a component relating to mental functioning and one relating to individuals' functional skills in their environment. IDD now commonly replaces the former term 'mental retardation' as a diagnostic term used to standardise a group of categories of sub-average mental functioning. The terms 'mentally challenged' or 'intellectual disability' are sometimes used.

Children with IDD tend to achieve developmental milestones (e.g., learning to sit up, crawl or walk) later than other children. Both adults and children with IDD exhibit delays in oral language development and in the development of adaptive behaviours such as self-help or self-care skills, deficits in memory skills, difficulties in learning social rules and problem-solving skills, and a lack of social inhibitors. According to the DSM-IV (APA 2000), three criteria must be met for a diagnosis of IDD: an IQ below 70, significant limitations in two or more areas of adaptive behaviour (as measured by an adaptive behaviour rating scale, i.e., communication, self-help skills, interpersonal skills and more) and evidence that the limitations became apparent before the age of 18.

The goal of most treatment programs for IDD is to develop intellectual and functional skills to the maximum possible level whether it is in special school programs or via mainstreaming. The emphasis is on the teaching of basic self-care skills such as bathing and feeding as well as vocational training toward independent living and job skills. Virtual environments offer a unique way in which to present functional tasks in a secure and gradable manner and have been used successfully to enable children with IDD to learn about and practice everyday tasks and behaviours. The Virtual City project comprised a series of task-based activities, situated in or outside the home, such as road crossing and going to a café and supermarket. The activities were displayed on a simple 2D desktop computer and monitor (Brown et al. 1998). Despite the use of simple graphics and mouse interaction, successful transfer of learning from use of a virtual supermarket to the real world was demonstrated (Cromby et al. 1996), and transfer of learning and increased engagement in the task were found following virtual environment training in travel, shopping and ordering food in a café (Cobb et al. 1998). Evidence of transfer of training has also been found, following VE training of kitchen skills, in students with learning disabilities attending a catering college (Rose et al. 1998, 2000).

The IREX (Interactive Rehabilitation and Exercise) video capture system has been shown to provide opportunities for children (Reid 2002) and young adults (Weiss et al. 2003; Yalon-Chamovitch and Weiss 2008) with IDD to engage in non-sedentary recreational activities. This system has also been shown to be effective as a physical fitness training program. A study of adults with IDD is presented later to illustrate VR's potential for fitness training. Although the participants were not children, the results of this study are included here because the level of games would be similar to those used for paediatric populations. A research group (n = 30; mean age = 52.3 years) with moderate IDD was matched for age, IDD level and functional abilities with a control group (n = 30, mean age = 54.3) (Lotan et al. 2009). A 5- to 6-week fitness program consisting of two 30-min sessions per week included game-like exercises provided by the Sony PlayStation II EyeToy VR system. Changes in physical fitness were monitored by the Energy Expenditure Index (EEI), the modified 12-min walk/run (Cooper test) and the Total Heart Beat Index (THBI). Significant ($p < 0.05$) improvements in physical fitness were demonstrated for the research group in comparison to the control group for the modified Cooper test and the THBI but not for the EEI test. VR technology intervention was suitable for adults with IDD and resulted in significant improvements in the physical fitness levels of the participants.

A more recent use of virtual interactions between people, electronic mentoring (e-mentoring) refers to a dyadic relationship in which a mentor, a senior person in age or experience, provides guidance and support to a less experienced or younger person, the protégé, via computer-mediated communication (Single, Muller and Cunningham 1999). E-mentoring is included in this chapter on VR because it provides an opportunity for 'virtual' interaction between individuals. More advanced manifestations of e-mentoring (e.g., Second Life; www.secondlife.com) use avatars and other VR-like simulations for interaction. Mentors perform a number of key functions for their protégés including vocational or instrumental support, psychological support through counselling, friendship, and encouragement and by serving as a role model by demonstrating appropriate behaviour (Ensher et al. 2003). Finn (1999) analyzed messages sent by people with physical and mental disabilities to an online discussion group over a 3-month period. He found that about half of the messages fell into socioemotional categories, such as expressing feelings, providing support and offering empathy. Rousso (2001) evaluated a community-based project that sought to strengthen the educational, vocational and social aspirations of adolescent girls with disabilities; most of the protégés were inspired by their mentors and began to take steps toward greater interdependence. Shpigelman et al. (2008) evaluated an e-mentoring intervention program based on mutual self-disclosure and friendship for youth with special needs including IDD. Using qualitative methods, the study characterised the e-mentoring process and its contributions to this population. Results provided support for the socioemotional potential of computer-mediated communication for youth with special needs, although some barriers were found in terms of their prior familiarity with computer-based technologies.

As indicated, children with IDD have relatively few opportunities to engage in non-sedentary recreational activities. Similar to children with ASD, they also need opportunities to practice functional skills in a safe setting. VR appears to meet both needs.

CEREBRAL PALSY

While the field of VR in medical rehabilitation has grown immensely in recent years, much of the research on its use for individuals with physical disabilities is focused on adult rehabilitation, particularly in relation to stroke rehabilitation (Deutsch et al. 2007; Henderson et al. 2007). While the paediatric literature presents a wide range of VR applications for the alleviation of a variety of impairments and functional and social limitations of children with different sensorimotor disabilities, the majority of VR applications relate to the rehabilitation of children with cerebral palsy (CP). In the following section, we review the literature relating the use of VR for children with CP as a model for its applicability to children with physical disabilities. The section commences with a brief description of CP, followed by a review of studies relating the effectiveness of VR interventions to address two primary treatment goals: playfulness and motor control. The specific attributes of VR technology as they relate to these treatment goals are discussed.

CP is a well-recognised neurodevelopmental condition beginning in early childhood and persisting throughout the lifespan; it is the most frequently reported diagnosis of children who receive rehabilitation treatment (Hayes et al. 1999). To encompass recent developments in the understanding of the neurobiology and pathology associated with brain development, and to adapt to the International Classification of Function (ICF 2001), CP was recently redefined by an international task force as follows: 'CP describes a group of disorders of the development of movement and posture causing activity limitations that are attributed to non-progressive disturbances that occurred in the developing fetal or infant brain' (Bax et al. 2005). The motor disorders of CP are often accompanied by disturbances of sensation, cognition, communication, perception and/or behaviour, and/or a seizure disorder (Bax et al. 2005). As this definition covers a wide range of clinical presentations and degrees of activity limitation, individuals with CP are usually categorised into subgroups. Traditional classification schemes have focused principally on the distribution pattern of the affected limbs (e.g., hemiplegia, dipelgia and quadriplegia). Additionally, modifiers are used to describe the primary tonal abnormality (e.g., hypertonia or hypotonia) as well as the dominant type of movement disorder present (e.g., spasticity, ataxia, dystonia or athetosis).

Physical rehabilitation of children with CP entails addressing specific impairments, such as spasticity, weakness, reduced range of motion, and sensory and perceptual deficits, as well as motor learning enabling the acquisition of functional skills. A variety of rehabilitation approaches are used to overcome the impairments and functional disabilities associated with CP, which include the neurodevelopmental treatment approach (Butler and Darrah 2001), strengthening exercises (Mockford and Caulton 2008) and task-related training such as constraint-induced movement therapy and treadmill exercise (Damiano and DeJong 2009; Taub et al. 2004). Much research is still necessary to determine the most appropriate therapeutic approaches for the diverse presentations of CP (Anttila et al. 2008).

The ability to engage in play is well accepted as necessary for normal child development. Exploration through play not only contributes to the development of spatial-motor control, but also is a key element in the development of the child's cognitive abilities, self-efficacy and social skills (Floery 1981; Slade and Palmer Wolf 1994). Children with sensory and/or motor disabilities that affect voluntary movement or mobility may often experience limited opportunities to engage in play activities (Miller and Reid 2003). Thus, children with disabilities tend to engage in more solitary play than do their peers without disabilities (Hestenes and Carroll 2000), leading to the development of a 'passive' personality (Missiuna and Pollock 1991), increased dependence on others and poor social skills (Howard 1996). As VR technology may offer opportunities for children with disabilities to experience play activities that are otherwise inaccessible to them, studies have explored the contribution of VR interventions to playfulness in children with CP.

Miller and Reid (2003) conducted focused interviews with 19 participants with CP, aged 8 to 13 years, following a VR play intervention with the Gesture Xtreme IREX VR system. The children's response to a single session indicated that it was an enjoyable experience that appeared to increase their self-competence and self-efficacy. The children reported a sense of control and mastery over the game, which provided them a safe way to explore and challenge their abilities. Furthermore, they indicated that involvement in VR play increased their acceptance by both family and peers.

In-depth interviews with the mothers of six children with physical disabilities (due to CP, spinal muscular atrophy and spina bifida) were conducted to determine the feasibility and the effects of a virtual game that was developed to encourage movement in response to music in the home environment (Tam et al. 2007). Prior to the interviews, families were given 10 min of training and a member of the research team visited each family at home to ensure proper system set-up. Additionally, each child attended six to eight weekly sessions, structured to develop the child's ability to interact with music, at the rehabilitation centre. All the children were able to play with the system in their 'free time.' It also provided opportunities to play with many different people such as friends, siblings, parents and grandparents. This induced changes in family dynamics with siblings and parents voluntarily spending more time with the child. The children's mothers also reflected that the VR system provided their children with opportunities to explore new skills that were not previously possible because of their physical limitations. Thus, while one mother was surprised by the musicality her child demonstrated, others commented on the improved concentration, body function, self-esteem and general exercise activity. Finally, and no less important, all the mothers commented on their child's satisfaction with the experience. As stated by one mother, 'anything that makes him happy makes me happy.'

To determine the degree of motivation elicited by VR play and to further delineate the key elements of VR treatment that promote volition during play, Harris and Reid (2005) observed and videotaped 16 children with CP during eight 1-hour play sessions using the IREX system. Each session began with the same game (Birds and Balls), after which the children were free to select the games they wanted to play with, leading to the use of between five and ten environments per session. Assessment using the Paediatric Volitional Questionnaire (Basu 2002) allowed quantification of behavioural indicators of volition by monitoring activities such as tries to solve problems, expresses pleasure or seeks challenges. Overall, the volitional scores indicated that VR intervention was a motivating activity. Moreover, several environmental elements were identified as crucial for increasing volitional activity. The first element was game variability, with greater variability leading to higher motivation. The second important element of the game related to how challenging it was. Children were particularly engaged in activities that were slightly above their skill level, thus offering a challenge while not being too frustrating. This is further supported by another study which demonstrated that VEs that are too unpredictable and frustrating for children with CP do not foster playfulness (Reid 2004). Finally, competitive games, whether involving competition with a robot or with a partner, induced greater volitional activity. Thus, VR play may also serve as a safe initiation into increased social participation for a child with disabilities.

A key factor in the evaluation of the effectiveness of any VR intervention is the degree to which attained skills transfer to the 'real world.' In a recent case study series, the transfer of increased playfulness achieved via VR play to the real world was assessed in three children with CP, ages 5 to 7 years (Weintraub et al. 2008). The intervention included three stages: pre- and post-test stages, consisting of eight 15-min sessions of free play in the children's classroom; and the experimental stage, consisting of ten 15-min sessions in which each child played with a partner with the Sony PlayStation 2 EyeToy system. All the sessions were videotaped and the children's performance was assessed using the Test of Playfulness (Bundy 2003). The results demonstrated that VR play could enhance playfulness even in young children. More importantly, the results indicated that play skills acquired via VR play were also transferred to the real world and improved the engagement of children in free play and social participation.

In conclusion, VEs can indeed provide opportunities for play to children whose ability to engage in social as well as solitary play is limited. Play within VR may offer not only a fun pastime, but also an opportunity to develop the cognitive and social/psychological skills attributed to play activities. Furthermore, play within the protected virtual world may enhance the ability of disabled children to explore play opportunities in the real world as well.

VR attributes may be particularly suited to the achievement of effective motor learning [see reviews by Holdern (2005) and Sveistrup (2004)]. The old adage 'practice makes perfect' is supported by a growing body of research indicating that changes in motor behaviour and neural plasticity are dependent on intensity of training and number of task-specific repetitions (Deluca et al. 2006; Kwakkel et al. 2004; Nudo et al. 2001; Van Peppen et al. 2004). Additional factors that are important for motor learning are the feedback provided regarding movement performance (i.e., the kinematics of the movement) and movement results (i.e., success in achieving the movement goal) (Thorpe and Valvano 2002), as well as the timing and frequency of the feedback (Austermann Hula et al. 2008). The significance of VR technology in this context is related to the motivation it provides to perform multiple task-oriented repetitions (Page et al. 2002). This is most important for children who are often not compliant in following a conventional exercise program because they find the exercises to be meaningless and uninteresting (Campbell 2000). VR technology also enables the presentation of multimodal feedback on performance and results, which can be presented at the frequency and timing most conducive to motor learning. Furthermore, the visually displayed sensory feedback received during the VR therapy may facilitate internalization of the motor representation of the target behaviour, which in turn enhances motor learning (You et al. 2005).

Examples of VR applications presented in the literature that address the rehabilitation of discrete movement control as well as upper and lower extremity functional movement in children with CP follow. A primary problem in CP is the child's difficulty in selective control of muscle activity, which results in inappropriate sequencing and co-activation of synergists and antagonists (Campbell 2000). For example, teaching the child to effectively control the tibialis anterior muscle, thereby preventing planter flexion contractures and the need for Botulinum toxin injections and/or surgical interventions, is often an important objective of motor rehabilitation (Campbell 2000). To determine whether a VR intervention can be used to selectively and effectively exercise ankle voluntary movements, Bryanton et al. (2006) compared the effectiveness of two applications of the IREX system with conventional exercise in ten children (ages 7 to 17 years) with CP. Both the conventional and VR protocols encouraged ankle dorsiflexion during chair-sitting and long-sitting (i.e., with the knees extended). The VR intervention achieved this goal by scoring the success of either ejecting a coconut from the child's toes or by causing a 'ninja' to jump, with the degree of dorsiflexion determining the score. The games' sensitivity could be adjusted to the child's control, allowing each child to reach the maximum score. All the children reported more fun with the VR exercises and their parents indicated a higher likelihood that the child would exercise at home with the VR system than with a conventional intervention. Moreover, kinematic analysis of the movements indicated that, while more repetitions were performed during the conventional exercises, the VR intervention induced greater mean ankle range of motion and longer hold times. Thus, this study suggested that VR can be used even by young children to improve isolated muscle control.

While treatment of specific impairments such as range of motion or muscle strength are important components in the treatment of children with CP, as indicated previously, repetitive task-oriented movements are imperative for the rehabilitation of functional movements (Harvey 2009). However, to date, the use of VR for the rehabilitation of gait and posture in children with CP has received very little attention. In a recent in-depth case study, Deutsch et al. (2008) examined the effects of VR intervention, using the low-cost commercially available Nintendo Wii system, on visual-perceptual processing, postural control and functional mobility of a 13-year-old boy with spastic diplegia. Using a client-centred approach, the games selected were based on the child's interest as well as on the therapeutic goals. These included sport games such as tennis, boxing and bowling. Each game had different motor control and visual-spatial demands, and the child's position (sitting vs. standing) and tasks were varied based on observation of performance. Following 11 VR sessions (each 60 to 90 min long), the child demonstrated improvements in all tested domains. Visual-perceptual processing improved, with the greatest improvement noted for visual discrimination, placing the child within the normal range in this domain. Lower extremity weight distribution became more symmetrical, and postural sway decreased indicating increased stance stability. Functional mobility, as determined by ambulation distance with forearm crutches, increased during training from 4.6 m to 45.7 m and continued to increase to 76.2 m during the 3-month follow-up period. This marked improvement had not been achieved or maintained by the child prior to the VR intervention. In addition to these marked improvements, the multiple player capability of the system facilitated social interaction and unexpected therapeutic effects. Since the patient expressed reduced interest in the game during the ninth session, a playmate with no physical disabilities was introduced in the tenth session. Turn taking, strategy sharing and encouragement were observed during this session. Furthermore, on the basis of this interaction, the patient decided to change his bowling strategy to match his partner's. This modelling probably explained the marked improvement in game score noted immediately in the next session.

Much of the VR literature has focused on upper extremity performance. The effects of VR treatments on functional reaching were examined in a pilot study with four children (Reid 2002), which was later extended to a randomised trial of 19 children with CP (ages 8 to 11) receiving a VR intervention and 12 children with CP (of the same age) receiving standard care (Reid and Campbell 2006). Each child participated in eight 1.5-hour sessions delivered once a week. The VR intervention utilised IREX technology, with each session designed so that approximately 15 min were spent with each game application. The majority of the virtual environments encouraged arm movements, while three elicited controlled trunk movements. Pre- and post-intervention assessments were carried out with a variety of observational assessment instruments (e.g., the Quality of Upper Extremity Skills Test) and self-perception tests (e.g., the Self-Perception Profile for Children). The results suggested that VR training may motivate children with CP to engage in repeated practice of reaching movements. However, only limited efficacy was demonstrated, due in part to the large drop-out of children in the control group. While these results are encouraging, the outcome measures used were not sensitive enough to capture an improvement in reaching movement.

To address this issue and to determine whether VR interventions also have a long-term effect, Chen et al. (2007) investigated the training effects of a VR intervention on kinematic variables of reaching behaviours. The testing procedure consisted of repeated baseline tests conducted during a 2-week period prior to the intervention, a 4-week intervention period with two to three treatment sessions per week, and follow-up testing 2 and 4 weeks following the intervention. Both specific movement impairments and functional abilities were assessed using kinematic movement analysis of reaching (toward targets placed in three directions) and the Fine Motor Domain of the Peabody Developmental Motor Scale (to assess grasping and visual motor integration specifically). Four children (ages 4.8 to 8.6 years) with spastic CP used eight commercially available games on the EyeToy system, which encouraged them to reach as quickly as possible toward virtual objects. Additionally, a VR system utilizing a sensor glove was employed to practice grasping activities within a VE. Following training, three out of the four children showed some improvement in the quality of reaching performance, demonstrating that even a simple off-the-shelf VR system could contribute to enhanced motor control. More importantly, the treatment demonstrated the ability to achieve some long-term effects as the gains made during training were partially maintained 4 weeks after the intervention.

Long-term effects of VR training are further substantiated by an in-depth case study of an 8-year-old child with hemiparetic CP, in which the effects of VR therapy on cortical reorganization were examined (You et al. 2005). Following an intensive VR intervention using the IREX VR system (training for 60 min a day, 5 days a week, for 4 weeks), functional magnetic resonance imaging (fMRI) demonstrated neuroplastic changes wherein the dominant bilateral primary sensorimotor cortical (SMC) activation and the ipsilateral supplementary motor area activation were replaced by contralateral SMC activation. These changes were accompanied by very substantial functional changes manifested in the greater amount of use made by the hand as well as in improved quality of movement.

In conclusion, while the number of studies implementing VR technology in the treatment of children with CP is limited and the research methodology of many of these studies is not sufficiently rigorous (e.g., small sample size, lack of control group), the available data suggest exciting prospects for the use of VR in the rehabilitation of children with physical disabilities. The current review focused on the treatment of children with CP. Similar studies on the benefits of VR interventions for the enhancement of motor control and functional abilities in adults with neurological impairments as a result of a stroke (Deutsch et al. 2007; Henderson et al. 2007) and traumatic brain injury (Thornton et al. 2005) lend strong support to the findings of the presented review, especially if one considers that playing comes more naturally to children than to adults. Furthermore, positive results have been reported with other medical conditions afflicting children such as traumatic brain injury (Sveistrup et al. 2004) and developmental coordination disorder (Eliasson et al. 2003). In some of these studies, additional treatment objectives have also been successfully addressed using VR technology, including the improvement of spatial skills necessary for navigation (see review by Stanton et al. 1998), the ability to operate a powered wheelchair (Hasdai et al. 1998), and the achievement of a general increase in physical activity and expenditure (Lotan et al. 2009).

PAIN RELIEF DURING BURN CARE

The use of VR interventions for the alleviation of pain perception in children has been determined by studies in which children experienced procedural pain due to medical procedures such as intravenous placement (Gold et al. 2006) and cancer treatment (Sander and Wint 2002; Windich-Biermeier et al. 2007; Wolitzky et al. 2005). In the present section we focus primarily on the integration of VR technology in the treatment of children who have suffered coetaneous burns, since this aetiology requires, in addition to painful wound care procedures, intensive physical rehabilitation.

Burn wound care consists of frequent dressing changes and is known to entail excruciating pain despite the administration of the maximum allowable dose of opioid analgesics (Perry and Heidrich 1982). Additionally, rehabilitation of patients with coetaneous burn wounds necessitates aggressive and often painful physical therapy which consists primarily of stretching exercises in an effort to increase the elasticity of the healing skin in order to maintain normal range of motion and function (Ward

1998). The pain associated with the initial trauma as well as the pain and distress endured during dressing changes and physical therapy often elevate the patients' anxieties, which further exacerbates their perception of pain. This, in turn, limits patients', and in particular children's, ability to cooperate during treatment and may lead to additional impairments such as joint contractures or the need for further surgery (Herndon 2007). Avoidance behaviour and resistance to treatment may be particularly problematic for effective wound care and physical therapy treatments in children who are unable to comprehend the long-term implications of their condition.

While opioid analgesics are considered the cornerstone of burn pain management, their partial effectiveness during wound care treatment and their extensive side effects limit their usefulness (Hoffman et al. 2001b). Since pain perception has a strong psychological component and requires attention (Chapman and Nakamura 1998), distracting attention from the painful stimulus is emerging as a viable intervention for adults and children undergoing acute painful medical procedures including burn wound treatment [see reviews by Dahlquist et al. (2007) and Patterson (1995)]. VR interventions may be particularly effective for pain distraction because they require considerable conscious attention and active participation, and involve multisensory input (Dahlquist et al. 2007). The neural correlates of VR-induced analgesia have been studied with fMRI, demonstrating that immersion in VR significantly reduces pain-related brain activity in all brain regions determined as active during painful stimulation (Hoffman et al. 2004a).

Recent studies have consistently shown that VR can function as a strong non-pharmacological pain reduction technique for both adults and children during burn wound care [see reviews by Mahrer and Gold (2009) and Wismeijer and Vingerhoets (2005)]. For example, Das et al. (2005) showed, in a small, randomised trial with seven children ages 5 to 18 years who acted as their own control, that self-rated pain intensity during wound dressing using medication only was 4.1 (on a 10-point scale), while the addition of VR significantly reduced pain severity to 1.3. Both the nurse administering the wound care and the parents concurred with the observation that the children's anxiety was markedly reduced during the VR sessions. Similarly, a within-patient design was utilised with 88 subjects, ages 6 to 65 years (75% of whom were younger than 18 years), to determine the effectiveness of VR immersion during painful physical therapy exercises. The exercise protocol was carefully controlled to ensure the same treatment duration and number of exercise repetitions during treatment with and without VR, while pain medication was held constant. The addition of VR distraction resulted in a significant 20% reduction in the subjects' worst pain intensity, a 26% reduction in pain unpleasantness, and a 37% reduction in the time spent thinking about the pain (Sharar et al. 2007). Furthermore, a study with seven subjects, ages 9 to 32 years, indicated that the analgesic effectiveness of VR does not diminish with three repeated interventions (Hoffman et al. 2001b).

The majority of VR studies done with children during post-burn care employed an HMD that blocks the view of the surrounding environment (i.e., the wound area and treatment equipment). Although some patients, particularly adults, reported that blocking the view lends to a lack of control and increased anxiety (van Twillert et al. 2007), the opposite was claimed for most patients, and particularly for children who regarded the surrounding environment as most stressful (Chan et al. 2007; Das et al. 2005; Gold et al. 2006; Hoffman et al. 2008; Sharar et al. 2007; van Twillert et al. 2007). Nausea, which, in the past, was a side effect attributed to the use of an HMD, was not a major issue in any of the studies with patients post-burn [see review by Wismeijer and Vingerhoets (2005)]. The highest rate of nausea was reported by Sharar et al. (2007) and occurred during post-burn physical therapy; 15% of the participants reported nausea as mild (15 on a 0 to 100 scale), while the remaining 85% reported no nausea.

In some cases, the use of an HMD may not be feasible or appropriate. Such is the case, for example, when on-going communication between the patient and the health provider is vital, or when the facial/head areas are burnt (van Twillert et al. 2007). Furthermore, special adaptations may be needed during wound care conducted while patients are submerged in a hydrotank in order to accommodate an HMD (Hoffman et al. 2008). While the effectiveness of VR displayed by an HMD has been shown to go beyond the effect of just blocking the view of the treatment environment (Gold et al. 2005), the application of HMD has not been compared with other VR platforms for pain alleviation. However, Mott et al. (2008) recently demonstrated that an augmentative VR system, which encouraged interaction with 3D animated characters displayed on a screen positioned in front of the child, was also more effective for pain reduction than other forms of distraction such as attention-distraction, positive reinforcement, relaxation and age-appropriate video programs.

VR simulations used during burn care generally encourage the children's active participation. For example, in the *SnowWorld* VE, children have the illusion of flying through an icy 3D environment depicting a virtual canyon, a river and waterfalls. During the interaction, the children shoot snowballs in various directions, at snowmen and igloos, while receiving appropriate visual and sound feedback (Hoffman et al. 2001b, 2008a,b; Sharar et al. 2007). However, the effect of the degree of immersion in the VE on pain alleviation is not yet clear. Sharar et al. (2007) examined the effectiveness of VR during post-burn physical therapy and determined that, while children provided higher subjective reports of 'presence' and 'realness' of the VE than did adults, age did not affect the analgesic effects of VR distraction. In contrast, in a study using experimental thermal pain, young adults (aged 18 to 20 years) who were exposed to two levels of immersive VR reported more pain reduction during the high immersion environment, with the amount of pain reduction positively and significantly correlated with the level of presence as reported by the subjects (Hoffman et al. 2004). Similarly, in a study of 11 patients (aged 9 to 40 years) whose wounds were treated with and without VR distraction, significant reductions in worst pain and pain unpleasantness were reported only by the six patients with the highest presence rating. In contrast, the five patients whose presence ratings were below the mean showed no significant changes in pain ratings. The study, however, did not report whether these differences may have been related to participant age (Hoffman et al. 2008).

As in other areas of VR research, the major methodological limitation of the reported studies concerns the use of small samples. However, because pain associated with burns is generally extremely high, burn patients are thought to be less easily distracted. Therefore, if VR interventions are significantly helpful in these situations, it is likely that they will work in less extreme conditions as well. In summary, the studies presented suggest that VR distraction is beneficial in alleviating children's pain without any significant side effects and can therefore serve as a viable adjunctive tool during the treatment of children undergoing painful therapeutic interventions.

SUMMARY AND CONCLUSIONS

As reviewed in this chapter, VR is now widely used as an educational tool for children, both as a means for imparting knowledge via active participation and as an opportunity to practice skills such as road crossing in preparation of participation in the actual task. Its use as an evaluation tool, for example, with children with ADHD, has been shown to surpass traditional paper-and-pen and computer-based tools due to its ability to engage children during the assessment. VR's inherent characteristic of playfulness has been used as a means to enhance social and communication skills and in the presentation of a variety of functional tasks, including road crossing, bus travel and restaurant dining, to children with ASD and IDD, and has been shown to provide opportunities to repetitively practice these skills in non-threatening settings. Moreover, positive social behaviours have been encouraged in children with ASD under circumstances where these behaviours can be 'enforced' via the virtual technology. The ability of VEs to motivate and distract individuals has been used very effectively to enhance the physical fitness of young people with IDD and to help children cope with painful treatments such as burn wound care. VR has also been shown to be a useful tool for achieving diverse intervention goals such as the rehabilitation of physical impairments and functional abilities (e.g., reaching and walking).

Despite these very encouraging results, VR-based rehabilitation is still a young, interdisciplinary field that is threatened by the double peril of the Gartner Group's Technology Hype Cycle (2010) as described by Rizzo (2002) and illustrated in Figure 9.8. It first ascended the 'Peak of Inflated Expectations' when

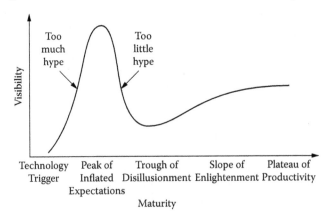

FIGURE 9.8 Gartner's Technology Hype Cycle showing the progression of emerging technologies from 'inflated expectations' to 'disillusionment' to 'enlightenment' and to 'productivity'. (Figure adapted from Weiss, P.L. and H. Ring. 2007. Commentary on virtual reality in stroke rehabilitation: Still more virtual than real. *Disability and Rehabilitation* 29:1147–1149.)

TABLE 9.1

Examples of Rehabilitation Technologies Illustrating Progress from the Recent Past (mid-1990s to early 2000s) to the Present (mid-2000s to 2010) and to the Likely Near Future (next 5 to 10 years)

	VR Applications for Paediatrics
Recent Past (mid-1990s to early 2000s)	VR primarily for assessment and recreation
	Computer games
	2D desktop and video capture simulations
	Cumbersome equipment (e.g., large and heavy HMDs and haptic devices)
Present (mid-2000s to 2010)	VR as an assessment and intervention tool
	Customized and off-the-shelf interactive 2D simulations with some 3D simulations available
	Size and weight of interface equipment considerably reduced
	Emergence of intelligent agents that act as therapists or mediators
Future (next 5 to 10 years)	VR for all
	Fully interactive 3D simulations with full feedback modes (visual, auditory, haptic, vestibular, olfactory)
	Ambient intelligence for wireless any time, any place accessibility for cooperative interactions
	Intelligent personal agents who are reliable and autonomous
	Tele-evaluation online analysis with feedback to patient

the media (and some researchers) over-rated the technology's potential applications. Therapists who viewed the level of simulation achieved in Hollywood movies and science museums considered whether VR could, in fact, be used clinically. However, images of children with ASD wearing massive HMDs (Strickland 1996) caused VR technology to quickly plummet into the 'Trough of Disillusionment.' At that point in time (as little as 5 to 10 years ago), due to technological limitations in both hardware and software, many therapists became frustrated by the lack of inexpensive, clinically relevant and readily available applications.

Table 9.1 highlights some of the key recent past, present and future applications of VR for children, indicating the progression of VR from a primarily 2D assessment tool to a more interactive 3D assessment and intervention tool. VR-based rehabilitation is now progressing along the Hype Cycle toward the 'Slope of Enlightenment' and in some clinical applications, notably, distraction therapy for pain and recreational opportunities for people with IDD, has even reached the 'Plateau of Productivity' where VR's assets are widely demonstrated and accepted (Rizzo and Kim 2005; Weiss and Ring 2007).

The paediatric VR intervention literature base remains small and limited from a methodological viewpoint. The early VR studies were clearly and necessarily focused on the development of novel applications and the demonstration of system feasibility with small numbers of participants belonging to a variety of populations. Moreover, most studies that examined effectiveness did not use robust control groups wherein VR-based intervention was compared to conventional therapy (Weiss and Ring 2007). Given the rapid development of VR technologies, on-going work will continue to be an essential contribution to the literature.

In applications of paediatric rehabilitation for both motor and cognitive deficits, the main focus of much of the early exploratory research was on the investigation of VR as an assessment tool. However, in the 2000s, the emphasis of research has shifted to also include clinical intervention studies with larger samples sizes. For example, Sharar et al. (2007) conducted a randomised control trial investigating the effect of VR distraction analgesia during physical therapy (n = 88 participants). The exercise protocol was carefully controlled to ensure the same treatment duration and number of exercise repetitions during treatment with and without VR, while pain medication was held constant. The addition of VR distraction resulted in significant reductions in the patients' worst pain intensity, pain unpleasantness, and time spent thinking about the pain. New studies are being published on a regular basis and are contributing to a growing body of evidence in support of VR-based rehabilitation; for example, see our own recent papers on applications of VEs for children with ASD (Josman et al. 2008; Gal et al. 2009).

Three recent papers have reviewed the state of VR in paediatric rehabilitation. Parsons et al. (2009) published a general review of VR applications in paediatric rehabilitation. Sandlund et al. (2009) evaluated the evidence on the effect of interactive computer play in children with sensorimotor disorders. This review included studies utilizing both traditional computer games as well as VR applications, applied as therapeutic intervention tools. Laufer and Weiss (submitted) evaluated the evidence from all studies published in English language peer-reviewed journals pertaining to the application of VR technology to the assessment and treatment of children with sensorimotor deficits. All three reviews conclude that the evidence to date is both positive and encouraging but that further, controlled studies are necessary.

RECOMMENDATIONS

To date the VEs used in paediatric rehabilitation are primarily (1) single-user (i.e., designed for and used by only one clinical client at a time) and (2) used locally within a clinical or educational setting. More recently, researchers have begun the development of new and more complex VR-based approaches according to two dimensions: the number of users and the distance between the users. Driven by a technology push and clinical pull phenomenon, the original approach has now expanded to three additional avenues: multiple users in co-located settings, single users in remote locations, and multiple users in remote locations. As a result, the VR paediatric rehabilitation research community needs to address the new concerns that are associated with such novel VEs.

There are several key issues that need to be addressed as VEs expand from being primarily supportive of single users in local locations, toward accommodating multiple users in local and remote locations. One important concern is user perspective; additional research is necessary to determine the importance of providing children with first, third or bird's eye perspectives. Such decisions, in the past, were typically driven by the technology selected to render the VE. In the future, such decisions should depend more upon the therapeutic needs of children with varying disabilities and the optimal presentation of therapeutic goals. Furthermore, the need to achieve a high level of virtual presence has generally been assumed in order to stimulate motivation and performance. This assumption needs to be more directly tested using outcome measures that are sensitive to this construct.

Another essential issue to consider is the availability of inexpensive and technically simple software and hardware. One cannot expect a remote, or even a typical, clinical setting to have access to high-end equipment nor to a team of programmers and technicians to provide support. The debate between the use of off-the-shelf vs. customised VR platforms continues to rage. Cheap and technically simple devices such as the Sony Playstation II EyeToy and the Nintendo Wii are highly attractive to clinicians. However, these devices have been designed for use with a wide population and are rarely adaptable for special needs. Although initial evidence demonstrates that they can be feasible and effective tools (Deutsch et al. 2008), they can also be misused if care is not taken to overcome their inherent limitations. For example, the desired therapeutic movements (e.g., shoulder abduction over a large range of motion) can be mimicked by compensatory movements (e.g., shoulder flexion over a smaller range of motion) without the VR system recognizing the substitution (Rand et al. 2008). Moreover, the easiest levels of games often require skills beyond the abilities of many patients.

Finally, it is important to recognise that the most functional VEs have been customised by specific research groups, and thus are often unavailable to other clinical researchers or, when available, are not readily customizable for other applications (e.g., for use in other languages or for different clinical populations). The recently publicised NeuroVR initiative (2007) provides a cost-free VE editor that allows non-expert users to easily set up and tune VEs including a supermarket, apartment, park, office, high school, university and restaurant. These VEs can then be run on the NeuroVR Player. Both are downloadable at no cost.

In conclusion, the rapid development of VR-based technologies over the past 15 years has been both an asset and a challenge for paediatric rehabilitation. As this review has illustrated, the availability of novel technologies that provide interactive, functional simulations with multimodal feedback enables clinicians to achieve traditional therapeutic goals that would be difficult, if not impossible, to attain via conventional therapy.

REFERENCES

American Psychiatric Association (APA). 2000. *Diagnostic and statistical manual of mental disorders (4th Edition-Text Revision)*. Arlington, VA: American Psychiatric Association.

Andonian, B., W. Rauch, and V. Bhise. 2003. Driver steering performance using joystick vs. steering wheel controls. *Human Factors in Driving, Seating, & Vision* (SP-1772). http://brianandonian.com/Documents/2003-01-0118.pdf (accessed May 27, 2009).

Anttila, H., J. Suoranta, A. Malmivaara, M. Mäkelä, and I. Autti-Rämö. 2008. Effectiveness of physiotherapy and conductive education interventions in children with cerebral palsy: A focused review. *Am J Phys Med Rehabil* 87(6):478–501.

Austermann Hula, S.N., D.A. Robin, E. Maas et al. 2008. Effects of feedback frequency and timing on acquisition, retention, and transfer of speech skills in acquired apraxia of speech. *J Speech Lang Hear Res* 51(5):1088–1113.

Bailey, F. and M. Moar. 2001. The vertex project: Children creating and populating 3D virtual worlds. *Jade* 20(1):19–30.

Barkley, R.A. 1990. *Attention deficit hyperactivity disorder: A handbook for diagnosis and treatment.* New York: Guilford Press.

Barkley, R.A. 1997. Behavioral inhibition, sustained attention, and executive functions: Constructing a unifying theory of ADHD. *Psychological Bulletin* 121(1):65–94.

Baron-Cohen, S. and P. Howlin. 1998. *Teaching children with autism to mind-read: A practical guide for teachers and parents.* New York: Wiley.

Bart, O., N. Katz, P.L. Weiss, and N. Josman. 2008. Street crossing by typically developed children in real and virtual environments. *OTJR: Occupation, Participation and Health* 28(2):89–96.

Basu, S. 2002. *The pediatric volitional questionnaire: A psychometric study.* Chicago: University of Illinois.

Bauminger, N. 2002. The facilitation of social-emotional understanding and social interaction in high-functioning children with autism: Intervention outcomes. *Journal of Autism and Developmental Disorders* 32:283–298.

Bax, M., M. Goldstein, P. Rosenbaum, A. Leviton, N. Paneth, B. Dan, B. Jacobsson, and D. Damiano. 2005. Proposed definition and classification of cerebral palsy, April 2005. *Developmental Medicine and Child Neurology* 47(8):571–576.

Bordnick, P., K.M. Graap, H.L. Copp, J.S. Brooks, M. Ferrer, and B. Logue. 2004. Utilizing virtual reality to standardize nicotine craving research: A pilot study, *Addictive Behaviors* 29:1889–1894.

Bowman, D.A., L.F. Hodges, D. Allison, and J. Wineman. 1999. The educational value of an information-rich virtual environment. *Presence* 8(3):317–331.

Brown, D.J., H.R. Neale, S.V.G. Cobb, and H. Reynolds. 1999. Development and evaluation of the virtual city. *International Journal of Virtual Reality* 4:28–41.

Bryanton, C., J. Bosse, M. Brien, J. McLean, A. McCormick, and H. Sveistrup. 2006. Feasibility, motivation, and selective motor control: Virtual reality compared to conventional home exercise in children with cerebral palsy. *Cyberpsychology and Behavior* 9(2):123–128.

Bundy, A.C. 2003. *Test of playfulness (ToP)* Vol. Ver. 4.0. Sydney, Australia: University of Sydney.

Butler, C. and J. Darrah. 2001. Effects of neurodevelopmental treatment (NDT) for cerebral palsy: An AACPDM evidence report. *Developmental Medicine and Child Neurology* 43(11):778–790.

Campbell, S.K. 2000. *Physical therapy for children.* Philadelphia: WB Saunders Co.

Cassell, J. 2004. Towards a model of technology and literacy development: Story listening systems. *Journal of Applied Developmental Psychology* 25(1):75–105.

Cassell, J. and T. Bickmore. 2003. Negotiated collusion: Modeling social language and its relationship effects in intelligent agents. *User Modeling and User-Adapted Interaction* 13(1–2):89–132.

CAVE. 2001. The CAVE virtual reality system. http://www.evl.uic.edu/pape/CAVE/ (accessed December 16, 2009).

Chakrabarti S. and E. Fombonne. 2001. Pervasive developmental disorders in preschool children. *Journal of the American Medical Association* 285(24):3093–3099.

Chan, E.A., J.W. Chung, T.K. Wong et al. 2007. Application of a virtual reality prototype for pain relief of pediatric burn in Taiwan. *Journal of Clinical Nursing* 16(4):786–793.

Chapman, C.R. and Y. Nakamura. 1998. Hypnotic analgesia: A constructivist framework. *International Journal of Clinical and Experimental Hypnosis* 46(1):6–27.

Chen, Y.P., L.J. Kang, T.Y. Chuang, J.L. Doong, S.J. Lee, M.W. Tsai, S.F. Jeng, and W.H. Sung. 2007. Use of virtual reality to improve upper-extremity control in children with cerebral palsy: A single-subject design. *Physical Therapy* 87(11):1441–1457.

Christiansen, C., B. Abreu, K. Ottenbacher, K. Huffman, B. Massel, and R. Culpepper. 1998. Task performance in virtual environments used for cognitive rehabilitation after traumatic brain injury. *Archives* 79:888–892.

Clancy, T.A., J.J. Rucklidge, and D. Owen. 2006. Road-crossing safety in virtual reality: A comparison of adolescents with and without ADHD. *Journal of Clinical Child and Adolescent Psychology* 35(2):203–215.

Cobb, S.V.G., H.R. Neale, and H. Reynolds. 1998. An emergent testing methodology for the evaluation of virtual learning environments. *Proceedings of Second European Conference on Disability, Virtual Reality & Associated Technologies*, ECDVRAT, September 1998, Skovde, Sweden, 17–23.

Cobb, S., L. Beardon, R. Eastgate, T. Glover, S. Kerr, H. Neale, S. Parsons, S. Benford, E. Hopkins, P. Mitchell, G. Reynard, and J.R. Wilson. 2002. Applied virtual environments to support learning of social interaction skills in users with Asperger's Syndrome. *Digital Creativity*, 13:11–22.

Cromby, J.J., P.J. Standen, and D.J. Brown. 1996. The potentials of virtual environments in the education and training of people with learning disabilities. *Journal of Intellectual Disability Research* 40:489–501.

Dahlquist, L.M., K.D. McKenna, K.K. Jones et al. 2007. Active and passive distraction using a head-mounted display helmet: Effects on cold pressor pain in children. *Health Psychology* 26(6):794–801.

Damiano, D.L., and S.L. DeJong. 2009. A systematic review of the effectiveness of treadmill training and body weight support in pediatric rehabilitation. *Journal of Neurologic Physical Therapy* 33(1):27–44.

Das, D.A., K.A. Grimmer, A.L. Sparnon et al. 2005. The efficacy of playing a virtual reality game in modulating pain for children with acute burn injuries: A randomized controlled trial [ISRCTN87413556]. *BMC Pediatrics* 5(1):1.

Dautenhahn, K. and I. Werry. 2002. A quantitative technique for analysing robot-human interactions. *IEEE/RSJ International Conference on Intelligent Robots and Systems*, Lausanne, Switzerland, 1132–1138.

Deluca, S.C., K. Echols, C.R. Law, and S.L. Ramey. 2006. Intensive pediatric constraint-induced therapy for children with cerebral palsy: Randomized, controlled, crossover trial. *Journal of Child Neurology* 21(11):931–938.

Deutsch, J.E., A.S. Merians, G.C. Burdea, R. Boian, S.V. Adamovich, and H. Poizner. 2002. Haptics and virtual reality used to increase strength and improve function in chronic individuals post-stroke: Two case reports. *Neurology Report* 26:79–86.

Deutsch, J.E., M. Borbely, J. Filler, K. Huhn, and P. Guarrera-Bowlby. 2008. Use of a low-cost, commercially available gaming console (Wii) for rehabilitation of an adolescent with cerebral palsy. *Physical Therapy* 88(10):1196–1207.

Dietz, P.H. and D.L. Leigh. 2001. DiamondTouch: A multi-user touch technology. Paper presented at the *ACM Symposium on User Interface Software and Technology (UIST)*, New York.

Durfee, W. 2001. Multi-modal virtual environments or haptics does not stand alone. *Proceedings of the Haptics, Virtual Reality, and Human Computer Interaction, Institute for Mathematics and its Applications*, Minneapolis, MN.

Eliasson, A.C., B. Rosblad, and C. Hager-Ross. 2003. Control of reaching movements in 6-year-old prematurely born children with motor problems—and intervention study. *Advances in Physiotherapy* 5:33–48.

eMagin Corporation. 2010. www.emagin.com/ (accessed December 16, 2009).

Ensher, E.A., C. Heun, and A. Blanchard. 2003. Online mentoring and computer-mediated communication: New directions in research. *Journal of Vocational Behavior* 63:264–288.

Feintuch, U., L. Raz, J. Hwang, J. Yongseok, N. Josman, N. Katz, R. Kizony, D. Rand, A.A. Rizzo, M. Shahar, and P.L. Weiss. 2006. Integrating haptic-tactile feedback into a video-capture-based virtual environment for rehabilitation. *CyberPsychology and Behavior* 9:129–132.

Finn, J. 1999. An exploration of helping process in an online self-help group focusing on issues of disability. *Health & Social Work* 24:220–231.

Floery, L. 1981. Studies of play: Implications for growth, development, and for clinical practice. *American Journal Occupational Therapy* 25:275–280.

Foreman, N., S. Boyd-Davis, M. Moar, L. Korallo, and E. Chappell. 2008. Can virtual environments enhance the learning of historical chronology? *Instructional Science* 36:155–173.

Gal, E., N. Bauminger, D. Goren-Bar, F. Pianesi, O. Stock, M. Zancanaro, and P.L. Weiss. 2009. Enhancing social communication of children with high functioning autism through a co-located interface. *Artificial Intelligence & Society* 24:75–84.

Gartner Inc. 2010. Gartner's Group. www4.gartner.com (accessed December 16, 2009).

GestureTek's IREX VR system. www.questuretekhealth.com (accessed December 16, 2009).

Gold, J., G. Reger, A. Rizzo et al. 2005. Virtual reality in outpatient phlebotomy: Evaluating pediatric pain distraction during blood draw. *Journal of Pain* 6(3):S57–S57.

Gold, J.I., S.H. Kim, A.J. Kant et al. 2005. Effectiveness of virtual reality for pediatric pain distraction during i.v. placement. *Cyberpsychology & Behavior* 9(2):207–212.

Greenberg, L.M. and I. Waldman. 1993. Developmental normative data on the Test of Variables of Attention. *Journal of Child Psychology & Psychiatry* 34:1019–1030.

Grynszpan, O., J.C. Martin, and J. Nadel. 2005. Designing educational software dedicated to people with autism. In *Assistive Technology: From Virtuality to Reality*, A. Pruski and H. Knops, Eds. Proceedings of AAATE, Lille, France: IOS Press, 456–460.

Harris, K. and D. Reid. 2005. The influence of virtual reality play on children's motivation. *Canadian Journal of Occupational Therapy* 72(1):21–29.

Harvey, R.L. 2009. Improving poststroke recovery: Neuroplasticity and task-oriented training. *Current Treatmeent Options in Cardiovascular Medicine* 11(3):251–259.

Hasdai, A., A.S. Jessel, and P.L. Weiss. 1998. Use of a computer simulator for training children with disabilities in the operation of a powered wheelchair. *American Journal of Occupational Therapy* 52(3):215–220.

Hay, D.F., A. Payne, and A. Chadwick. 2004. Peer relations in childhood. *Journal of Child Psychology and Psychiatry* 45:84–108.

Hayes, M.S., I.R. McEwen, D. Lovett, M.M. Sheldon, and D.W. Smith. 1999. Next step: Survey of pediatric physical therapist's educational needs and perceptions of motor control, motor development and motor learning as they relate to services for children with developmental disabilities. *Pediatric Physical Therapy* 11(4):164–182.

Henderson, A., N. Korner-Bitensky, and M. Levin. 2007. Virtual reality in stroke rehabilitation: A systematic review of its effectiveness for upper limb motor recovery. *Top Stroke Rehabilitation* 14(2):52–61.

Herndon, D.N. *Total burn care.* 3rd ed. Saunders, London: Elsevier.

Hestenes, L.L. and D.E. Carroll. 2000. The play interactions of young children with and without disabilities: Individual and environmental influences. *Early Childhood Research Quarterly* 15(2):229–246.

Hoffman, H.G., J. Prothero, M.J. Wells, and J. Groen. 1998. Virtual chess: Meaning enhances users' sense of presence in virtual environments. *International Journal of Human-Computer Interaction* 10:251–263.

Hoffman, H.G., A. Garcia-Palacios, D.R. Patterson et al. 2001. The effectiveness of virtual reality for dental pain control: A case study. *Cyberpsychology & Behavior* 4(4):527–535.

Hoffman, H.G., D.R. Patterson, G.J. Carrougher, et al. 2001. Effectiveness of virtual reality-based pain control with multiple treatments. *Clinical Journal of Pain* 17(3):229–235.

Hoffman, H.G., D.R. Patterson, E. Seibel et al. 2008. Virtual reality pain control during burn wound debridement in the hydrotank. *Clinical Journal of Pain* 24(4):299–304.

Hoffman, H.G., D.R. Patterson, M. Soltani, et al. In press. Virtual reality pain control during physical therapy range of motion exercises for a patient with multiple blunt force trauma injuries. *Cyberpsychology & Behavior* 12(1):47–49.

Hoffman, H.G., T.L. Richards, B. Coda et al. 2004. Modulation of thermal pain-related brain activity with virtual reality: Evidence from fMRI. *Neuroreport* 15(8):1245–1248.

Hoffman, H.G., S.R. Sharar, B. Coda et al. 2004. Manipulating presence influences the magnitude of virtual reality analgesia. *Pain* 111(1–2):162–168.

Holden, M.K. 2005. Virtual environments for motor rehabilitation: Review. *Cyberpsychology & Behavior* 8(3):187–211; discussion 212–219.

Howard, L. 1996. A comparison of leisure time activities between able-bodied children and children with physical disabilities. *British Journal of Occupational Therapy* 59:570–574.

Inman, D.P., K. Loge, and J. Leavens. 1997. VR education and rehabilitation. *Communications ACM* 40:53–55.

InterSense Incorporated. 1996. Intersense InterTrax2. www.isense.com (accessed December 16, 2009).

IJsselsteijn, W.A., H. de Ridder, and J. Freeman. 2000. Avons SE Presence: Concept, determinants, and measurement. *Proceedings of the SPIE, Human Vision and Electronic Imaging V*. Presented at Photonics West, Human Vision and Electronic Imaging V, January 23–28, San Jose, CA, 3959–3976.

Jack, D., R. Boian, A.Merians, M. Tremaine, G.C. Burdea, S.V. Adamovich, M. Recce, and H. Poizner. 2001. Virtual reality-enhanced stroke rehabilitation. *IEEE Transactions of Neural Systems and Rehabilitation Engineering* 9:308–318.

Josman, N., H. Milika Ben-Chaim, S. Friedrich, and P.L. Weiss. 2008. Effectiveness of virtual reality for teaching street-crossing skills to children and adolescents with autism. *International Journal on Disability and Human Development* 7:49–56.

Kaplan, E.F., H. Goodglass, and S. Weintraub. 1983. *The Boston naming test,* 2nd ed. Philadelphia, PA: Febiger.

Katz, N., H. Ring, Y. Naveh, R. Kizony, U. Feintuch, and P.L. Weiss. 2005. Effect of interactive virtual environment training on independent safe street crossing of stroke patients with unilateral spatial neglect. *Disability & Rehabilitation* 27:1235–1243.

Keshner, E.A. and R.V. Kenyon. 2009. Postural and spatial orientation driven by virtual reality. In *Advanced technologies in neurorehabilitation*, A. Gagglioli, E.A. Keshner, P.L. Weiss, G. Riva, Eds. Amsterdam: IOS Press, 209-229.

Kim, P. 2006. Effects of 3D virtual reality of plate tectonics on fifth grade students' achievement and attitude towards science. *Interactive Learning Environments* 14(1):25–34.

Kizony, R., N. Katz, and P.L. Weiss. 2003. Adapting an immersive virtual reality system for rehabilitation. *Journal of Visualization and Computer Animation* 14:261–268.

Kwakkel, G., R. van Peppen, R.C. Wagenaar, S. Wood Dauphinee, C. Richards, A. Ashburn, K. Miller, N. Lincoln, C. Partridge, I. Wellwood, and P. Langhorne. 2004. Effects of augmented exercise therapy time after stroke: A meta-analysis. *Stroke* 35(11):2529–2539.

Landa, R. 2000. Social language use in Asperger syndrome and in high-functioning autism. In *Asperger syndrome*, A. Klin, F.R. Volkmar, and S.S. Sparrow, Eds. New York: Guilford Press, 121–155.

Lord, C., M. Rutter, and A. LeCouteur. 1994. Autism diagnostic interview-revised: A revised version of a diagnostic interview for caregivers of individuals with possible pervasive developmental disorders. *Journal of Autism & Developmental Disorders* 19:185–212.

Lotan, M., S. Yalon-Chamovitz, and P. L. Weiss. 2009. Improving physical fitness of individuals with intellectual and developmental disability through a virtual reality intervention program. *Research in Developmental Disabilities* 30(2):229–239.

Mahrer, N.E. and J.I. Gold. 2009. The use of virtual reality for pain control: A review. *Current Pain and Headache Reports* 13(2):100–109.

Mania, K. and A. Chalmers. 2001. The effects of levels of immersion on memory and presence in virtual environments: A reality centered approach. *CyberPsychology & Behavior* 4:247–264.

Mantovani, F. and G. Castelnuovo. 2003. Sense of presence in virtual training: Enhancing skills acquisition and transfer of knowledge through learning experience in virtual environments. In *Being There: Concepts, Effects and Measurement of User Presence in Synthetic Environments*, G. Riva, F. Davide, W.A. IJsselsteijn, Eds. Amsterdam, the Netherlands: IOS Press.

McComas, J., M. MacKay, and J. Pivik. 2002. Effectiveness of virtual reality for teaching pedestrian safety. *CyberPsychology & Behavior* 5(3):185–190.

Miller, S. and D. Reid. 2003. Doing play: Competency, control, and expression. *Cyberpsychology & Behavior* 6(6):623–632.

Missiuna, C. and N. Pollock. 1991. Play deprivation in children with physical disabilities; the role of the occupational therapist in presenting secondary disability. *American Journal of Occupational Therapy* 45:882–888.

Mitchell, P., S. Parsons, and A. Leonard. 2007. Using virtual environments for teaching social understanding to adolescents with autistic spectrum disorders. *Journal of Autism and Developmental Disorder* 37: 589–600.

Mockford, M. and J.M. Caulton. 2008. Systematic review of progressive strength training in children and adolescents with cerebral palsy who are ambulatory. *Pediatric Physical Therapy* 20(4):318–333.

Motek Medical. 1994. Motek's CAREN. www.motekmedical.com/ (accessed December 16, 2009).

Mott, J., S. Bucolo, L. Cuttle et al. 2008. The efficacy of an augmented virtual reality system to alleviate pain in children undergoing burns dressing changes: A randomised controlled trial. *Burns* 34(6):803–808.

Murray, D.K.C. 1997. Autism and information technology: Therapy with computers. In *Autism and Learning: A Guide to Good Practice*, S. Powell and R. Jordan, Eds. London: David Fulton Publishers.

Nash, E.B., Edwards, G.W., Thompson, J.A., and W. Barfield. 2000. A review of presence and performance in virtual environments. *International Journal of Human-Computer Interaction* 12:1–41.

Neale, H.R., S.V. Cobb, S. Kerr, and A. Leonard. 2002. Exploring the role of virtual environments in the special needs classroom. *Proceedings of the 4th International Conference on Disability, Virtual Reality and Associated Technologies* (ICDVRAT), September 2002, Veszprem, Hungary, 259–266.

NeuroVR. 2007. NeuroVR Initiative. www.neurovr.org (accessed December 16, 2009).

Nintendo. 2006. Nintendo Wii. http://www.nintendo.com/wii (accessed December 16, 2009).

Novint Technologies. 2010. Novint's Falcon. http://home.novint.com (accessed December 16, 2009).

Nudo, R.J., E.J. Plautz, and S.B. Frost. 2001. Role of adaptive plasticity in recovery of function after damage to motor cortex. *Muscle & Nerve* 24(8):1000–1019.

Page, S.J., P. Levine, S. Sisto, Q. Bond, and M. V. Johnston. 2002. Stroke patients' and therapists' opinions of constraint-induced movement therapy. *Clinical Rehabilitation* 16(1):55–60.

Parker, J.G., K.H. Rubin, J.M. Price, and M.E. DeRosier. 1995. Peer relationships, child development, and adjustment: A developmental psychopathology perspective. In *Developmental Psychopathology*, D. Cicchetti and D.J. Cohen, Eds. New York: Wiley, 96–161.

Parsons, S., L. Beardon, H.R. Neale, G. Reynard, R. Eastgate, J.R. Wilson, S.V. Cobb, S. Benford, P. Mitchell, and E. Hopkins. 2000. Development of social skills amongst adults with Asperger's Syndrome using virtual environments: The AS Interactive project. *Proceedings of the 3rd International Conference on Disability, Virtual Reality and Associated Technologies*, Sardinia, 163–170.

Parsons, S. 2001. Social conventions in virtual environments: Investigating understanding of personal space amongst people with autistic spectrum disorders. *Robotic & Virtual Interactive Systems in Autism Therapy.* University of Hertfordshire, Hatfield, U.K.

Parsons, S., P. Mitchell, and A. Leonard. 2004. The use and understanding of virtual environments by adolescents with autistic spectrum disorders. *Journal of Autism and Developmental Disorders* 34: 449–466

Parsons, S., P. Mitchell, and A. Leonard. 2005. Do adolescents with autistic spectrum disorders adhere to social conventions in virtual environments? *Autism* 9: 95–117.

Parsons, S., A. Leonard, and P. Mitchell. 2006. Virtual environments for social skills training: Comments from two adolescents with autistic spectrum disorder. *Computers & Education* 47:186–206.

Parsons, T.D., T. Bowerly, J. Galen Buckwalter, and A.A Rizzo. 2007. A controlled clinical comparison of attention performance in children with ADHD in a virtual reality classroom compared to standard neuropsychological methods. *Child Neuropsychology* 13:363–381.

Parsons, T.D., A.A. Rizzo, S. Rogers, and P. York. 2009. Virtual reality in paediatric rehabilitation: A review. *Developmental Neurorehabilitation* 12(4):224–238.

Patterson, D.R. 1995. Non-opioid-based approaches to burn pain. *Journal of Burn Care & Rehabilitation* 16(3 Pt 2):372–376.

Perry, S. and G. Heidrich. 1982. Management of pain during debridement: A survey of U.S. burn units. *Pain* 13(3):267–280.

Pivik, J., J. McComas, I. MacFarlane, and M. LaFlamme. 2002. Using virtual reality to teach disability awareness. *Journal of Educational Computing Research* 26(2):203–218.

Pollak, Y., P.L. Weiss, A.A. Rizzo, V. Gross-Tsur, and R. Shalev. 2009. The utility of a continuous performance test embedded in virtual reality in measuring ADHD-related deficits. *Journal of Developmental and Behavioral Pediatrics* 30(1):2–6.

Pugnetti, L., L. Mendozzi, E. Attree, E. Barbieri, B.M. Brooks, C.L. Cazzullo, A. Motta, and F.D. Rose. 1998. Probing memory and executive functions with virtual reality: Past and present studies. *CyberPsychology & Behavior* 1:151–162.

Rand, D., R. Kizony, U. Feintuch, N. Katz, N. Josman, A.A. Rizzo, and P.L. Weiss. 2005. Comparison of two VR platforms for rehabilitation: Video capture versus HMD. *Presence, Teleoperators and Virtual Environments* 14:147–160.

Rand, D., N. Katz, R. Kizony, and P.L. Weiss. 2005. The virtual mall: A functional virtual environment for stroke rehabilitation. *Annual Review of CyberTherapy and Telemedicine: A Decade of VR* 3:193–198.

Rand, D., R. Kizony, and P.L. Weiss, P.L. 2008. The Sony PlayStation II EyeToy: Low-cost virtual reality for use in rehabilitation. *Journal of Neurologic Physical Therapy* 32:155–163.

Reid, D. 2002. The use of virtual reality to improve upper-extremity efficiency skills in children with cerebral palsy: A pilot study. *Technology and Disability* 14:53–61.

Reid, D. 2004. The influence of virtual reality on playfulness in children with cerebral palsy: A pilot study. *Occupational Therapy International* 11(3):131–144.

Reid, D. and K. Campbell. 2006. The use of virtual reality with children with cerebral palsy: A pilot randomized trial. *Therapeutic Recreation Journal* 40(4):255–268.

Reinkensmeyer, D.J., M.G. Iobbi, L.E. Kahn, D.G. Kamper, and C.D. Takahashi. 2003. Modeling reaching impairment after stroke using a population vector model of movement control that incorporates neural firing-rate variability. *Neural Computing* 15:2619–2642.

Rizzo, A.A., J.G. Buckwalter, and U. Neumann. 1997. Virtual reality and cognitive rehabilitation: A brief review of the future. *Journal of Head Trauma Rehabilitation* 12:1–15.

Rizzo, A.A. 2002. Virtual reality and disability: Emergence and challenge. *Disability & Rehabilitation* 24:567–569.

Rizzo, A.A., M.T. Schultheis, K. Kerns, and C. Mateer. 2004. Analysis of assets for virtual reality in neuropsychology. *Neuropsychology Rehabilitation* 14:207–239.

Rizzo, A.A., T. Bowerly, C. Shahabi, J. Galen Buckwalter, D. Klimchuk, and R. Mitura. 2004. Diagnosing attention disorders in a virtual classroom. *Computer* 87–89.

Rizzo, A.A. and G. Kim. 2005. A SWOT analysis of the field of virtual rehabilitation and therapy. *Presence: Teleoperators and Virtual Environments* 14:1–28.

Rizzo, A.A., T. Bowerly, J. Galen Buckwalter, D. Klimchuk, R. Mitura, and T.D. Parsons. 2006. A virtual reality scenario for all seasons: The virtual classroom. *CNS Spectrums* 11(1):35–44.

Robertson, J. and J. Good. 2005. Children's narrative development through computer game authoring. *TechTrends* 49(5):43–59.

Rose, F.D., E.A. Attree, B.M. Brooks, D.M. Parslow, P.R. Penn, and N. Ambihaipahan. 1998. Transfer of training from virtual to real environments. *Proceedings of 2nd European Conference on Disability, Virtual Reality & Associated Technologies*, ECDVRAT, September, Skovde, Sweden, 69–75.

Rose, F.D., B.M. Brooks, and E.A. Attree. 2000. Virtual reality in vocational training of people with learning disabilities. *Proceedings of the 3rd International Conference on Disability, Virtual Reality and Associated Technologies* (ICDVRAT), September 23–25, Sardinia, 129–135.

Rousso, H. 2001. What do Frida Kahlo, Wilma Mankiller, and Harriet Tubman have in common? Providing role models for girls with (and without) disabilities. In *Double jeopardy: Addressing gender equity in special education,* H. Rousso, and M. Wehmeyer, Eds. Albany, NY: State University of New York Press, 337–360.

Ryokai, K., C. Vaucelle, and J. Cassell. 2003. Virtual peers as partners in storytelling and literacy learning. *Journal of Computer Assisted Learning* 19(2):195–208.

Sander Wint, S., D. Eshelman, J. Steele et al. 2002. Effects of distraction using virtual reality glasses during lumbar punctures in adolescents with cancer. *Oncology Nursing Forum* 29 (1):E8–E15.

Sandlund, M., S. McDonough, and C. Hager-Ross. 2009. Interactive computer play in rehabilitation of children with sensorimotor disorders: A systematic review. *Developmental Medicine & Child Neurology* 51(3):173–179.

Schultheis, M.T. and A.A. Rizzo. 2001. The application of virtual reality technology for rehabilitation. *Rehabilitation Psychology* 46:296–311.

Schuemie, M.J., P. van der Straaten, M. Krijn, and C.A.P.G. van der Mast. 2001. Research on presence in virtual reality: A survey. *Cyberpsychology & Behavior* 4:183–201.

Schwebel, D.C., J. Gaines, and J. Severson. 2008. Validation of virtual reality as a tool to understand and prevent child pedestrian injury. *Accident Analysis and Prevention* 40:1394–1400.

Sharar, S.R., G.J. Carrougher, D. Nakamura et al. 2007. Factors influencing the efficacy of virtual reality distraction analgesia during postburn physical therapy: Preliminary results from 3 ongoing studies. *Archives of Physical Medicine and Rehabilitation* 88(12 Suppl 2):S43–49.

Sheridan, T.B. 1992. Musings on telepresence and virtual presence. *Presence: Teleoperators and Virtual Environments* 1:120–125.

Shpigelman, C., S. Reiter, and P.L. Weiss. 2008. E-mentoring for youth with special needs: Preliminary results. *CyberPsychology & Behavior* 11:196–200.

Sigman, M. and E. Ruskin. 1999. Continuity and change in the social competence of children with autism, Down Syndrome, and developmental delays. *Monographs of the Society for Research in Child Development* 64(1), Serial No. 256.

Silver, M. and P. Oakes. 2001. Evaluation of a new computer intervention to teach people with autism or Asperger syndrome to recognize and predict emotions in others. *Autism* 5(3):299–316.

Single, P.B. C.B. Muller and C.M. Cunningham. (1999). MentorNet: Lessons Learned from electronic communities for women engineers. *Proceedings of the Institute of Electrical and Electronics Engineers (IEEE) International Symposium on Technology and Society* (pp. 376–43), New Brunswick,NJ.

Slade, A. and D. Palmer Wolf. 1994. *Children at play: Clinical and developmental approaches to meaning and representation.* Oxford: Oxford University Press.

Slater, M. 1999. Measuring presence: A response to the Witmer and Singer questionnaire. *Presence: Teleoperators and Virtual Environments* 8:560–566.

Slater, M. 2003. A note on presence terminology. *Presence-Connect* 3.

Slater, M., C. Guger, and G. Edinger. 2006. Analysis of physiological responses to a social situation in an immersive virtual environment. *Presence: Teleoperators and Virtual Environments* 15:553–569.

Stanney, K.M., R.R. Mourant, and R.S. Kennedy.1998. Human factors issues in virtual environments: A review of the literature. *Presence* 7:327–351.

Stanton, D., N. Foreman, and P.N. Wilson. 1998. Uses of virtual reality in clinical training: Developing the spatial skills of children with mobility impairments. In *Virtual environments in clinical psychology and neuroscience*, G. Riva, B.K. Wiederhold, and E. Molinari, Eds. Amsterdam, the Netherlands: IOS Press.

Strickland, D., L.M. Marcus, G.B. Mesibov, and K. Hogan. 1996. Brief report: Two case studies using virtual reality as a learning tool for autistic children. *Journal of Autism and Developmental Disorder* 26:651–659.

Sun, K., Y. Lin, and C. Yu. 2008. A study on learning effect among different learning styles in a web-based lab of science for elementary school students. *Computers and Education* 50:1411–1422.

Sveistrup, H. 2004. Motor rehabilitation using virtual reality. *Journal of Neuroengineering and Rehabilitation* 1(1):10. www.pubmedcentral.nih.gov/articlerender.fcgi?artid=546406

Sveistrup, H., M. Thornton, C. Bryanton et al. 2004. Outcomes of intervention programs using flatscreen virtual reality. *Conference Proceedings IEEE Engineering in Medicine and Biology Society* 7:4856–4858.

Tam, C., H. Schwellnus, C. Eaton, Y. Hamdani, A. Lamont, and T. Chau. 2007. Movement-to-music computer technology: A developmental play experience for children with severe physical disabilities. *Occupational Therapy International* 14(2):99–112.

Taub, E., S.L. Ramey, S. DeLuca, and K. Echols. 2004. Efficacy of constraint-induced movement therapy for children with cerebral palsy with asymmetric motor impairment. *Pediatrics* 113(2):305–312.

Thornton, M., S. Marshall, J. McComas et al. 2005. Benefits of activity and virtual reality based balance exercise programmes for adults with traumatic brain injury: Perceptions of participants and their caregivers. *Brain Injury* 19(12):989–1000.

Thorpe, D.E. and J. Valvano. 2002. The effects of knowledge of performance and cognitive strategies on motor skill learning in children with cerebral palsy. *Pediatric Physical Therapy* 14(1):2–15.

Van Peppen, R.P., G. Kwakkel, S. Wood-Dauphinee, H.J. Hendriks, P.J. Van der Wees, and J. Dekker. 2004. The impact of physical therapy on functional outcomes after stroke: What's the evidence? *Clinical Rehabilitation* 18(8):833–862.

van Twillert, B., M. Bremer, and A.W. Faber. 2007. Computer-generated virtual reality to control pain and anxiety in pediatric and adult burn patients during wound dressing changes. *Journal of Burn Care & Research* 28(5):694–702.

Virtual Research Systems. 1998. Virtual V8. http://www.virtualresearch.com/products/v8 (accessed December 16, 2009).

Vogel, J.J., A. Greenwood-Ericksen, J. Cannon-Bowers, and C.A. Bowers. 2006. Using virtual reality with and without gaming attributes for academic achievement. *Journal of Research on Technology in Education* 39:105–118.

Ward, R.S. 1998. Physical rehabilitation. In *Burn Care and Therapy*, G. J. Carrougher, Ed. St. Louis, MO: Mosby.

Wiederhold, B.K. and M.D. Wiederhold. 1998. A review of virtual reality as a psychotherapeutic tool: *CyberPsychology & Behavior* 1(1):45–52.

Wiederhold, B.K. and M.D. Wiederhold. 2004. *Virtual healing: Human stories of success.* San Diego, CA: Interactive Media Institute.

Wiederhold, B.K., D.P. Jang, R.G. Gevirtz et al. 2002.The treatment of fear of flying: A controlled study of imaginal and virtual reality graded exposure therapy. *IEEE Transactions on Information Technology in Biomedicine* 6:218–223.

Weintraub, N., Y. Wyssocky, and U. Feintuch. 2008. Playing in a make-believe world: VR intervention for increasing playfulness of children with cerebral palsy. Paper presented at the annual conference of the American Occupational Therapy Association, Long Beach, CA.

Weiss, P.L. and A.S. Jessel. 1998. Virtual reality applications to work. *Work* 11:277–229.

Weiss, P.L., P. Bialik, and K. Kizony. 2003. Virtual reality provides leisure time opportunities for young adults with physical and intellectual disabilities. *CyberPsychology & Behavior* 6:335–342.

Weiss, P.L., D. Rand, N. Katz, and R. Kizony. 2004. Video capture virtual reality as a flexible and effective rehabilitation tool. *Journal of Neuroengineering and Rehabilitation* 1:12. http://www.jneuroengrehab.com/content/1/1/12

Weiss, P.L. and H. Ring. 2007. Commentary on virtual reality in stroke rehabilitation: Still more virtual than real. *Disability and Rehabilitation* 29:1147–1149.

WHO. 2001. International Classification of Functioning, Disability and Health (ICF). World Health Organization. Geneva, Switzerland.

Windich-Biermeier, A., I. Sjoberg, J.C. Dale et al. 2007. Effects of distraction on pain, fear, and distress during venous port access and venipuncture in children and adolescents with cancer. *Journal of Pediatric Oncology Nursing* 24(1):8–19.

Wismeijer, A.A. and A.J. Vingerhoets. 2005. The use of virtual reality and audiovisual eyeglass systems as adjunct analgesic techniques: A review of the literature. *Annals of Behavioral Medicine* 30(3):268–278.

Witmer, B.G. and M.J. Singer.1998. Measuring presence in virtual environments: A presence questionnaire. *Presence: Teleoperators and Virtual Environments* 7:225–240.

Wolitzky, K., R. Fivush, E. Zimand, et al. 2005. Effectiveness of virtual reality distraction during a painful medical procedure in pediatric oncology patients. *Psychology and Health* 20(6):817–824.

Yalon-Chamovitz, S. and P.L. Weiss. 2008. Virtual reality as a leisure activity for young adults with physical and intellectual disabilities. *Research in Developmental Disabilities* 29:273–287.

You, S.H., S.H. Jang, Y.H. Kim, M. Hallett, S.H. Ahn, Y.H. Kwon, J.H. Kim, and M.Y. Lee. 2005. Virtual reality-induced cortical reorganization and associated locomotor recovery in chronic stroke: An experimenter-blind randomized study. *Stroke* 36(6):1166–1171.

Zancanaro M., F. Pianesi, O. Stock, P. Venuti, A. Cappelletti, G. Iandolo, M. Prete, and F. Rossi. 2007. Children in the museum: An environment for collaborative storytelling. In *PEACH: Intelligent interfaces for museum visits*, O. Stock and M. Zancanaro, Eds. Berlin: Springer.

Index

Printed and bound by CPI Group (UK) Ltd, Croydon, CR0 4YY

21/10/2024

01777044-0008